MW

T

TP9404122

MBCSBN

ANNALS OF
THE NEW YORK ACADEMY
OF SCIENCES

Volume 691

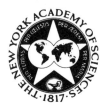

EDITORIAL STAFF

Executive Editor
BILL BOLAND

Managing Editor
JUSTINE CULLINAN

Associate Editor
COOK KIMBALL

The New York Academy of Sciences
2 East 63rd Street
New York, New York 10021

CAROTENOIDS
IN HUMAN HEALTH

ANNALS OF THE NEW YORK ACADEMY OF SCIENCES

Volume 691

CAROTENOIDS
IN HUMAN HEALTH

*Edited by Louise M. Canfield,
Norman I. Krinsky, and James A. Olson*

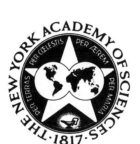

*The New York Academy of Sciences
New York, New York
1993*

Library of Congress Cataloging-in-Publication Data

Carotenoids in human health/edited by Louise M. Canfield, Norman I. Krinsky, and James A. Olson.
    p. cm.—(Annals of the New York Academy of Sciences, ISSN 0077-8923; v. 691)
    Includes bibliographical references and index.
    ISBN 0-89766-827-8 (cloth : alk. paper). —ISBN 0-89766-828-6 (paper : alk. paper)
    1. Carotenoids—Physiological effect—Congresses. 2. Carotenoids—Health aspects—Congresses. I. Canfield, Louise M. II. Krinsky, Norman I. III. Olson, James A. IV. Series.
    [DNLM: 1. Carotenoids—physiology—congresses. 2. Carotenoids—therapeutic use—congresses. W1 AN626YL v. 691 1993/QU 110 C2934 1993]
Q11.N5 vol. 691
[QP671.C35]
500 s—dc20
[612'.01528]
DNLM/DLC
for Library of Congress

93-43193
CIP

Bi-Comp/PCP
Printed in the United States of America
√ **ISBN 0-89766-827-8** (cloth)
ISBN 0-89766-828-6 (paper)
ISSN 0077-8923

ANNALS OF THE NEW YORK ACADEMY OF SCIENCES

Volume 691

December 31, 1993

CAROTENOIDS IN HUMAN HEALTH[a]

Editors and Conference Chairs

LOUISE M. CANFIELD, NORMAN I. KRINSKY, AND JAMES A. OLSON

CONTENTS

[a] The papers in this volume were presented at a conference entitled Carotenoids in Human
Health, which was held by the New York Academy of Sciences in San Diego, California
on February 6–9, 1993.

Financial assistance was received from:

Major funders
- HENKEL CORPORATION

Supporters
- BASF CORPORATION
- HOFFMANN-LA ROCHE INC.

Contributors
- BETATENE LIMITED
- HALL LABORATORIES, INC.
- KRAFT GENERAL FOODS
- MEAD JOHNSON RESEARCH CENTER
- SANDOZ PHARMACEUTICAL CORPORATION

Preface

In April of 1990, seventeen scientists met in Atlanta for breakfast to discuss mutual interests in carotenoid research. We ranged in experience in working with carotenoids from more than 20 years to less than 2 years and represented fields as diverse as analytical chemistry and epidemiology. It was an exhilarating time for carotenoid research. Peto's landmark paper[1] suggesting the possible link between carotenoids and cancer had inspired clinical and epidemiological trials. These were just beginning to result in laboratory data. Our discussions in that meeting centered on appropriate quantitation and analysis of carotenoids, interpretation of clinical data and the exciting possibility that β-carotene might have new biological actions independent of its function as a precursor of vitamin A.

Interest in carotenoid research has soared in the intervening four years. Enthusiasm generated at our 1990 meeting has resulted in yearly pre-FASEB meetings, a newsletter, a Gordon Conferences series and the meeting that has resulted in this volume. In addition, during this time, two volumes of *Methods in Enzymology*[2,3] have been devoted to carotenoid analysis and several other meetings on the subject, including the triennial International Symposium on Carotenoids, have been held.

Concurrent with the growth in the numbers of workers interested in carotenoid research, the knowledge base in the field has increased. Today we recognize the possible biological significance of carotenoids other than β-carotene and of metabolites other than vitamin A. Widespread use of HPLC-photodiode array spectroscopy provides the capability of identifying carotenoids and their metabolites based on subtle differences in their UV spectra. Our improved understanding of the chemical reactions of carotenoids with active oxygen species as well as their interactions with other biological antioxidants such as vitamins E and C has allowed us to better predict their reactions *in vivo*. Improved mass spectral techniques have provided us with the identification of new metabolites, and the use of radiolabelled carotenoids will allow us to precisely trace carotenoid absorption and metabolism *in vivo*. Using improved HPLC techniques, we have quantitated the major carotenoids in our food supply and therefore can more accurately assess our dietary intake. The powerful techniques of molecular biology have yielded exciting new data which is providing insight into previously unrecognized biological actions of carotenoids.

In spite of these impressive recent gains in better understanding of the carotenoids, their *in vivo* action remains an enigma. At the time of this writing, carotenoid supplementation had yet to demonstrate a significant effect on human disease processes. On the other hand, carotenoids effectively inhibit tumorigenesis and improve immune status in a variety of animal and cellular models, and their application to some human precancerous lesions results in remission. Carotenoids prevent lipid oxidation *in vitro* and diets rich in carotenoid-containing foods appear to lower the risk of heart disease. Conversely, it has not yet been possible to demonstrate a protective effect of β-carotene supplementation on lipoprotein oxidation *in vivo*. As in any rapidly developing field, emerging research appears to raise as many, if not more, questions than it answers. How are cellular levels and transport of carotenoids regulated? Are metabolites of carotenoids important, and if so, among the many hundreds possible, which ones are biologically significant and in which systems do they act? Do carotenoids work independently of other antioxidants? Is there a biological requirement for carotenoids which cannot be satisfied by another dietary lipid or antioxidant? Clearly, there is much to be learned.

This conference brought together international experts in diverse areas of carotenoid research with the hope that important clues to the action of carotenoids in human health would emerge and creative approaches for future research would be developed. As will be apparent by reading this volume, our objectives were well met. It is our hope that this document will provide new insight into the biological actions of carotenoids, thereby stimulating creative new research activities germane to the relationship between carotenoids and human health.

Louise M. Canfield

DEDICATION

This volume is dedicated to the members of the Carotenoid Research Interaction Group (CaRIG) for their dedication to fostering an atmosphere of collaborative research activities based on a free exchange of ideas and observations.

Louise M. Canfield
Norman I. Krinsky
James A. Olson

REFERENCES

1. PETO, R., R. DOLL, J. D. BUCKLEY & M. B. SPORN. 1981. Can carotenoids materially reduce cancer rates? Nature (London) **290:** 201–208.
2. PACKER, L., Ed. 1992. Carotenoids, Part A, Chemistry, Separation, Quantitation and Antioxidation. Methods in Enzymology, Vol. 213. Academic Press. San Diego.
3. PACKER, L., Ed. 1993. Carotenoids, Part B, Metabolism, Genetics and Biosynthesis. Methods in Enzymology, Vol. 214. Academic Press. San Diego.

Physical and Chemical Properties of Carotenoids[a]

HARRY A. FRANK

Department of Chemistry
University of Connecticut
215 Glenbrook Road
Storrs, Connecticut 06269-3060

INTRODUCTION

Of the many important questions concerning the structure and function of carotenoids, the following are the most pressing: What are the structures of carotenoids *in vivo*? How do the structures determine their biological activities? What are the mechanisms of radical reactions with carotenoids? What is the nature of the interaction between carotenoids and biological antioxidants? What is the mechanism by which carotenoids quench active oxygen species? Undoubtedly, the answers to these questions lie in understanding the molecular features of carotenoids that control their structures, electronic states and distributions, and the dynamics of the intra- and intermolecular processes they can undergo. Our approach to analyzing carotenoid properties has been the application of physical chemical methodology to systematic series of carotenoids.[1] In this manner, clear trends in the properties of these molecules will emerge. The techniques used include absorption,[2] fluorescence,[3] resonance Raman (rR),[4] nuclear magnetic resonance (NMR),[5] electron paramagnetic resonance (EPR),[6] and fast-transient optical spectroscopies,[7] as well as X-ray diffraction[8] and computational methods.[9] This paper summarizes some of the recent accomplishments in this area.

Absorption Spectroscopy

Energy Levels

The bright visible coloring associated with carotenoids is their most distinguishing feature. This readily observed, prominent, characteristic of carotenoids, however, masks the complicated nature of their energy state level complexion. It is now known that carotenoids (and polyenes) possess two low-lying electronic excited singlet states that account for many of their optical properties.[10,11] These states are denoted 1^1B_u and 2^1A_g according to the idealized group theoretical (C_{2h} point group) designations. The ground state designation is 1^1A_g. The pronounced absorption in the visible regions that is characteristic of all carotenoids is attributable to a strongly allowed transition from the ground 1^1A_g state to the 1^1B_u state. Lying below the 1^1B_u state is the 2^1A_g state into which absorption from the ground state is symmetry forbidden. The presence of the 2^1A_g state has been verified by

[a] This work is supported in the author's laboratory by grants from the National Institutes of Health (GM-30353) and the University of Connecticut Research Foundation.

1

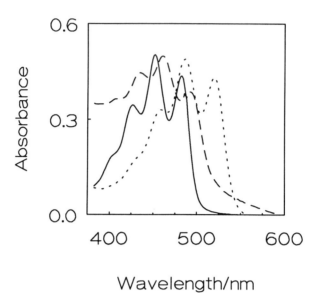

FIGURE 1. Solvent-induced shifts of the absorption spectrum of spheroidene in petroleum ether (*solid line*), Triton X-100 detergent micelles (*dashed line*), and CS_2 (*dotted line*).

absorption, emission, and dynamics measurements.[1] Indeed, the existence of a low-lying 2^1A_g state is now widely accepted as a general feature of all carotenoid molecules.

Solvent Effects

Owing to dispersion forces, the $1^1A_g \rightarrow 1^1B_u$ transition frequency may undergo a pronounced shift to lower energy when the highly polarizable carotenoids are dissolved in nonpolar solvents of increasing refractive index[10,12] (FIG. 1). The spectral shift does not depend on the solvent polarity, but rather on the solvent polarizability.[10] Experimentally, the $1^1A_g \rightarrow 1^1B_u$ transition frequency follows a linear dependence with the ratio $(n^2 - 1)/(n^2 + 2)$, where n is the solvent refractive index.[10,12–15] This ratio is directly proportional to the solvent polarizability.

Solvent-induced shifts of the $1^1A_g \rightarrow 2^1A_g$ absorption or the $2^1A_g \rightarrow 1^1A_g$ emission frequency are also expected, although the magnitude of these is smaller than for transitions involving the 1^1B_u state because the interaction is proportional to the electronic dipole moment of the transition.[10] This dipole moment is small owing to the forbidden nature of the transitions between the 2^1A_g state and the ground state.

Molecular Orbital Theoretical Calculations

Molecular orbital theory calculations using semiempirical methods yield reasonable descriptions of the energy of the 1^1B_u state and the oscillator strength of the $1^1A_g \rightarrow 1^1B_u$ transition.[9,10,16] The proper implementation of molecular orbital methods requires first that the geometric coordinates of the molecule be optimized to yield the minimum energy conformation. This has been done using an AM1 Hamiltonian and standard minimization techniques of the MOPAC program.[17] Simple molecular orbital theory calculations are not well suited, however, for a quantitative description of the 2^1A_g state, although, in principle, they should succeed with sufficient configuration interaction. Qualitatively correct trends in the energy levels of polyenes have been observed with double (or higher) excitations included in the configuration interaction.[18] It should be emphasized, however, that the energies of the 2^1A_g states for the very long-chain carotenoids (>10 carbon-carbon double bonds) are still the subject of some controversy. The positions of the 2^1A_g states in these molecules have not been well described either theoretically or experimentally.

"cis-Peaks"

Absorption spectroscopy provides a convenient means of identifying the presence of different stereochemical isomers of carotenoids. A so-called "cis-peak" is well-known to occur at shorter wavelengths than the primary visible absorption band of carotenoids. The cis-peak signifies a change in the linear all-trans structure of the carotenoid to a cis configuration. For example, the cis-peak for the change of β-carotene from its all-trans configuration to its 15-15'-cis configuration occurs at approximately 140 nm below the longest wavelength vibronic band of the strong, visible-absorption[19] (FIG. 2). An HPLC analysis of spheroidene using a normal phase, silica column procedure separates the different geometrical isomers (FIG. 3). In general, the cis-peak arises because of less stringent singlet state absorption selection rules when the symmetry of the molecule is lowered. It usually appears at the expense of some intensity in the main absorption bands. The intensity of the cis-peak is highest for central-cis-stereochemical isomers. However, recent

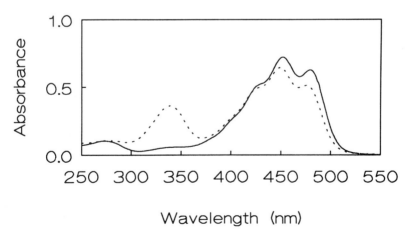

FIGURE 2. The absorption spectra of 15-15'-cis-β-carotene (*dotted line*) and all-*trans*-β-carotene (*solid line*) in hexane.

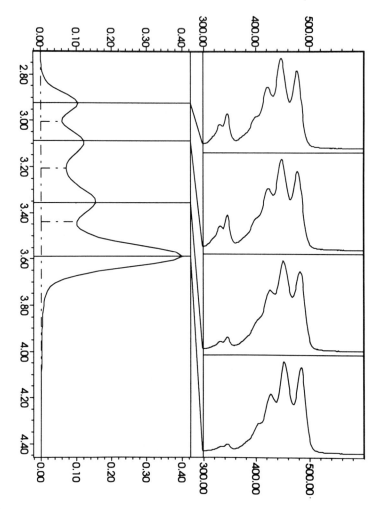

FIGURE 3. Normal phase, silica column HPLC chromatogram of the carotenoid, spheroidene. The *left hand panel* shows the HPLC separation of different geometric isomers of spheroidene over a 2.80–4.40-minute column retention time interval. The *horizontal axis* of this panel is calibrated in absorbance units. The *right hand panel* shows the absorption spectrum of each of the different geometric isomers. The *horizontal axis* of this panel is in nanometer units.

theoretical calculations have suggested that if twisting at the ends of the carotenoid conjugated π-electron chain are present in a central *cis* geometrical isomer, the intensity of the *cis*-peak may be greatly attenuated.[9] Therefore, although the presence of a *cis*-peak in the absorption spectrum of a carotenoid is indicative of a *cis*-geometric isomeric structure, the absence of a *cis*-peak cannot be taken as evidence that the molecule is in a *trans* configuration.

Fluorescence Spectroscopy

2^1A_g and 1^1B_u Emission

Owing to advances in the methodology for the isolation and purification of carotenoids, particularly high performance liquid chromatography (HPLC) techniques, weak fluorescence has been unambiguously observed from carotenoids.[3,20-26] The fluorescence yields are typically very low ($\sim 10^{-4}$ or less). Thus, great care must be taken to eliminate impurities in the solution that have plagued previous measurements of carotenoid fluorescence spectra.

Because of the importance of the position of the 2^1A_g state in elucidating energy transfer by carotenoids in photosynthetic pigment-protein complexes, a significant experimental effort by numerous groups has gone into attempting to establish values for the 2^1A_g state energies of various carotenoids.[19] The techniques used include Raman, absorption, fluorescence and fluorescence excitation spectroscopies applied to carotenoids having varying extents of π-electron conjugation.[19] Fluorescence has been the primary tool used in the most recent studies. Carotenoids and polyenes having eight or less conjugated carbon-carbon double bonds display fluorescence that is significantly "Stokes-shifted" from the absorption spectrum.[3,23,27,28] This fluorescence originates from the low-lying 2^1A_g state. Carotenoids having more than eight carbon-carbon double bonds display fluorescence that originates from the 1^1B_u state and has a very small Stokes shift. The crossover from the "1^1B_u" to "2^1A_g" emission at a conjugated chain length of eight is qualitatively understood by the fact that rapid internal conversion to the 2^1A_g state competes favorably with fluorescence for deactivation of the 1^1B_u state in the shorter chain length molecules.[3] Because the longer carotenoids do not fluoresce from their 2^1A_g states it is difficult to determine the energies of the lowest singlet states in these molecules. To a first approximation one can extrapolate the energies of the 2^1A_g states of the shorter polyene and carotenoid molecules to the longer conjugated systems.[3] The trends observed for the state energies indicate that while both the 1^1B_u and 2^1A_g state energies decrease with extent of π-electron conjugation, the 1^1B_u–2^1A_g energy gap increases.[3] This is at least partly the reason for the change in internal conversion behavior that leads to the crossover from 2^1A_g emission to 1^1B_u emission with increasing extent of π-electron conjugation.

Triplet States

Once the energy of the 2^1A_g state of a carotenoid has been established, it is possible to deduce the energy (E_T) of its lowest lying triplet state from a rule-of-thumb that derives from a valence bond theory description of the 2^1A_g states of polyenes.[10] Very little is known about the positions of triplet states in carotenoids and what their role is in quenching active oxygen species (e.g. the $^1\Delta_g$ singlet state of oxygen). In the valence bond theory model, the triplet state energy of a carotenoid is approximated by about one-half the energy of the 2^1A_g state. If one compares the 2^1A_g state energies of some representative carotenoids determined by fluorescence methods with the triplet energies for the same conjugated chain length extrapolated from the triplet state determinations of short polyenes[29-31] (TABLE 1), it is evident that the $E_T \sim \frac{1}{2}E_2 1_{Ag}$ rule-of-thumb holds reasonably well.

Transient Optical Spectroscopy

Energy Gap Law

The lifetimes of the lowest excited singlet states of carotenoids depend on the energy gap between this state and the ground state. This so-called "energy gap law"[32] is expressed by the equation

$$k_{ic} = c \cdot \exp(-\gamma \Delta E / \hbar \omega_M)$$

where k_{ic} is the internal conversion rate constant, approximated by the inverse of the lifetime of the first excited singlet state. This approximation is reasonably good because k_{ic} for carotenoids is much larger than the radiative rate constant, $k_f \sim 10^9$ s^{-1}. ΔE is the 1^1A_g to 2^1A_g energy difference, c is a pre-exponential constant, $\hbar \omega_M$ is the energy of the high frequency "acceptor" modes, and γ is related to the relative displacement of the potential surfaces in the two electronic states. For linear polyenes, the C-C stretching vibrations $\hbar \omega_M \sim 1300$–1600 cm^{-1} are thought to be the appropriate acceptor modes for internal conversion.[33] FIGURE 4 shows that the dependence of the natural logarithm of the decay rate constant for a series of spheroidene molecules is linear with respect to their $2^1A_g \rightarrow 1^1A_g$ transition energies. The energies of the states were determined by the fluorescence experiments described above.[3] The rate constants were measured by subpicosecond transient absorption techniques.[34] The transition energy for spheroidene (10 carbon-carbon double bonds) is not known because fluorescence has not yet been detected from the S_1 state of that molecule. A computer-generated fit of the logarithm of the energy gap law expression to the rate constants associated with the other three compounds yielded a value of 14,100 cm^{-1} for the 2^1A_g energy of

TABLE 1. Singlet and Triplet State Energies of Carotenoids (cm^{-1} Units)[a]

Number of Conjugated Carbon-Carbon Double Bonds	1^1B_u State Energies	2^1A_g State Energies	T_1 Triplet State Energies
1			≤28,700
2			20,830
3			16,450
4			13,750
5			(11,670)
6			(10,170)
7	23,600	18,400	(9,010)
8	22,500	16,700	(8,090)
9	21,500	15,300	(7,340)
10	20,800	(14,100)	(6,710)
11			(6,190)
12			(5,740)
13			(5,350)

[a] The triplet state energies in parentheses were extrapolated from data taken on short polyenes (also in the table but not in parentheses).[29–31] The 1^1B_u and 2^1A_g state energies were determined from fluorescence studies on a series of homologous spheroidene molecules.[3] The 2^1A_g energy value in parentheses was determined by subpicosecond transient absorption techniques.[34]

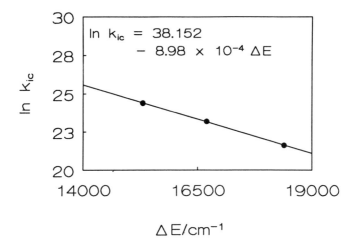

FIGURE 4. A linear least-squares fit of the natural logarithm of the S_1 state decay rate constants, k_{ic}, $\sim 1/\tau$ plotted versus the S_1 state spectral origins (ΔE) of 3,4,5,6-tetrahydrospheroidene, 3,4,7,8-tetrahydrospheroidene and 3,4-dihydrospheroidene, deduced from fluorescence studies. The best fit to the equation, $ln\ k_{ic} = ln c - \gamma \Delta E / \hbar \omega_M$ yielded values of 8.98×10^{-4} cm for $\gamma / \hbar \omega_M$ and 38.152 for $ln c$.

spheroidene.[34] This value is in good agreement with the value determined by extrapolation ($\sim$14,000 cm^{-1}).[3] Longer carotenoids are expected to have even shorter 2^1A_g lifetimes corresponding to even lower 2^1A_g excited state energies. Hence, the energy gap law provides an indirect method for determining the 2^1A_g state energies of carotenoids via transient optical spectroscopy. If the dynamics of the excited singlet states can be determined via fast transient absorption techniques, the 2^1A_g energies of these nonfluorescent molecules may be readily determined.

CONCLUSIONS

This brief overview has demonstrated that spectroscopic techniques can reveal the structures, energy state distributions, and dynamics of the intramolecular processes of carotenoids. Advances in this area of carotenoid research are progressing at such a rapid pace that many of the ambiguities in the determinations of carotenoid structures and electronic states are likely to be resolved in the very near future.

ACKNOWLEDGMENTS

The author would like to thank Professor Ronald L. Christensen, Ms. Beverly DeCoster, Dr. Michael R. Wasielewski, Dr. David Gosztola, Dr. Ronald Gebhard, Professor Johan Lugtenburg, Professor Robert Connors, Professor Richard Cogdell, Ms. Roya Farhoosh, and Ms. Agnes Cua for their substantial contributions to the experiments described herein.

REFERENCES

1. COGDELL, R. J. & H. A. FRANK. 1987. How carotenoids function in photosynthetic bacteria. Biochim. Biophys. Acta **895:** 63–79.
2. FRANK, H. A., B. W. CHADWICK, S. TAREMI, S. KOLACZKOWSKI & M. BOWMAN. 1986. Singlet and triplet absorption spectra of carotenoids bound in the reaction centers of *Rhodopseudomonas sphaeroides* R-26. FEBS Lett. **203:** 157–163.
3. DECOSTER, B., R. L. CHRISTENSEN, R. GEBHARD, J. LUGTENBURG, R. FARHOOSH & H. A. FRANK. 1992. Low-lying electronic states of carotenoids. Biochim. Biophys. Acta **1102:** 107–114.
4. ROBERT, B. & H. A. FRANK. 1988. A resonance Raman investigation of the effect of lithium dodecyl sulfate on the B800-850 light-harvesting protein of *Rhodopseudomonas acidophila* 7750. Biochim. Biophys. Acta **934:** 401–405.
5. GEBHARD, R., K. VAN DER HOEF, C. A. VIOLETTE, H. J. M. DE GROOT, H. A. FRANK & J. LUGTENBURG. 1991. ^{13}C Magic angle spinning NMR evidence for a 15,15'-Z configuration of the spheroidene chromophore in the *Rhodobacter sphaeroides* reaction center. Pure Appl. Chem. **63:** 115–122.
6. FRANK, H. A. 1992. Electron paramagnetic resonance studies of carotenoids. *In* Methods in Enzymology Carotenoids, Part A. Chemistry, Separation, Quantitation and Antioxidation. L. Packer, Ed. Vol. 213: 305–312. Academic Press. New York, NY.
7. FRANK, H. A. & C. A. VIOLETTE. 1989. Monomeric bacteriochlorophyll is required for triplet energy transfer between the primary donor and the carotenoid in photosynthetic bacterial reaction centers. Biochim. Biophys. Acta **976:** 222–232.
8. FRANK, H. A., S. S. TAREMI & J. R. KNOX. 1987. Crystallization and preliminary X-ray and optical spectroscopic characterization of the photochemical reaction center from *Rhodobacter sphaeroides* strain 2.4.1. J. Mol. Biol. **198:** 139–141.
9. CONNORS, R. E., D. S. BURNS, R. FARHOOSH & H. A. FRANK. Unpublished results.
10. HUDSON, B. S., B. E. KOHLER & K. SHULTEN. 1982. Linear polyene electronic structure and potential surfaces. *In* Excited States. E. C. Lim, Ed. Vol. 6: 22–95. Academic Press. New York, NY.
11. BIRGE, R., J. A. BENNETT, H. L.-B. FANG & G. E. LEROI. 1978. The two-photon spectroscopy of all-trans retinal and related polyenes. *In* Springer Series in Chem. Phys. A. H. Zewail, Ed. Vol. 3: 347–354. Springer. Berlin.
12. ANDERSSON, P. O., T. GILLBRO, L. FERGUSON & R. J. COGDELL. 1991. Absorption spectral shifts of carotenoids related to medium polarizability. Photochem. Photobiol. **54:** 353–360.
13. ANDREWS, J. R. & B. S. HUDSON. 1978. Environment effects on radiative rate constants with application to linear polyenes. J. Chem. Phys. **68:** 4587–4594.
14. BASU, S. 1964. Theory of solvent effects on molecular electronic spectra. Adv. Quantum Chem. **1:** 145–169.
15. LEROSEN, A. L. & C. E. REID. 1952. An investigation of certain solvent effects in absorption spectra. J. Chem. Phys. **20:** 233–236.
16. ZHANG, C.-F., C. A. VIOLETTE, H. A. FRANK & R. R. BIRGE. 1989. Electronic states of isolated and reaction center-bound carotenoids. Biophys. J. **55:** 223a.
17. STEWART, J. J. P. Quantum Chemistry Program Exchange Program 455, V. 5. 1988, Indiana University.
18. TAVAN, P. & K. SCHULTEN. 1979. The $2^1A_g - 1^1B_u$ energy gap in the polyenes: an extended configuration interaction study. J. Chem. Phys. **70:** 5407–5413.
19. H. A. FRANK & R. J. COGDELL. Photochemistry and functions of carotenoids in photosynthesis. *In* Carotenoids in Photosynthesis. Ch. 8. A. Young & G. Britton, Eds. Springer-Verlag. London. In press.
20. SNYDER, R., E. ARVIDSON, C. FOOTE, L. HARRIGAN & R. L. CHRISTENSEN. 1985. Electronic energy levels in long polyenes: $S_2 \rightarrow S_0$ emission in all-trans-1,2,5,7,9,11,13-tetradecaheptaene. J. Am. Chem. Soc. **107:** 4117–4122.

21. WATANABE, J., S. KINOSHITA & T. KUSHIDA. 1987. Effects of nonzero correlation time of system-reservoir interaction on the excitation profiles of second-order optical processes in β-carotene. J. Chem. Phys. **87:** 4471–4477.

22. GILLBRO, T. & R. J. COGDELL. 1989. Carotenoid fluorescence. Chem. Phys. Lett. **158:** 312–316.

23. COSGROVE, S. A., M. A. GUITE, T. B. BURNELL & R. L. CHRISTENSEN. 1990. Electronic relaxation in long polyenes. J. Phys. Chem. **94:** 8118–8124.

24. SHREVE, A. P., J. K. TRAUTMAN, T. G. OWENS & A. C. ALBRECHT. 1991. Determination of the S_2 lifetime of β-carotene. Chem. Phys. Lett. **178:** 89–96.

25. SHREVE, A. P., J. K. TRAUTMAN, H. A. FRANK, T. G. OWENS & A. C. ALBRECHT. 1991. Femtosecond energy-transfer processes in the B800-850 light-harvesting complex of *Rhodobacter sphaeroides* 2.4.1. Biochim. Biophys. Acta **1058:** 280–288.

26. BONDAREV, S. L., S. M. BACHILO, S. S. DVORNIKOV & S. A. TIKHOMIROV. 1989. $S_2 \rightarrow S_0$ fluorescence and transient $S_n \leftarrow S_1$ absorption of all-trans-β-carotene in solid and liquid solutions. J. Photochem. Photobiol. A: Chemistry **46:** 315–322.

27. MIMURO, M., Y. NISHIMURA, I. YAMAZAKI, T. KATOH & U. NAGASHIMA. 1991. Fluorescence properties of the allenic carotenoid fucoxanthin: analysis of the effect of keto carbonyl group by using a model compound, all-trans-beta-apo-8'-carotenal. J. Lumin. **50:** 1–10.

28. SHREVE, A. P., J. K. TRAUTMAN, T. G. OWENS & A. C. ALBRECHT. 1991. A femtosecond study of *in vivo* and *in vitro* electronic state dynamics of fucoxanthin and implications for photosynthetic carotenoid-to-chlorophyll energy transfer mechanisms. Chem. Phys. **154:** 171–178.

29. EVANS, D. F. 1960. Magnetic perturbation of single-triplet transitions. Part IV. Unsaturated compounds. J. Chem. Soc. **1960:** 1735–1745.

30. EVANS, D. F. 1961. Magnetic perturbation of singlet-triplet transitions. Part VI. Octa-1,3,5,7-tetraene. J. Chem. Soc. **1961:** 2566–2569.

31. BENSASSON, R., E. J. LAND & B. MAUDINAS. 1976. Triplet states of carotenoids from photosynthetic bacteria studied by nanosecond ultraviolet and electron pulse irradiation. Photochem. Photobiol. **23:** 189–193.

32. ENGLMAN, R. & J. JORTNER. 1970. The energy gap law for radiationless transitions in large molecules. Mol. Phys. **18:** 145–164.

33. WASIELEWSKI, M. R., D. G. JOHNSON, E. G. BRADFORD & L. D. KISPERT. 1989. Temperature dependence of the lowest excited singlet-state lifetime of all-trans-β-carotene and fully deuterated all-trans-β-carotene. J. Chem. Phys. **91:** 6691–6697.

34. FRANK, H. A., R. FARHOOSH, R. GEBHARD, J. LUGTENBURG, D. GOSZTOLA & M. R. WASIELEWSKI. Unpublished results.

Physical Quenching of Singlet Oxygen and *cis-trans* Isomerization of Carotenoids[a]

WILHELM STAHL AND HELMUT SIES

Institut für Physiologische Chemie I
Universität Düsseldorf
Postfach 101007
D-4000 Düsseldorf, Germany

INTRODUCTION

Beyond their function as vitamin A precursors, carotenoids have been shown to exhibit additional biological activities,[1-3] enhancing intracellular communication[4-7] and efficiently scavenging reactive oxygen species.[8-11] Quenching of $^1O_2$ and reactions with oxygen-centered radicals have been studied. Carotenoids occur in different geometrical forms (*trans*- and *cis*-isomers), which are interconverted by light, thermal energy or chemical reactions.[12] Although numerous geometrical configurations are possible, only a limited number of these are formed preferentially.

β-Carotene predominantly exists in the all-*trans*, 9-*cis*, 13-*cis* and 15-*cis* forms (FIG. 1). Recently, the geometrical isomers of these carotenoids attracted attention because of the suggestion of isomer-specific functions. Specific geometrical isomers of retinoic acid are known to be active in the regulation of gene expression.[13-15]

Physical Quenching of $^1O_2$

Normal aerobic metabolism is associated with the production of reactive oxygen species. Singlet oxygen is a biologically occurring excited state of ground state (triplet) oxygen.

Singlet oxygen can be generated when a sensitizer is excited to its first excited state and then undergoes intersystem crossing to a metastable triplet state:

$$\text{Sens} \xrightarrow{h\nu} {}^1\text{Sens} \longrightarrow {}^3\text{Sens} \tag{1}$$

$$^3\text{Sens} + {}^3O_2 \longrightarrow \text{Sens} + {}^1O_2 \tag{2}$$

Triplet states can initiate further reactions, *e.g.*, with ground state oxygen to form singlet oxygen.

Porphyrins, chlorophylls, bilirubin, and riboflavin are examples of endogenous sensitizers in biological systems. Exogenous compounds such as psoralen, anthra-

[a] This work was supported by the National Foundation for Cancer Research, Bethesda, MD; the Ministerium für Wissenschaft und Forschung, Nordrhein-Westfalen; and the Bundesministerium für Forschung und Technologie, Bonn.

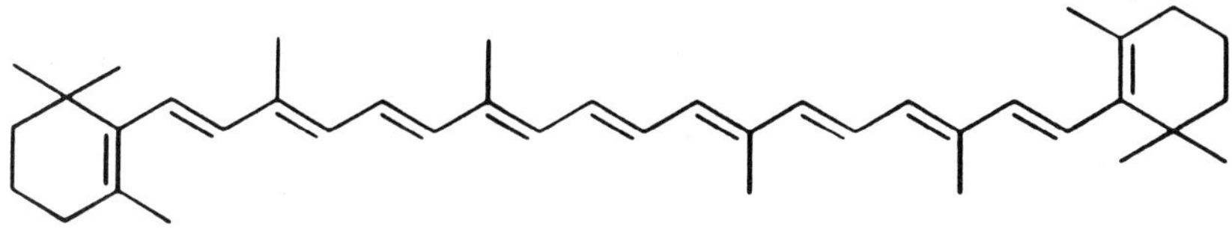

all−trans ß−Carotene

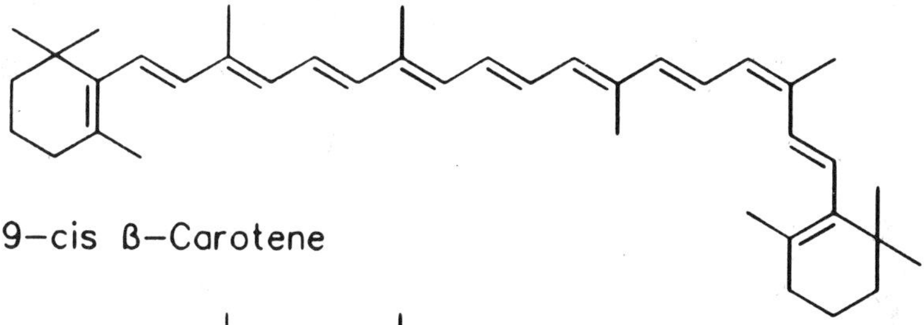

9−cis ß−Carotene

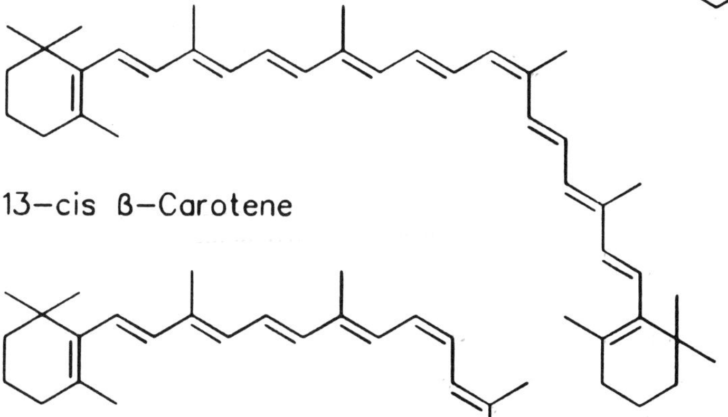

13−cis ß−Carotene

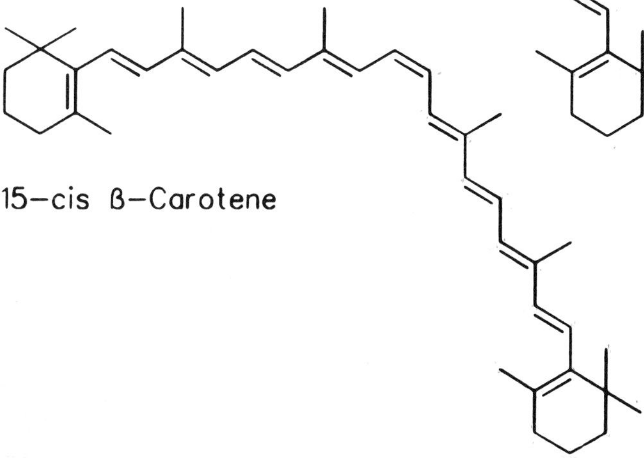

15−cis ß−Carotene

FIGURE 1. Structures of all-*trans* and the main mono-*cis* isomers of β-carotene.

cene, rose bengal, and methylene blue can act as sensitizing agents producing $^1O_2$ when irradiated with light.

Quenching of Singlet Oxygen by Carotenoids

Singlet oxygen can interact with other molecules generally in two different ways, chemical reactions or energy transfer reactions, leading to the deactivation of singlet oxygen.

β-Carotene has been known as an efficient quencher of $^1O_2$ since the study by Foote and Denny.[9,16] By means of a variety of techniques (reviewed in[17]), quenching rate constants have been determined for the biological carotenoids and xanthophylls, and they fall within a range close to diffusion control.

The deactivation of $^1O_2$ by carotenoids results predominantly from physical quenching, a process involving transfer of excitation energy from $^1O_2$ to the carotenoid and resulting in the formation of ground state oxygen ($^3O_2$) and triplet excited carotenoid ($^3C^*$) (Reaction 3). The energy is dissipated through rotational and vibrational interactions between $^3C^*$ and the solvent to recover ground state carotenoid (Reaction 4).

$$^1O_2 + C \rightarrow {}^3O_2 + {}^3C^* \qquad\qquad\qquad (3)$$

$$^3C^* \rightarrow C + \text{thermal energy} \qquad\qquad\qquad (4)$$

The carotenoid can thus be considered to act as a "catalyst" for deactivation of potentially harmful $^1O_2$.[18]

It is generally accepted that an increasing number of conjugated double bonds is associated with more efficient quenching ability against $^1O_2$.[18-20] Recently, Di Mascio *et al.*[20] and Truscott and co-workers[21,22] studied the $^1O_2$ quenching abilities of carotenoids with similar numbers of conjugated double bonds, revealing differences in their $^1O_2$ quenching abilities, *e.g.*, for β-carotene and lycopene, which may be taken as an indication of a role for the end groups.

To examine whether the different behavior could be due to structural differences of the end groups, a number of new carotenoids were studied.[23]

The singlet molecular oxygen quenching activity of carotenoids and newly synthesized polyene polyketones (Fig. 2) and capsorubin isomers was examined using the thermodissociable endoperoxide of 3,3'-(1,4-naphthylene) dipropionate (NDPO$_2$) as $^1O_2$ source and a germanium diode to monitor $^1O_2$ photoemission. C_{28}-polyene tetrone exhibits the highest physical quenching rate constant with $^1O_2$ ($k_q = 16 \times 10^9$ $M^{-1}s^{-1}$). For comparison, the rate constant for the most efficient biological carotenoid, lycopene, is $k_q = 9 \times 10^9$ $M^{-1}s^{-1}$ and that of β-carotene $k_q = 5 \times 10^9$ $M^{-1}s^{-1}$. The presence of two oxalyl chromophores at the ends of the polyene chain seems to enhance the $^1O_2$ quenching ability in the C_{28}-polyene tetrone. C_{28}-polyene tetrone diacetal ($k_q = 9 \times 10^9$ $M^{-1}s^{-1}$) and C_{40}-epiisocapsorubin ($k_q = 8 \times 10^9$ $M^{-1}s^{-1}$) also have high $^1O_2$ quenching abilities.

While carotenoids are the most efficient biological quenchers of $^1O_2$ yet tested, the extent to which they play a role in protecting cells against $^1O_2$-related biological damage remains a challenging question. Singlet oxygen is known to be capable of damaging DNA[24-26] detected as plasmid DNA strand breaks and resulting in loss of biological activity and mutagenesis;[27] lipids[28,29] and enzymes, resulting in their inactivation.[30] Singlet oxygen can be generated *in vivo* by photosensitization reactions[31] and during phagocytosis.[32]

β-Carotene and related carotenoids were reported to be effective scavengers of free radicals under physiological conditions.[33-35] The interaction of carotenoids with radicals results in oxidation products. Autoxidation of β-carotene leads to the formation of epoxides at the β-ionone ring and to ketones (β-apo-carotenones) and aldehydes (β-apo-carotenals) of different chain lengths, including retinal.[36]

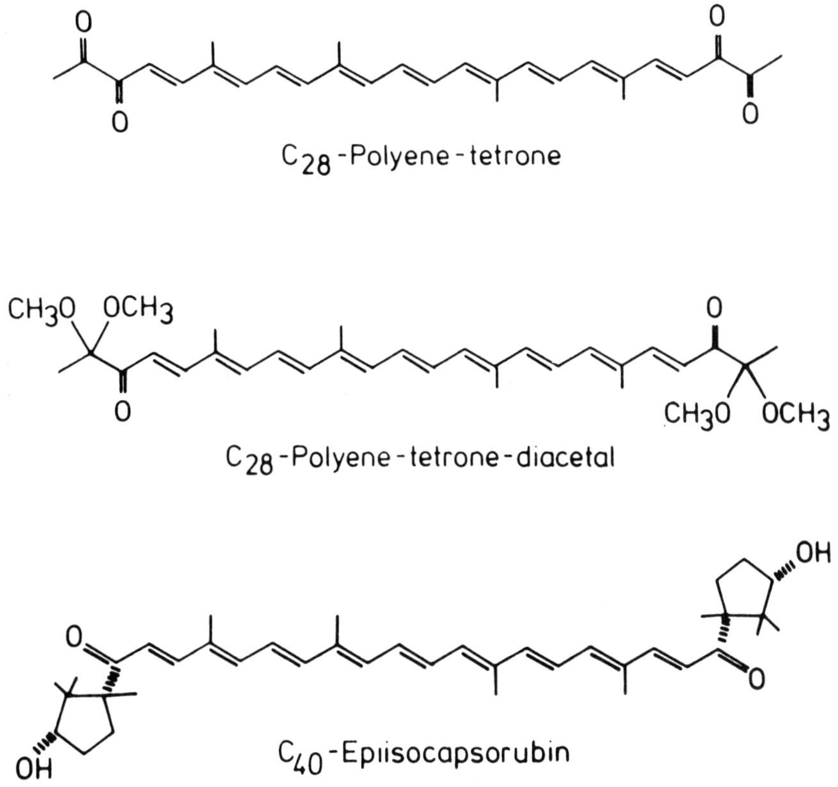

C_{28}-Polyene-tetrone

C_{28}-Polyene-tetrone-diacetal

C_{40}-Epiisocapsorubin

FIGURE 2. Structures of synthetic carotenoids (see also text).

cis-trans *Isomers of Carotenoids*

Carotenoids are micronutrients and are absorbed via the gut and further transported in chylomicrons within the lymphatic system to the liver. During lipoprotein assembly they are incorporated mainly into LDLs, the major transport form of carotenoids in human blood.[37,38] Different organs contain various amounts of carotenoids.[39,40] Liver, adrenal glands and testes contain higher amounts of carotenoids than kidney, ovary or fat tissue.

Carotenoids may undergo *trans-* or *cis-*isomer interconversion by quenching singlet oxygen and photochemical or thermal processes. Several *cis-*isomers of carotenoids have been detected in human serum and various fruits and vegetables.[41–45] Little is known, however, about the formation, distribution and biological relevance of the *cis-*isomers in human tissues.

Isomers of carotenoids (especially *cis* and *trans* isomers of β-carotene) might exhibit different biological functions. Considering recent results on the biological specificity of retinoic acid isomers their possible role as stereospecific precursors of retinoids might be discussed.[46]

cis-trans *Isomers of β-Carotene and Lycopene in Human Serum and Tissues*

β-Carotene and lycopene are the most abundant carotenoids in human serum and tissues and have been shown to consist of a mixture of geometrical isomers.[40,45,47] FIGURE 3A shows the HPLC chromatogram of a human serum sample. 9-*cis* β-Carotene is present only in trace amounts. The other geometrical isomer present is 13-*cis* β-carotene. 15-*cis* β-Carotene, however, was not detected.

Although the individual β-carotene serum levels might vary several-fold, the contribution of 13-*cis* to total β-carotene, does not exceed 7% of total β-carotene. In tissue samples, however, two mono-*cis* isomers of β-carotene are present in significant amounts (9-*cis* and 13-*cis*); 15-*cis* β-carotene is found in trace amounts (FIG. 3B).

At least six geometrical isomers of lycopene are found in human serum and tissues (FIG. 3A,B). Similar results were obtained by Krinsky *et al.*[45] who observed at least 4–5 geometrical isomers in the chromatogram of a human plasma sample. The isomers directly eluting after the all-*trans* peak should be *cis-*isomers with the double bond located near the terminal positions of the molecule as determined by UV-VIS-spectroscopy. They are present in considerable amounts in serum and tissues. The *cis-*isomers of lycopene contribute more than 50% to total lycopene in human serum and tissue. In contrast to the β-carotene isomer pattern, human serum and tissue do not differ substantially in their composition of lycopene isomers.

Absorption of β-Carotene Geometrical Isomers

It is not yet known whether the absence of 9-*cis* β-carotene in serum is due to its low concentration compared to all-*trans* in dietary fruits and vegetables or as a result of specific biochemical mechanisms such as stereospecific uptake or *in vivo* isomerization.

After application of a natural mixture of all-*trans* and 9-*cis* β-carotene geometrical isomers (extract from *Dunaliella salina*) human serum samples were analysed for their β-carotene isomer pattern (FIG. 4). Only all-*trans* β-carotene appeared in serum, indicating that the composition of geometrical isomers in the diet is not responsible for the observed low level of 9-*cis* in human serum.[48] All-*trans* β-carotene shows a biokinetics similar to that described by other authors.[49]

In contrast to β-carotene, the *cis-*isomers of lycopene are absorbed when present in a dietary source.[50] There are different possibilities to explain the lack of 9-*cis* β-carotene in human serum. The *cis-*isomer might not be absorbed from the intestine, which would require specific discrimination mechanisms between geometrical isomers; alternatively, the *cis-*isomer is absorbed but very rapidly distributed into tissues. This would require distribution mechanisms working more

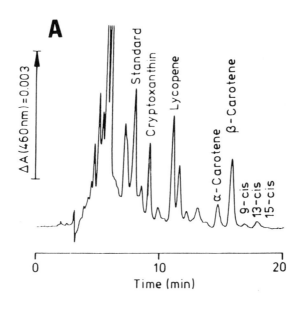

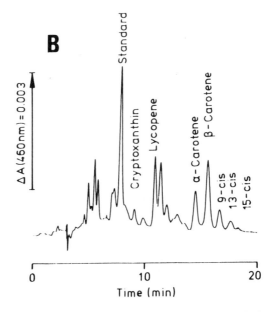

FIGURE 3. HPLC-chromatograms of a human serum (**A**) and testis tissue (**B**) sample.

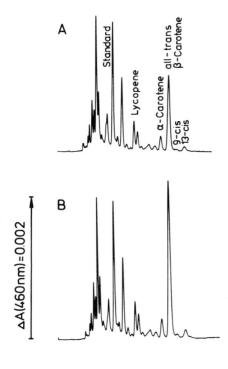

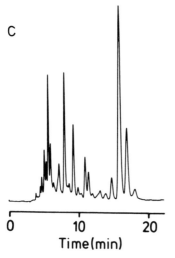

FIGURE 4. HPLC-chromatograms of human serum samples; before **(A)** and 48 h after **(B)** application of a natural mixture of all-*trans* and 9-*cis* β-carotene. **(C)** 48-h sample spiked with original 9-*cis* β-carotene.

rapidly than uptake. Furthermore, isomerases to produce all-*trans* β-carotene or enzymes processing 9-*cis* β-carotene to other products such as 9-*cis* retinoic acid could be operative.

REFERENCES

1. COMSTOCK, G. W., T. L. BUSH & K. HELZLSOUER. 1992. Serum retinol, beta-carotene, vitamin E, and selenium as related to subsequent cancer of specific sites. Am. J. Epidemiol. **135:** 115–121.
2. PETO, R., R. DOLL, J. D. BUCKLEY & M. B. SPORN. 1981. Can dietary beta-carotene materially reduce human cancer rates? Nature (London) **290:** 201–208.
3. ZIEGLER, R. G. 1989. A review of epidemiologic evidence that carotenoids reduce the risk of cancer. J. Nutr. **119:** 116–122.
4. BERTRAM, J. S., A. PUNG, M. CHURLEY, J. KAPPOCK, L. R. WILKENS & R. V. COONEY. 1991. Diverse carotenoids protect from chemically-induced neoplastic transformation. Carcinogenesis **12:** 671–678.
5. PUNG, A., J. E. RUNDHAUG, C. N. YOSHIZAWA & J. S. BERTRAM. 1988. β-Carotene and canthaxanthin inhibit chemically and physically induced neoplastic transformations in 10T1/2 cells. Carcinogenesis **9:** 1533–1539.
6. WOLF, G. 1992. Retinoids and carotenoids as inhibitors of carcinogenesis and inducers of cell-cell communication. Nutr. Rev. **50:** 270–274.
7. ZHANG, L. X., R. V. COONEY & J. S. BERTRAM. 1991. Carotenoids enhance gap junctional communication and inhibit lipid peroxidation in C3H/10T1/2 cells: relationship to their cancer chemopreventive action. Carcinogenesis **12:** 2309–2314.
8. BURTON, G. W. & K. U. INGOLD. 1984. β-Carotene: an unusual type of lipid antioxidant. Science **224:** 569–573.
9. FOOTE, C. S. & R. W. DENNY. 1968. Chemistry of singlet oxygen. VII. Quenching by β-carotene. J. Am. Chem. Sci. **90:** 6233–6235.
10. KRINSKY, N. I. 1989. Antioxidant functions of carotenoids. Free Radical Biol. Med. **7:** 617–635.
11. SIES, H., W. STAHL & A. R. SUNDQUIST. 1992. Antioxidant functions of vitamins (vitamins E and C, beta-carotene, and other carotenoids). In Beyond Deficiency: New Views on the Function and Health Benefits of Vitamins. H. E. Sauberlich & L. J. Machlin, Eds. Vol. 669: 7–20. Ann. N.Y. Acad. Sci.
12. ZECHMEISTER, L. 1962. *Cis-trans* Isomeric Carotenoids, Vitamin A, and Arylpolyenes. Springer Verlag. Vienna.
13. HEYMAN, R. A., D. J. MANGELSDORF, J. A. DYCK, R. B. STEIN, G. EICHELE, R. M. EVANS & C. THALLER. 1992. 9-*cis* Retinoic acid is a high affinity ligand for the retinoic X receptor. Cell **68:** 397–406.
14. LEVIN, A. A., L. J. STURZENBECKER, S. KAZMER, T. BOSAKOWSKI, C. HUSELTON, G. ALLENBY, J. SPECK, CL. KRATZEISEN, M. ROSENBERGER, E. LOVEY & J. F. GRIPPO. 1992. 9-*cis* Retinoic acid stereoisomer binds and activates the nuclear receptor RXR. Nature **355:** 359–361.
15. KLIEWER, S. A., K. UMESONO, D. J. NOONAN, R. A. HEYMAN & R. M. EVANS. 1992. Convergence of 9-*cis* retinoic acid and peroxisome proliferator signalling pathways through heterodimer formation of their receptors. Nature **358:** 771–774.
16. FOOTE, C. S., Y. C. CHANG & R. W. DENNY. 1970. Chemistry of singlet oxygen. XI. *Cis-trans* isomerization of carotenoids by singlet oxygen and a probable quenching mechanism. J. Am. Chem. Soc. **92:** 5218–5219.
17. DI MASCIO, P., A. R. SUNDQUIST, T. P. A. DEVASAGAYAM & H. SIES. 1992. Assay of lycopene and other carotenoids as singlet oxygen quenchers. Methods Enzymol. **213:** 429–438.
18. KRINSKY, N. I. 1979. Carotenoid protection against oxidation. Pure Appl. Chem. **51:** 649–660.
19. MATHIS, P. & C. SCHENCK. 1982. The function of carotenoids in photosynthesis. In

Carotenoid Chemistry & Biochemistry. G. Britton & T. W. Goodwin, Eds. 339–351. Pergamon Press. Oxford.

20. DiMascio, P., P. S. Kaiser & H. Sies. 1989. Lycopene as the most efficient biological carotenoid singlet oxygen quencher. Arch. Biochem. Biophys. **274:** 532–538.
21. Truscott, T. G. 1990. The photophysics and photo-chemistry of carotenoids. J. Photochem. Photobiol. B: Biol. **6:** 359–371.
22. Conn, P. F., W. Schalch & T. G. Truscott. 1991. The singlet oxygen and carotenoid interaction. J. Photochem. Photobiol. B: Biol. **11:** 41–47.
23. Devasagayam, T. P. A., T. Werner, H. Ippendorf, H. D., Martin & H. Sies. 1992. Synthetic carotenoids, novel polyene polyketones and new capsorubin isomers as efficient quenchers of singlet molecular oxygen. Photochem. Photobiol. **55:** 511–514.
24. Piette, J. 1991. Biological consequences associated with DNA oxidation mediated by singlet oxygen. J. Photochem. Photobiol. **11:** 241–260.
25. Epe, B. 1991. Genotoxicity of singlet oxygen. Chem. Biol. Interact. **80:** 239–260.
26. Sies, H. & C. F. M. Menck. 1992. Singlet oxygen induced DNA damage. Mutat. Res. **275:** 367–375.
27. Wefers, H., D. Schulte-Frohlinde & H. Sies. 1987. Loss of transforming activity of plasmid DNA (pBR322) in E. coli caused by singlet oxygen. FEBS Lett. **211:** 49–52.
28. Kulig, M. J. & L. L. Smith. 1973. Sterol metabolism. XXV. Cholesterol oxidation by singlet molecular oxygen. J. Org. Chem. **38:** 3639.
29. Kalyanaraman, B., J. B. Feix, F. Sieber, J. P. Thomas & A. W. Girotti. 1987. Photodynamic action of merocyanine 540 on artificial and natural cell membranes: involvement of singlet molecular oxygen. Proc. Nat. Acad. Sci. **84:** 2999.
30. Tsai, C. S., R. P. Godin & A. J. Wand. 1985. Dye sensitized photo-oxidation of enzymes. Biochem. J. **225:** 203.
31. Kanofsky, J. R. 1989. Singlet oxygen production in biological systems. Chem. Biol. Interact. **70:** 1–28.
32. Steinbeck, M. J., A. U. Kahn & M. J. Karnovsky. 1992. Intracellular singlet oxygen generation by phagocytosing neutrophils in response to particles coated with a chemical trap. J. Biol. Chem. **267:** 13425–13433.
33. Packer, J. E., J. S. Mahood, V. O. Mora-Arellano, T. F. Slater, R. L. Willson & B. S. Wolfenden. 1981. Free radicals and singlet oxygen scavengers: reaction of a peroxy-radical with β-carotene, diphenyl furan and 1,4-diazobicyclo(2,2,2)-octane. Biochem. Biophys. Res. Commun. **98:** 901–909.
34. Burton, G. W. & K. U. Ingold. 1984. β-carotene: an unusual type of lipid antioxidant. Science **224:** 569–573.
35. Kennedy, T. A. & D. C. Liebler. 1992. Peroxyl radical scavenging by β-carotene in lipid bilayers. J. Biol. Chem. **267:** 4658–4663.
36. Handelman, G. J., F. J. G. M. van Kuijk, A. Chatterjee & N. I. Krinsky. 1991. Characterization of products formed during the autoxidation of β-carotene. Free Radical Biol. Med. **10:** 427–437.
37. Parker, R. S., 1989. Carotenoids in human blood and tissues. J. Nutr. **119:** 101–104.
38. Krinsky, N. I., D. G. Cornwell & J. L. Oncley. 1958. The transport of vitamin A and carotenoids in human plasma. Arch. Biochem. Biophys. **73:** 233–246.
39. Kaplan, L. A., J. M. Lau & E. A. Stein. 1990. Carotenoid composition, concentration and relationships in various human organs. Clin. Physiol. Biochem. **8:** 1–8.
40. Stahl, W., W. Schwarz, A. R. Sundquist & H. Sies. 1992. Cis-trans isomers of lycopene and β-carotene in human serum and tissues. Arch. Biochem. Biophys. **294:** 173–177.
41. Jensen, C. D., T. W. Howes, G. A. Spiller, T. S. Pattison, J. H. Whittam & J. Scala. 1987. Observations on the effects of ingesting cis- and trans-beta-carotene isomers on human serum concentration. Nutr. Rep. Int. **35:** 413–422.
42. Chandler, L. A. & S. J. Schwartz. 1987. HPLC separation of cis-trans carotene isomers in fresh and processed fruits and vegetables. J. Food Sci. **52:** 669–672.
43. Sowell, A. L., D. L. Huff, E. W. Gunter & W. J. Driskell. 1988. Identification of cis-carotenoids in human sera analyzed by reversed phase high performance liquid chromatography with diode array detection. J. Chromatogr. **431:** 424–430.

44. KHACHIK, F., G. R. BEECHER & W. R. LUSBY. 1989. Separation, identification, and quantification of the major carotenoids in extracts of apricots, peaches, cantaloupe, and pink grapefruit by liquid chromatography. J. Agric. Food Chem. **37:** 1465–1473.
45. KRINSKY, N. I., M. D. RUSSETT, G. J. HANDELMAN & D. M. SNODDERLY. 1990. Structural and geometrical isomers of carotenoids in human plasma. J. Nutr. **120:** 1654–1662.
46. LEVIN, A. A., L. J. STURZENBECKER, S. KAZMER, T. BOSAKOWSKI, C. HUSELTON, G. ALLENBY, J. SPECK, CL. KRATZEISEN, M. ROSENBERGER, A. LOVEY & J. F. GRIPPO. 1992. A new pathway for vitamin A: understanding the pleiotropic effects of retinoids. *In* Beyond Deficiency. H. E. Sauberlich & L. J. Machlin, Eds. Vol. 669: 70–86. Ann. N.Y. Acad. Sci.
47. BIERI, J. G., E. D. BROWN & J. C. SMITH. 1985. Determination of individual carotenoids in human plasma by high performance liquid chromatography. J. Liq. Chromatogr. **8:** 473–484.
48. STAHL, W., W. SCHWARZ & H. SIES. 1993. Human serum concentrations of all-*trans* β- and α-carotene but not 9-*cis* β-carotene increase upon ingestion of a natural isomer mixture obtained from *Dunaliella salina* (Betatene). J. Nutr. **123:** 847–851.
49. BROWN, E. D., M. S. MICOZZI, N. E. CRAFT, J. G. BIERI, G. BEECHER, B. K. EDWARDS, A. ROSE, P. R. TAYLOR & J. C. SMITH. 1989. Plasma carotenoids in normal men after a single ingestion of vegetables or purified β-carotene. Am. J. Clin. Nutr. **49:** 1258–1265.
50. STAHL, W. & H. SIES. 1992. Uptake of lycopene and its geometrical isomers is greater from heat-processed than from unprocessed tomato juice in humans. J. Nutr. **122:** 2161–2166.

Antioxidant Reactions of Carotenoids[a]

DANIEL C. LIEBLER

Department of Pharmacology and Toxicology
College of Pharmacy
University of Arizona
Tucson, Arizona 85721

The carotenoid antioxidant hypothesis postulates that carotenoids prevent cancer and degenerative diseases by preventing biological oxidative damage.[1-4] In this context, the term "antioxidant" broadly refers to any reaction that consumes oxidants. Carotenoids indeed are versatile antioxidants—they prevent both singlet oxygen- and free radical-mediated damage. Foote and colleagues first demonstrated the exceptional singlet oxygen quenching action of β-carotene (**1**, FIG. 1) in 1968.[5] Burton and Ingold later documented the peroxyl radical scavenging properties of β-carotene.[6] Several other groups have described β-carotene-dependent inhibition of lipid peroxidation.[7-13] β-Carotene is the most widely studied antioxidant carotenoid and is a prototype for many other carotenoids, which display similar antioxidant properties.[14] The biological relevance of carotenoid antioxidant actions in humans was affirmed by the work of Mathews-Roth and colleagues, who employed β-carotene to treat erythropoietic porphyria, in which photosensitizer-generated singlet oxygen and free radicals cause oxidative skin damage.[15] The evident promise of carotenoids as preventive agents for cancer[2,16] and atherosclerosis[4] suggests an even broader human health significance for carotenoid antioxidant chemistry.

Do carotenoids act as antioxidants *in vivo*? If so, how can the carotenoid antioxidant hypothesis be tested experimentally? One might measure oxidative damage in relevant *in vitro* and *in vivo* models and attempt to modulate the damage by manipulating tissue carotenoid levels. This certainly presents a daunting analytical challenge, not only because oxidative damage is inherently difficult to measure, but also because modulation of damage may reflect actions of other antioxidants or other processes (*e.g.*, repair). An alternate approach is to identify specific products of carotenoid antioxidant reactions that may serve as markers for antioxidant function. Measurement of marker products in systems where carotenoids suppress oxidative damage would provide convincing evidence for biologically relevant antioxidant function. Implementation of this approach requires an understanding of carotenoid-oxidant reaction chemistry and the development of sensitive analytical methods to detect reaction products. Here I summarize our current understanding of carotenoid antioxidant chemistry and discuss the potential utility of specific products as markers for carotenoid antioxidant actions.

Antioxidant and Autoxidation Reactions

Burton and Ingold demonstrated that β-carotene inhibits lipid peroxidation primarily by trapping peroxyl radicals and is thus a *chain-breaking antioxidant*.[6]

[a] This work was supported in part by United States Public Health Service Grant CA 56875.

Chain-breaking antioxidants react primarily with peroxyl radicals, which propagate radical chain reactions[17] (Eq. 1).

$$LOO^\bullet + LH \rightarrow LOOH + L^\bullet \tag{1}$$

The antioxidant reaction is depicted in Eq. (2), in which the antioxidant traps a peroxyl radical to form an antioxidant-derived radical intermediate.

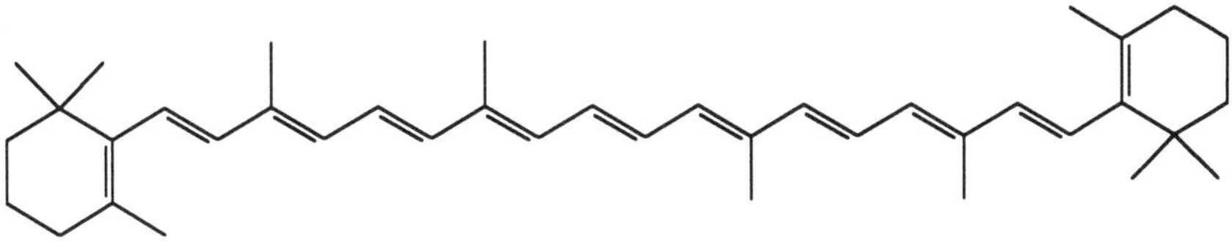

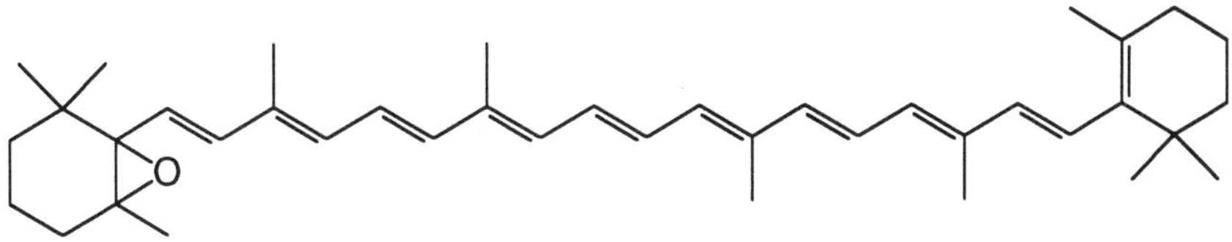

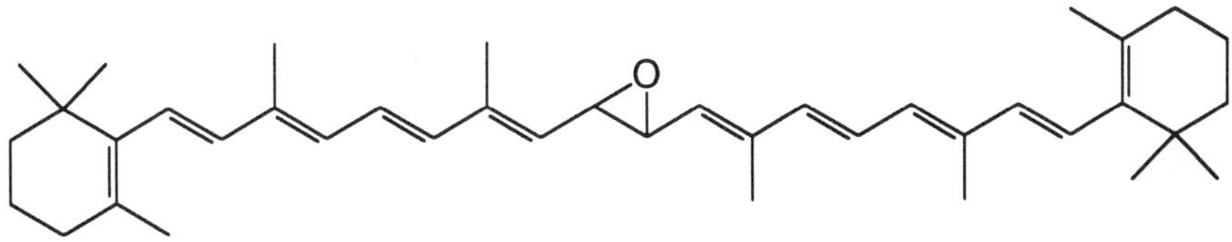

FIGURE 1. Structures of β-carotene and its epoxide and endoperoxide oxidation products.

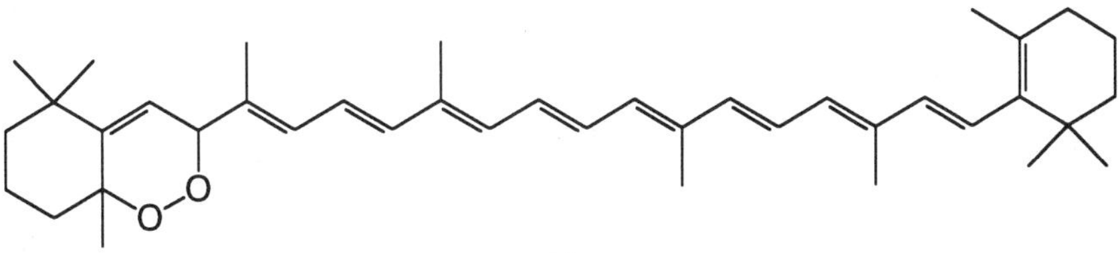

$$LOO^\bullet + antioxidant \rightarrow \text{"radical intermediate"} \tag{2}$$

To be biologically effective chain-breaking antioxidants, carotenoids must preferentially intercept peroxyl radicals, even when other oxidizable substrates are present in great excess. In other words, reaction 2 must be *much* faster than reaction 1. Nature's best chain-breaking antioxidant, α-tocopherol (vitamin E), does this with ease. One α-tocopherol molecule typically protects 1000 membrane phospholipids,[18,19] because it reacts with peroxyl radicals 100–1000 times faster than do phospholipid-bound polyunsaturated fatty acids.[20,21] β-Carotene, too, is exceptionally reactive towards peroxyl radicals[22] and might be expected to be as potent an antioxidant as α-tocopherol.

However, *in vitro* experiments in solution, detergent micelles, and in lipid bilayer systems indicate that β-carotene does not suppress lipid peroxidation nearly as well as α-tocopherol at equal concentrations.[12,23] The reason for this difference, as Burton and Ingold demonstrated, is that the "radical intermediate" formed from β-carotene in reaction 2 behaves somewhat differently from that formed from α-tocopherol, the tocopheroxyl radical.[6] Both intermediates may trap a second peroxyl radical to form a nonradical product (Eq. 3).

$$\text{"radical intermediate"} + LOO^{\bullet} \rightarrow \text{nonradical product(s)} \qquad (3)$$

In a competing reaction, both radical intermediates react *reversibly* with oxygen to form a peroxyl radical (Eq. 4).

$$\text{"radical intermediate"} + O_2 \leftrightarrow \text{antioxidant-OO}^{\bullet} \qquad (4)$$

For the tocopheroxyl radical, the equilibrium in reaction 4 lies far to the left and the tocopheroxyl radical is consumed mainly by reaction 3.[24] However, for the β-carotene-derived radical intermediate, the equilibrium in reaction 4 lies much farther to the right. Moreover, the equilibrium is pushed further to the right as the oxygen tension is increased.[6] Reaction 4 generates a peroxyl radical, which continues a radical chain.

Reaction pathways such as (reaction 2 $\rightarrow$ reaction 3) consume radicals and are referred to here as *antioxidant reactions*. In contrast, reaction pathways such as (reaction 2 $\rightarrow$ reaction 4) consume antioxidants without consuming radicals and are *autoxidation reactions*. Antioxidant effectiveness depends on the balance between antioxidant reactions, which trap radicals, and autoxidation reactions, which drain antioxidants from the system. Burton and Ingold demonstrated that for β-carotene this balance is highly dependent on oxygen tension and that β-carotene antioxidant performance decreases at high oxygen tensions.[6] Others have confirmed this oxygen effect,[9,12,13] and it seems likely that the lower antioxidant potency of β-carotene in some *in vitro* experiments reflects β-carotene autoxidation (*i.e.*, reaction 4). However, low antioxidant potency may also reflect the way in which β-carotene is incorporated into the experimental system used as discussed below. Based on their model studies of the oxygen effect in homogeneous solution, Burton and Ingold suggested that β-carotene should be most effective as an antioxidant in tissues with lower oxygen tensions.[6] Our studies in a liposome model indicated that β-carotene provided essentially equal antioxidant protection under an air atmosphere (150 torr O_2) as under a 15 torr O_2 atmosphere,[9] which is similar to the oxygen tension in many tissues.[25] We did observe that β-carotene was consumed faster under air than under 15 torr O_2, even though β-carotene provided similar antioxidant protection under both conditions.[9] More rapid depletion under air presumably reflected greater β-carotene autoxidation under air than under 15 torr O_2. β-Carotene therefore should provide antioxidant protection even to more highly oxygenated tissues, although concomitant autoxidation reactions may waste a greater fraction of the β-carotene in these tissues.

Reactions of β-Carotene with Peroxyl Radicals

Application of modern analytical techniques has yielded valuable information on the oxidative fate of β-carotene in peroxyl radical reactions. Peroxyl radicals derived from the azo initiators 2,2′-azobis(2,4-dimethylvaleronitrile) (AMVN) in hexane[26] or 2,2′-azobis(isobutyronitrile) in toluene[27] yielded 5,6-epoxy-β,β-carotene (**2**, FIG. 1), and two isomers of a previously unreported product, 15,15′-epoxy-β,β-carotene (**3**). The oxidations in toluene also yielded several chain cleavage products, including β-apo-10′-carotenal (**4**, FIG. 2), β-apo-12′-carotenal (**5**), β-apo-14′-carotenal (**6**), retinal (**7**), and β-apo-13′-carotenone (**8**). Peroxyl radicals apparently mediated β-carotene "autoxidation" in toluene,[27] benzene,[28] and carbon tetrachloride[28] without an azo initiator, since essentially the same products were formed. Extended oxidation in these systems yields an increasingly complex product distribution, as all of the primary products undergo further oxidation.[26,28]

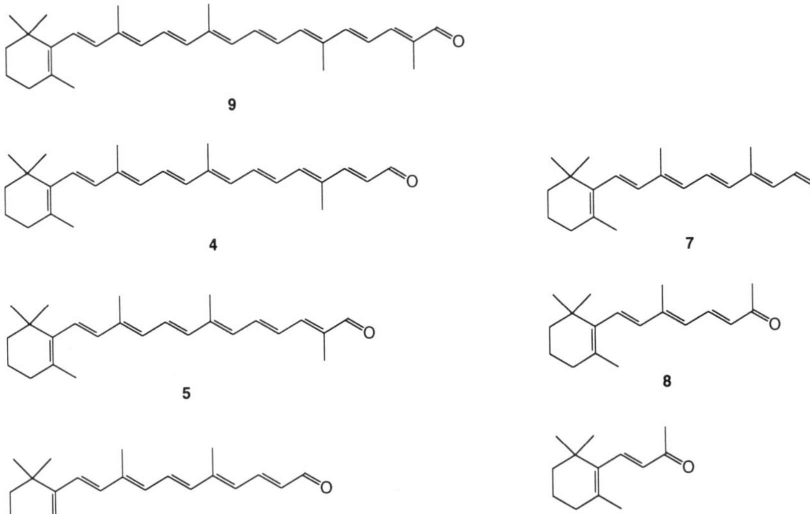

FIGURE 2. Structures of β-carotene chain-cleavage products.

Peroxyl radicals are thought to react with carotenoids and related polyenes by addition.[6] Addition to the 5,6-double bond followed by elimination of an alkoxyl radical thus yields epoxides **2** and **3**[26,29] (FIG. 3, pathway A). Peroxyl radical addition to the polyene chain may also initiate the formation of apocarotenal and apocarotenone chain cleavage products. Addition of a peroxyl radical to any of the polyene double bonds would form a resonance-stabilized radical adduct (FIG. 3, pathway B). Addition of a second peroxyl radical would form a *bis*-peroxyl adduct, which then would decompose to carbonyl-containing products. The adducts themselves have not been identified as products, but their existence has been inferred from the formation of carbonyl products. Although addition of the

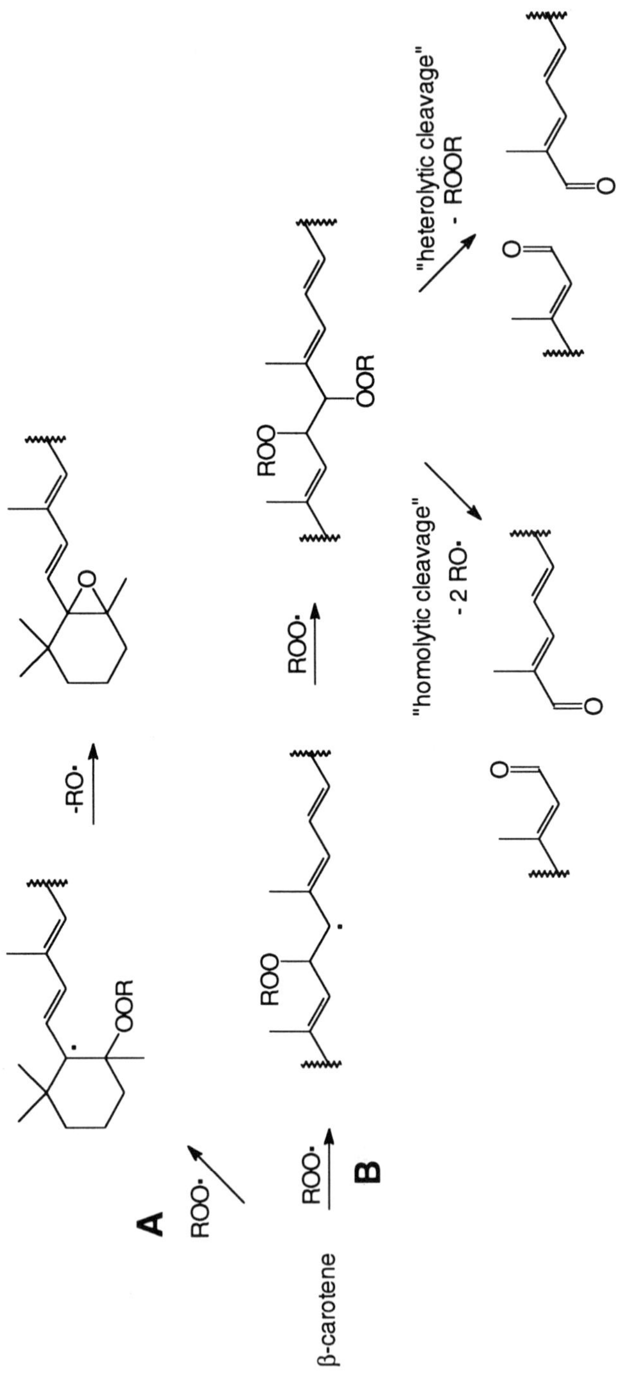

FIGURE 3. Reaction pathways for peroxyl radical-dependent β-carotene oxidation via radical addition (see text for discussion).

second peroxyl radical in FIGURE 3 is depicted as occurring vicinal (*i.e.*, immediately adjacent) to the first, addition could occur at other positions on the polyene, because this radical is resonance-delocalized. Indeed, addition to other positions may be favored if steric hindrance between bulky peroxyl substituents retards vicinal addition. However, the polyunsaturated dialdehydes expected from decomposition of these "nonvicinal" *bis*-peroxyl adducts have not yet been identified as β-carotene oxidation products. Another mechanism for cleavage of the β-carotene polyene to carbonyl products may involve formation of dioxetane intermediates, which would decompose readily to the observed carbonyl products. Although dioxetanes most likely are intermediates in singlet oxygen-dependent oxidations (see below), there is no evidence for their involvement in peroxyl radical-mediated oxidations.

Peroxyl radicals may react with β-carotene by mechanisms other than addition. For example, peroxyl radicals are sufficiently strong oxidants to remove an electron from the electron-rich β-carotene polyene[30,31] (Eq. 5).

$$\beta\text{-carotene} + ROO^{\bullet} \rightarrow \beta\text{-carotene}^{+\bullet} + ROO^{-} \qquad (5)$$

The resulting β-carotene cation radical displays a characteristic near-infrared absorption at approximately 955 nm.[22,30] Although this resonance-stabilized radical is reported not to react readily with oxygen, it appears to be a strong enough oxidant to accept electrons from other electron donors.[32] In this regard, it seems possible that carotenoid cation radicals, if formed in biological systems, could be reduced back to carotenoids by α-tocopherol, ubiquinol, or other lipophilic electron donors.

Carotenoids apparently do not react with peroxyl radicals by hydrogen abstraction. Samaokyszyn and Marnett indicated that the prostaglandin synthetase-dependent co-oxidation of 13-*cis*-retinoic acid yielded a 4-hydroxy product and a 5,6-epoxide analogous to product **2** formed from β-carotene.[29] The 4-hydroxy product, which was thought to arise via abstraction of the allylic 4-hydrogen followed by oxygen addition, hydrogen abstraction, and hydroperoxide reduction, was formed only in oxidations mediated by the enzyme and was not produced by peroxyl radicals.[29] Moreover, 4-hydroxy derivatives have not been reported as products of β-carotene autoxidation.

Relationship of Product-Forming Reactions to Antioxidant Effects

The potential relevance of the product-forming mechanisms discussed above is that they may indicate which β-carotene oxidation products arise from antioxidant (*i.e.*, radical trapping) reactions as opposed to autoxidation reactions. Of the products discussed above, epoxides **2** and **3** are formed by the most straightforward mechanism[26,29] (FIG. 3, pathway A). However, the epoxide-forming reaction releases an alkoxyl radical, which reduces the net consumption of radicals to zero. Oxidation of β-carotene to epoxides thus would not be expected to produce an antioxidant effect.

The other predominant reaction of β-carotene with peroxyl radicals yields carbonyl products (FIG. 3, pathway B). Whether this reaction sequence results in an antioxidant effect depends on how the postulated *bis*-peroxyl adducts decompose. Homolytic cleavage of the alkyldioxy moieties, as suggested by Mordi *et al.*[28] would form carbonyl products, but also would release two alkoxyl radicals, which would continue radical chains. This would result in no net radical consumption and no antioxidant effect. On the other hand, heterolytic cleavage of the vicinal alkyldioxy moieties would yield carbonyl fragments and a dialkyl peroxide or other nonradical products. β-Carotene oxidation to carbonyl products by this pathway would then consume two peroxyl radicals and produce an antioxidant effect.

Although all of the above reaction products are formed under conditions that favor β-carotene autoxidation (*e.g.*, high oxygen tension), no data document variations in relative product yields with oxygen tension. Studies examining product distributions at different oxygen tensions may help to differentiate autoxidation products (formed preferentially at high oxygen tension) from antioxidant reaction products (formed at low oxygen tension).

Reaction products other than those derived from peroxyl radical addition may also reflect antioxidant reactions. Peroxyl radicals may oxidize β-carotene to a cation radical, as discussed above. Grant *et al.* reported that carotenoid cation radicals formed in tetrahydrofuran reacted immediately with this solvent[30] and it seems reasonable to suspect that cation radicals formed in biological media could yield unique products. Identification of products formed by one-electron oxidation of β-carotene would indicate whether unique products result from one-electron oxidations or whether previously identified products may also result from one-electron oxidations. As with products of radical addition, assignment of one-electron oxidation products as antioxidant-specific would be based on the mechanism and oxygen tension-dependence of product formation.

Oxidation of β-Carotene by Singlet Oxygen

Carotenoids were the first singlet oxygen quenchers to be characterized and remain among the most effective quenchers known.[5,33] The predominant quenching mechanism is a "physical quenching" reaction, in which the carotenoid converts singlet oxygen to triplet (ground state) oxygen by absorbing and then thermally dispersing excess excited state energy.[33] Physical quenching is accompanied by a chemical reaction that destroys the carotenoid.[14,34] Although a single β-carotene molecule may quench up to 1000 singlet oxygen molecules before becoming oxidized,[5] irreversible oxidation ultimately limits this antioxidant capacity. The antioxidant impact of this "chemical quenching" reaction undoubtedly is negligible. However, the reaction is of potential interest because it may generate specific marker products for β-carotene-singlet oxygen interactions.

To investigate this possibility, we studied the photooxidation of β-carotene in homogeneous toluene/methanol solutions.[35] Oxidations were done by irradiating oxygenated solutions containing β-carotene, Rose Bengal bis(trimethylammonium) salt with a quartz halogen lamp at 4°C. Products were isolated from the reaction mixture and analyzed by reverse phase and normal phase HPLC with diode array detection and by direct probe mass spectrometry or gas chromatography-mass spectrometry. Products of the reaction included β-apo-8'-carotenal (**9**), β-apo-10'-carotenal (**4**), β-apo-14'-carotenal (**6**), and β-ionone (**10**) (FIG. 2). In addition to these chain cleavage products, a unique oxygen-addition product was identified as β-carotene-5,8-endoperoxide (**11**) (FIG. 1).

Photooxidations may involve free radical (Type I) reactions as well as singlet oxygen (Type II) reactions.[14] Free radical oxidation might be suspected in this system, as apocarotenal products are formed by free radical oxidations (see above). However, free radicals apparently did not mediate product formation in our photooxidation system. The photooxidation did not produce either 5,6-epoxide **2** or

15,15′-epoxide **3**, which are peroxyl radical oxidation products of β-carotene[26] and are formed by AMVN-initiated oxidation in the same solvent. Moreover, product yields were not affected in photooxidations containing β-carotene and equimolar α-tocopherol. α-Tocopherol at this concentration completely suppressed AMVN-initiated oxidation. These results indicate that β-carotene photooxidation was mediated by singlet oxygen rather than by free radicals.

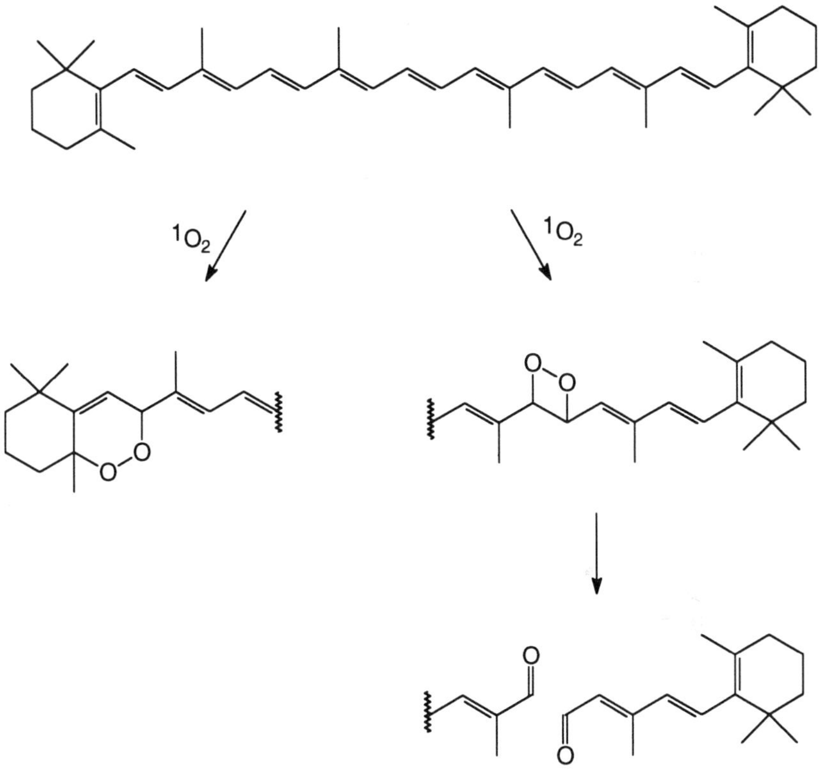

FIGURE 4. Reaction pathways for singlet oxygen-dependent β-carotene oxidation (see text for discussion).

The formation of both the carbonyl products and endoperoxide can be attributed to well-known reactions of singlet oxygen (FIG. 4). Chain cleavage may result from addition of singlet oxygen to the polyene to form labile dioxetanes, which then decompose to carbonyl products.[36] Interestingly, not all bonds were cleaved. The observed product pattern indicated attack at the 7,8-, 9,10-, 11,12-, and 13,14-double bonds. We have no explanation for this apparent selectivity. Formation of the endoperoxide represents singlet oxygen addition to the *cis* form of the 5,6,7,8-diene. This reaction has been observed previously in photooxidations of structurally analogous retinoids.[37,38]

Endoperoxide **11** (FIG. 1) is unique among known β-carotene oxidation products in that it has been identified only in oxidations mediated by singlet oxygen. Further investigations in more biologically relevant model systems will be required to establish the validity of endoperoxide **11** or a structurally unique decomposition product as a specific marker for the reaction of β-carotene with singlet oxygen. If singlet oxygen does oxidize carotenoids to endoperoxides in biological systems, *cis* isomers of β-carotene and other carotenoids may yield analogous products. Moreover, estimation of partition ratios between physical singlet oxygen quenching and endoperoxide formation may permit quantitative estimates of singlet oxygen quenching in tissues through product analysis.

Antioxidant Effectiveness of β-Carotene in Vitro

An important intermediate objective in the search for antioxidant-specific products of β-carotene oxidation is the development of appropriate experimental models for *in vitro* studies. These models can be used to characterize the relationships between formation of specific products and the expression of antioxidant effects under defined conditions. The ability to accurately manipulate β-carotene concentrations in such systems is critical to defining its antioxidant role. Incorporation of β-carotene into biological membranes *in vitro* clearly would be easier than manipulation of β-carotene concentrations through dietary supplementation. Moreover, *in vitro* incorporation could provide more precise control over carotenoid levels and would eliminate secondary variables related to nutrient absorption and distribution during β-carotene supplementation. Despite these advantages, incorporation of β-carotene into biological membranes *in vitro* has proved difficult.

Recent studies indicate that β-carotene inhibited AMVN-initiated peroxidation of phosphatidylcholine liposomes at concentrations of approximately 0.1–0.5 mole percent (*i.e.*, 0.1–0.5 mol β-carotene per 100 mol phospholipid).[9,12] These concentrations are similar to those of α-tocopherol in biological membranes.[18,19] In contrast, little or no inhibition of AMVN-initiated lipid peroxidation was detected in rat liver microsomes to which β-carotene had been added at 10 nmol per mg microsomal protein (approximately 1.5 mole percent based on microsomal phospholipid).[11] Other work indicated that 50 percent inhibition of iron-catalyzed microsomal lipid peroxidation required 50 nmol β-carotene per mg protein (approximately 7.5 mol percent).[13] These concentrations are 10–50-fold higher than needed to provide antioxidant protection in liposomes and might be above levels that could be achieved by dietary supplementation.

We postulated that these differences reflected differences in the physical incorporation and distribution of β-carotene in the microsomal and liposomal models studied. In the liposome systems, β-carotene was mixed with phospholipids prior to liposome formation.[9,12] This procedure apparently results in incorporation of β-carotene into the bilayer structure, although the exact orientation of the carotenoid remains uncertain. We refer here to β-carotene in this model as "incorporated" β-carotene. In contrast, microsomal membranes are preformed lipid bilayers to which β-carotene was added from stock solutions in chloroform[13] or absorbed from glassware used for microsome preparation.[11] How β-carotene is associated with these lipid bilayers is unclear and we refer here to β-carotene in these preparations as "added" β-carotene.

In order to distinguish differences in the antioxidant actions of "incorporated" and "added" β-carotene under controlled conditions, we employed dilinoleoyl-phosphatidylcholine liposomes to which β-carotene had been added by both methods. We incubated liposomes with 50 μM FeCl$_3$, xanthine, and xanthine oxidase and measured lipid peroxidation via the assay of conjugated dienes.[9] Peroxidation in liposomes containing 0.4 mole percent "incorporated" β-carotene was inhibited by approximately 80 percent (FIG. 5). In liposomes containing "added" β-carotene (from a stock solution in tetrahydrofuran), peroxidation was inhibited by only 10–20 percent. In experiments where peroxidation was initiated instead by AMVN or by the water-soluble azo initiator 2,2'-*bis*-(2-amidinopropane hydrochloride), similar results were obtained (data not shown). These results suggest that differences in the method of β-carotene incorporation into membrane preparations may drastically affect antioxidant activity. Similar results were observed previously in microsomes supplemented with α-tocopherol by addition of an ethanolic stock solution.[39] This procedure increased microsome-associated α-tocopherol several-fold, but did not increase antioxidant protection. In contrast, enhanced antioxidant

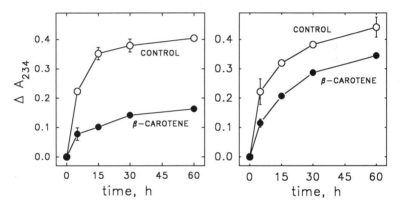

FIGURE 5. Inhibition of lipid peroxidation in dilinoleoylphosphatidylcholine liposomes by β-carotene. Small unilamellar liposome suspensions (0.5 mM phospholipid) were incubated with 50 μM FeCl$_3$, xanthine, and xanthine oxidase and oxidation was monitored by assay of conjugated dienes. Liposomes contained no antioxidant (*open symbols*) or 0.4 mole percent "incorporated" β-carotene (*left, filled symbols*) or 0.4 mole percent "added" β-carotene (*right, filled symbols*).

protection was provided by α-tocopherol generated *in situ* by microsomal esterase-catalyzed hydrolysis of α-tocopheryl succinate.[39] Ester hydrolysis presumably was accompanied by a more effective incorporation of the released α-tocopherol into the membranes.

The necessity of reliable methods to incorporate β-carotene into biological membranes or lipoproteins for *in vitro* studies seems clear, but the methods themselves remain to be identified. Bertram and co-workers found that carotenoids added to cultured cells from stock solutions in tetrahydrofuran inhibited lipid peroxidation,[40] neoplastic transformation[41] and enhanced connexin43 gene expression.[42] However, cells apparently are better able to incorporate solubilized carotenoids than are isolated membrane preparations. This may be due to the participation of cellular binding and transport proteins analogous to those that interact with α-tocopherol.[43,44] These proteins appear to facilitate the incorporation of

α-tocopherol into microsomal membranes *in vitro*.[45,46] We are currently investigating this and other approaches to incorporating β-carotene and other carotenoids into biological membranes.

ACKNOWLEDGMENTS

I thank Steve Stratton, Kathy Kaysen and Drs. William Schaefer and Thomas McClure for their contributions to this work.

REFERENCES

1. KRINSKY, N. I. 1989. Prev. Med. **18:** 592–602.
2. BYERS, T. & G. PERRY. 1992. Ann. Rev. Nutr. **12:** 139–159.
3. AMES, B. N. 1983. Science **221:** 1256–1264.
4. STEINBERG, D., J. A. BERLINER, G. W. BURTON, T. E. CAREW, A. CHAIT, G. M. CHISOLM, H. ESTERBAUER, A. M. FOGELMAN, P. L. FOX, C. D. FURBERG, J. M. GAZIANO, K. F. GEY, S. M. GRUNDY, W. R. HARLAN, R. J. HAVEL, C. H. HENNEKENS, H. F. HOFF, R. L. JACKSON, H. J. KAYDEN, A. KEECH, N. I. KRINSKY, J. MANSON, S. PARTHASARATHY, J. PROBSTFIELD, W. A. PRYOR, B. RIFKIND, E. R. STADTMAN, R. B. WALLACE, J. L. WITZUM, S. YLAHERTTUALA & S. YUSUF. 1992. Circulation **85:** 2338–2344.
5. FOOTE, C. S. & R. W. DENNY. 1968. J. Am. Chem. Soc. **90:** 6233–6235.
6. BURTON, G. W. & K. U. INGOLD. 1984. Science **224:** 569–573.
7. TERAO, J. 1989. Lipids **24:** 659–661.
8. KRINSKY, N. I. & S. M. DENEKE. 1982. J. Natl. Cancer Inst. **69:** 205–210.
9. KENNEDY, T. A. & D. C. LIEBLER. 1992. J. Biol. Chem. **267:** 4658–4663.
10. LIM, B. P., A. NAGAO, J. TERAO, K. TANAKA, T. SUZUKI & K. TAKAMA. 1992. Biochim. Biophys. Acta **1126:** 178–184.
11. PALOZZA, P., S. MOUALLA & N. I. KRINSKY. 1992. Free Radical Biol. Med. **13:** 127–136.
12. STOCKER, R., Y. YAMAMOTO, A. F. MCDONAGH, A. N. GLAZER & B. N. AMES. 1987. Science **235:** 1043–1046.
13. VILE, G. F. & C. C. WINTERBOURN. 1988. FEBS Lett. **238:** 353–356.
14. KRINSKY, N. I. 1989. Free Radical Biol. Med. **7:** 617–635.
15. MATHEWS-ROTH, M. M. 1986. Biochimie **68:** 875–884.
16. MALONE, W. F. 1991. Am. J. Clin. Nutr. **53:** 305S–313S.
17. PRYOR, W. A. 1984. *In* Free Radicals in Molecular Biology, Aging & Disease. D. Armstrong, R. S. Sohal, R. G. Cutler & T. F. Slater, Eds. 13–41. Raven Press. New York.
18. KORNBRUST, D. J. & R. D. MAVIS. 1980. Lipids **15:** 315–322.
19. SEVANIAN, A., A. D. HACKER & N. ELSAYED. 1982. Lipids **17:** 269–277.
20. BURTON, G. W. & K. U. INGOLD. 1981. J. Am. Chem. Soc. **103:** 6472–6477.
21. HOWARD, J. A. & K. U. INGOLD. 1967. Can. J. Chem. **45:** 793–802.
22. PACKER, J. E., J. S. MAHOOD, V. O. MORA-ARELLANO, T. F. SLATER, R. L. WILLSON & B. S. WOLFENDEN. 1981. Biochem. Biophys. Res. Commun. **98:** 901–906.
23. PRYOR, W. A., T. STRICKLAND & D. F. CHURCH. 1988. J. Am. Chem. Soc. **110:** 2224–2229.
24. DOBA, T., G. W. BURTON, K. U. INGOLD & M. MATSUO. 1984. J. Chem. Soc. Chem. Commun. 461–462.
25. KESSLER, M., J. HOPER, D. K. HARRISON, K. SKOLASINOKA, W. P. KLOVEKORN, F. SEBENING, H. J. VOLKHOLZ, I. BEIER, C. KERNBACH, C. RETTIG & H. RICHTER. 1984. *In* Oxygen Transport to Tissues-V, Adv. Exp. Biol. Med., Vol. 169. D. W. Lubbers, H. Acker, E. Lenger-Follert & T. K. Goldstick, Eds. 69–80. Plenum Press. New York.
26. KENNEDY, T. A. & D. C. LIEBLER. 1991. Chem. Res. Toxicol. **4:** 290–295.

27. HANDELMAN, G. J., F. J. G. M. VAN KUIJK, A. CHATTERJEE & N. I. KRINSKY. 1991. Free Radical Biol. Med. **10:** 427–437.
28. MORDI, R. C., J. C. WALTON, G. W. BURTON, L. HUGHES, K. U. INGOLD & D. A. LINDSAY. 1991. Tetrahedron Lett. **32:** 4203–4206.
29. SAMOKYSZYN, V. M. & L. J. MARNETT. 1987. J. Biol. Chem. **262:** 14119–14133.
30. GRANT, J. L., V. J. KRAMER, R. DING & L. D. KISPERT. 1988. J. Am. Chem. Soc. **110:** 2151–2157.
31. JOVANOVIC, S. V., I. JOVANOVIC & L. JOSIMOVIC. 1992. J. Am. Chem. Soc. **114:** 9018–9021.
32. SIMIC, M. G. 1992. Methods Enzymol. **213:** 444–453.
33. FOOTE, C. S. 1979. *In* Singlet Oxygen. H. H. Wasserman & R. W. Murray, Eds. 139–171. Academic Press. New York.
34. HASEGAWA, K., J. D. MACMILLAN, W. A. MAXWELL & C. O. CHICHESTER. 1969. Photochem. Photobiol. **9:** 165–169.
35. STRATTON, S. P., W. H. SCHAEFER & D. C. LIEBLER. 1993. Submitted.
36. BARTLETT, P. D. & M. E. LANDIS. 1979. *In* Singlet Oxygen. H. H. Wasserman & R. W. Murray, Eds. 244–286. Academic Press. London.
37. DALLE, J. P., M. MOUSSERON-CANET & J. C. MANI. 1969. Bull. Soc. Chim. Fr. 232–239.
38. OLIVE, J. L. & M. MOUSSERON-CANET. 1969. Bull. Soc. Chim. Fr. 3252–3257.
39. CARINI, R., G. POLI, M. U. DIANZANI, S. P. MADDIX, T. F. SLATER & K. H. CHEESEMAN. 1990. Biochem. Pharmacol. **39:** 1597–1601.
40. ZHANG, L. X., R. V. COONEY & J. S. BERTRAM. 1991. Carcinogenesis **12:** 2109–2114.
41. BERTRAM, J. S., A. PUNG, M. CHURLEY, T. J. KAPPOCK, IV, L. R. WILKINS & R. V. COONEY. 1991. Carcinogenesis **12:** 671–678.
42. ZHANG, L. X., R. V. COONEY & J. S. BERTRAM. 1992. Cancer Res. **52:** 5707–5712.
43. CATIGNANI, G. L. & J. G. BIERI. 1977. Biochim. Biophys. Acta **497:** 349–357.
44. MURPHY, D. J. & R. D. MAVIS. 1981. J. Biol. Chem. **256:** 10464–10468.
45. BEHRENS, W. A. & R. MADERE. 1982. Nutr. Res. **2:** 611–618.
46. ROBEY-BOND, S. M., R. D. MAVIS & J. N. FINKELSTEIN. 1989. *In* Vitamin E: Biochemistry and Health Implications. Ann. N.Y. Acad. Sci., Vol. 570. A. T. Diplock, L. J. Machlin, L. Packer & W. A. Pryor, Eds. 511–513. New York Academy of Sciences. New York.

The Photochemistry of Carotenoids

Some Photosynthetic and Photomedical Aspects[a]

DEVENS GUST,[b] THOMAS A. MOORE,[b] ANA L. MOORE,[b]
GIULIO JORI,[c] AND ELENA REDDI[c]

[b]Department of Chemistry and Biochemistry
Center for the Study of Early Events in Photosynthesis
Arizona State University
Tempe, Arizona 85287-1604
and
[c]Department of Biology
University of Padova
Via Trieste 75-35121
Padova, Italy

The occurrence of carotenoid polyenes in the human diet and the resulting health-related effects are a direct consequence of the fact that carotenoids are vital constituents of the photosynthetic apparatus of green plants and other organisms. World-wide, immense quantities of these materials are biosynthesized each year, and they find their way into the food chains of animals and humans through a variety of pathways. Carotenoids were selected by the evolving photosynthetic apparatus because of their unique photophysical properties. Thus, consideration of these properties and the ways in which photosynthetic organisms make use of them can help us understand some of the health-related roles of carotenes. This article will briefly review the photosynthetic functions of carotenoids and show how they can be mimicked in properly designed synthetic molecular systems. Finally, an illustration of how the results of these model system studies may be used to design medically useful carotenoid-containing agents will be presented.

Carotenoid Photophysics

This discussion applies to the genre of carotenoid pigments having nine or more conjugated double bonds including oxy- and hydroxy-substituted compounds, although there are, of course, small differences between pigments. The most obvious property of carotenes is their intense orange color, which results from absorption of light in the 400–550-nm region. Carotenes typically have very high extinction coefficients ($\varepsilon_{max} \sim 10^5$) in this region. This strongly electric dipole allowed transition is from the ground state (S_0) to the *second* excited singlet state, S_2, of the carotenoid. As one would expect for an upper excited singlet state, the S_2 species has a very short lifetime (on the order of 100 fs).[1] Because of the short

[a] This research was supported by the U.S. Department of Energy (DE-FG02-87ER13791) and the National Science Foundation (CHE-8903216). This is publication 153 from the Arizona State University Center for the Study of Early Events in Photosynthesis. The Center is funded by U.S. Department of Energy Grant DE-FG02-88ER13969 as part of the U.S. Department of Agriculture–Department of Energy–National Science Foundation Plant Science Center Program.

lifetime, the quantum yield of fluorescence emission from this state is very low ($\leq 10^{-4}$) in spite of the strongly allowed nature of the transition and its correspondingly large radiative rate constant ($\sim 10^9$ s^{-1}).[2]

The transition to the lowest-lying excited singlet state of carotenoids, S_1, is electric dipole forbidden,[3] and is not observed in the usual single-photon absorption experiment. The lifetime of the S_1 state, as measured by transient absorption techniques, is on the order of 10–40 ps for most carotenoids.[4,5] The state decays essentially exclusively via internal conversion. Fluorescence from S_1 is virtually undetectable (quantum yield $< 10^{-4}$), and intersystem crossing to the triplet state is not observed. Because the forbidden nature of the $S_0 \rightarrow S_1$ transition makes it very difficult to detect, the energy of the S_1 state has not been directly determined. The S_1 level of β-carotene was recently reported to lie at ~ 650 nm, based on experiments using nonlinear optical techniques.[6]

Although carotenoid triplet states are not formed by the usual intersystem crossing pathway, they can be produced via triplet-triplet energy transfer from other species (see below). Thus, their transient absorption characteristics are well known.[7] Typically, they have strong absorption maxima at about 540 nm ($\varepsilon_T - \varepsilon_G \sim 1 \times 10^5$ M^{-1}cm^{-1}). In most organic solvents in the absence of oxygen, carotenoid triplet states have lifetimes of 5–10 μs. Neither phosphorescence from these triplets nor $S_0 \rightarrow T_1$ absorption has been observed, and therefore the energies of the carotenoid triplet states have not been spectroscopically measured. Energy transfer studies have demonstrated that the energy of the lowest-lying carotenoid triplet is below that of singlet oxygen at ~ 1.0 eV. Results from our laboratory obtained using a calorimetric technique (photoacoustic spectroscopy) have located the lowest-lying triplet state of a representative carotenoid (see structure 7 below) at 0.65 ± 0.04 eV. Thus, the expected origin of the phosphorescence would be about 1900 nm.

Carotenoids in Photosynthesis

Antenna Function

Although the photosynthetic reaction centers of plants and other organisms are responsible for the conversion of light energy into chemical potential, the reaction center pigments actually absorb only a tiny fraction of the light. More than 99% is supplied to the reaction center by singlet-singlet energy transfer from antenna systems. The antenna pigments vary according to the conditions under which the organisms live, but carotenoid polyenes are responsible for a large fraction of the light absorbed and used by many species.[8] As far as is known, carotenoid singlet states transfer excitation to chlorophyll molecules (Eq. 1, 2), which then relay the excitation energy to the reaction center.

$$\text{Car} \xrightarrow{h\nu} {}^1\text{Car} \tag{1}$$

$$^1\text{Car} + \text{Chl} \rightarrow \text{Car} + {}^1\text{Chl} \tag{2}$$

Carotenes are well suited to this role in that they absorb light strongly in spectral regions where the extinction coefficients of chlorophyll molecules are relatively low. On the other hand, as will be discussed in more detail below, the short lifetimes and low fluorescence quantum yields of carotenoid polyenes impose stringent conditions upon efficient singlet-singlet energy transfer to chlorophylls.

In spite of this restriction, singlet-singlet energy transfer efficiencies in many organisms approach unity.

Carotenoid Photoprotection

Under certain conditions, most photosynthetic organisms unavoidably generate chlorophyll triplet excited states when exposed to light. Often, these are produced in the reaction center via recombination of charge-separated states. Chlorophyll triplet states are excellent sensitizers for formation of singlet oxygen from the oxygen ground-state triplet as per Equation 3.

$$^3Chl + {}^3O_2 \rightarrow Chl + {}^1O_2 \tag{3}$$

Singlet oxygen, with an energy ~ 1 eV above the ground state, is a highly reactive species which can react with and destroy lipid bilayer membranes and other vital components of an organism. Thus, singlet oxygen production in a photosynthetic species is potentially very injurious.[9–11] Such organisms have developed a two-pronged defense mechanism based upon the low energy of the carotenoid triplet state mentioned above. Carotenes can quench chlorophyll triplet states at a rate which precludes singlet oxygen generation via a triplet-triplet energy transfer process (Eq. 4). Alternatively, carotenoids can quench singlet oxygen itself through energy transfer (Eq. 5) or chemical reaction.

$$^3Chl + Car \rightarrow Chl + {}^3Car \tag{4}$$

$$^1O_2 + Car \rightarrow {}^3O_2 + {}^3Car \tag{5}$$

The carotenoid triplet state returns harmlessly to the ground state with the liberation of heat.

Carotenoid Regulation of Photosynthesis

It has been found that carotenoid polyenes are involved in a mechanism whereby some photosynthetic organisms dissipate excess chlorophyll singlet excitation energy. This mechanism comes into play at high light levels, and evidently helps protect the organism from light-induced damage.[12] The activation of this mechanism is signaled by the conversion of violaxanthin to zeaxanthin, but the details of the process are not as yet understood.

Mimicry of Carotenoid Photosynthetic Functions

The photosynthetic apparatus of an organism is exceedingly complex. For example, the reaction center of a photosynthetic bacterium contains on the order of 10,000 atoms. As a result, the study of synthetic model compounds which abstract certain features of natural photosynthesis into simpler systems is an attractive research area. Such studies can both help reveal the workings of the natural process and lead to the design of new applications, even photomedical applications, of the photosynthetic principles. We shall illustrate this concept with the results of a few model system investigations carried out in our laboratories.

Antenna Function

Chlorophyll molecules in the antenna systems of plants can readily exchange singlet excitation via the Förster mechanism, which is based upon a coulombic interaction between the transition dipoles of the donor and acceptor chromophores.[13] The Förster mechanism is most efficient for acceptors with large extinction coefficients and donors with high fluorescence quantum yields. As mentioned above, the fluorescence quantum yields of both the carotenoid S_1 and S_2 states are extremely low. This suggests that they will be poor singlet energy donors, and that there may be unusual structural requirements for antenna function. As we shall see, this is in fact the case.

STRUCTURES 1,2. Carotenoporphyrin esters.

The rate of singlet-singlet energy transfer by the Förster mechanism depends inversely upon the sixth power of the donor-acceptor separation. Carotenoids are such poor energy donors and have such short excited singlet state lifetimes that singlet transfer between carotenoids and chlorophyll or porphyrin acceptor molecules in solution is not observed, even at high concentrations of the pigments. A closer association of the two chromophores is necessary. One way to achieve such an association is to covalently tether the carotenoid donor to its cyclic tetrapyrrole acceptor. Some years ago, we prepared carotenoporphyrin **1** in order to investigate this possibility.[14] The molecule consists of a synthetic carotenoid polyene linked covalently to a tetraarylporphyrin, which is a synthetically accessible model for chlorophyll. The absorption spectrum of **1** is essentially identical to the sum of the spectra of related unlinked carotenoids and porphyrins, and there is no strong electronic coupling between the chromophores. The ester linkage constrains the edges of the carotenoid and porphyrin moieties to be within ~5 Å of one another. Thus, one might hope to observe singlet-singlet transfer between them. This possibility was investigated using fluorescence excitation spectroscopy. It was found that within experimental error (~5%), none of the light absorbed by the carotenoid led to fluorescence emission from the porphyrin. Energy transfer was not observed.

Clearly, a greater degree of electronic interaction between the donor and acceptor moieties is required. Nuclear magnetic resonance (NMR) studies indicated that although the edges of the carotenoid and porphyrin chromophores are constrained to be close to one another, the molecule exists in a linear, extended conformation in solution. Carotenoporphyrin **2** was designed and synthesized in order to achieve a closer interaction of the two species, while maintaining the same ester linkage.[15] NMR studies of **2** demonstrated[15] that as a result of the ortho attachment of the carotenoid to the porphyrin *meso* ring, the carotenoid folds back across the porphyrin so that the π-electron systems are essentially in van der Waals contact. The separation of the two stacked systems is ~4 Å. Fluorescence excitation experiments on this carotenoporphyrin revealed that singlet-singlet transfer from the carotenoid to the porphyrin occurs with a quantum yield of 25%.

The results for **1** and **2** show that significant singlet-singlet energy transfer requires relatively strong electronic interaction between the chromophores such as that provided by van der Waals contact. Increased electronic interactions between the carotenoid and tetrapyrrole moieties in a linked system can also be achieved by involving the linkage itself. This approach is illustrated by molecules **3** and **4**, which consist of carotenoid polyenes linked to pyropheophorbides (deriva-

STRUCTURES 3,4. Carotenopyropheophorbide dyads.

5: $R_2 = R_3 = H$, $R_1 =$

6: $R_1 = R_3 = H$, $R_2 =$

7: $R_1 = R_2 = H$, $R_3 =$

STRUCTURES 5-7. Carotenoporphyrin amides.

tives of natural chlorophylls).[17,18] In carotenopyropheophorbide dyad **3**, singlet-singlet transfer from the carotenoid to the tetrapyrrole was not detected ($\leq 5\%$) using either steady-state fluorescence excitation or time resolved methods. This result is as expected, given the findings for **1** discussed above, because the long saturated linkage keeps the chromophores well separated. In the case of **4**, however, singlet transfer efficiency was ~50%, as detected by both methods. In this case, the requisite electronic interaction is not provided by close approach through-space of the π-electron systems, as in **2**, but rather through interactions across the amide linkage between the chromophores. Indeed, the partial double bond nature of the amide linkage suggests that the linkage orbitals could play a role in the transfer process.

The potential involvement of the linkage bonds was investigated in a study of carotenoporphyrin dyads **5-7**.[19] This set of molecules consists of identical carotenoid and porphyrin moieties which are joined by amide linkages. However, the point of attachment of the carotenoid to the porphyrin *meso* aryl group is varied. The singlet-singlet energy transfer quantum yields for the three molecules, as measured by the fluorescence excitation method, were 0.17, 0.10 and 0.13 for **5**, **6** and **7**, respectively. A lower transfer quantum yield, and therefore a slower singlet energy transfer rate, was observed for meta compound **6** than for para molecule **7**, in spite of the fact that NMR and molecular mechanics calculations showed that the separation of the two chromophores was smaller for the meta carotenoporphyrin. These results are consistent with transfer mediated by the linkage bonds, rather than through-space interchromophore interactions.

The results for these model systems raise questions concerning the mechanism of the singlet-singlet energy transfer process. The Förster coulombic mechanism mentioned above should not be very efficient for donation from either the S_1 or the S_2 states of the carotenoids unless the interchromophore separation is very small. This is confirmed by the carotenoporphyrin studies, which show that significant transfer requires that the donor and acceptor approach one another to within a few angstroms. However, this spatial requirement and the observation that transfer quantum yields in some molecules correlate with the nature of the linkage between the chromophores suggests that donor-acceptor orbital overlap may be important. If this is the case, then electron exchange may play a role in the transfer process. The electron exchange mechanism for energy transfer can be visualized as a double electron transfer process between the two chromophores, and as such its rate is a function of the overlap between donor and acceptor orbitals. This overlap may occur through space (and decay approximately exponentially with distance), or with the help of the linkage bonds (through a superexchange interaction). The high quantum yield for singlet-singlet transfer in **4** and the dependence of the transfer quantum yield on substitution pattern in **5–7** are both consistent with an electron exchange contribution.[19] The relative contributions of the two mechanisms to carotenoid-to-tetrapyrrole singlet transfer in natural and synthetic systems and the identity of the donor state(s) (*i.e.*, S_1 or S_2) are active areas of research.

Regardless of the transfer mechanism, the results for model systems show that rapid singlet-singlet transfer requires close spatial proximity of the carotenoid and tetrapyrrole π-electron systems. This result led to a prediction that in photosynthetic organisms, carotenoids involved in singlet transfer would be found closely associated with their accepting chlorophylls.[17,20] A crystal structure determination of the reaction center from *Rb. sphaeroides* has since revealed that the reaction center carotenoid is in van der Waals contact with a bacteriochlorophyll monomer.[21]

Photoprotection

The most efficient mechanism for protection of photosynthetic organisms from singlet oxygen damage is quenching of the chlorophyll triplet state at a rate which is much faster than singlet oxygen sensitization. Thus, an understanding of the structural and energetic prerequisites for triplet-triplet energy transfer from tetrapyrroles to carotenoids (Eq. 4) is vital to understanding photoprotection. Triplet transfer usually occurs by an electron exchange mechanism, and thus requires orbital overlap between the donor and acceptor. Model system studies have shown that there are many ways to achieve this overlap. Some of these are illustrated in this section.

As the triplet states of chlorophylls and porphyrins can have lifetimes of ms, highly efficient quenching of tetrapyrrole triplets by carotenoids can be achieved even with slow transfer rates. However, efficient photoprotection requires triplet transfer at a rate which can compete with singlet oxygen sensitization. Rate constants for reaction of tetrapyrrole triplet states with oxygen can be $>1 \times$

10^9 $M^{-1}s^{-1}$ and oxygen concentrations in air-saturated solutions are typically in the millimolar range. Thus, efficient photoprotection requires relatively rapid carotenoid quenching of tetrapyrrole triplets. One way to achieve this in model systems is to employ covalent linkages which promote orbital overlap via through-bond (superexchange) interactions.

Carotenoporphyrin dyads **5–7** are examples.[19] Excitation of a deoxygenated toluene solution of meta isomer **6**, for example, with a 590-nm, ~10-ns pulse of laser light produces the porphyrin first excited singlet state C-^{1}P. This species undergoes normal intersystem crossing to give the porphyrin triplet C-^{3}P in high yield. This state may be monitored via its triplet-triplet absorption spectrum, which has a maximum at about 440 nm. In a typical tetraarylporphyrin, this state decays over a period of several hundred μs to a few ms, depending upon conditions. However, in dyad **6**, the transient absorbance of C-^{3}P decays with a lifetime of only 40 ns. An absorption with a maximum at ~550 nm rises with the same time constant. The spectrum of this transient shows that it is the carotenoid triplet state, ^{3}C-P. The ^{3}C-P absorption decays with a lifetime of 5.7 μs, as is typical for carotenoid triplets. Thus, the carotenoid of **6** efficiently quenches the attached porphyrin triplet state. The ortho and para isomers **5** and **7** display even more rapid triplet-triplet energy transfer, which occurs within the instrument response time, and may well be as fast or faster than intersystem crossing. The high rates of triplet transfer in these molecules and the dependence of the transfer rate upon substitution position, rather than through-space separation, are consistent with an electron exchange process mediated by the amide and other linkage bonds. The reduced rate of triplet transfer for the meta compound is consistent with the relative HOMO and LUMO orbital densities at the ortho, meta and para positions as determined by simple molecular orbital calculations, and thus with superexchange coupling through the π-electron system of the linkage.[19] This interpretation is bolstered by the fact that triplet-triplet transfer in these molecules occurs in a glassy matrix at 77 K with no appreciable change in rate.

Another way of mediating triplet-triplet energy transfer between carotenoids and porphyrins is illustrated by carotenoporphyrin **8**.[22] The long polymethylene linkage between the two moieties suggests that triplet transfer by a through-bond mechanism such as that found for **5–7** would be inefficient. Indeed, if the molecule is dissolved in a frozen glass at 77 K or a rigid plastic matrix, excitation of the porphyrin with a laser pulse yields a C-^{3}P state via normal intersystem crossing with the normal porphyrin triplet lifetime (ms). However, if **8** is dissolved in a fluid organic solvent such as benzene at room temperature, the results are quite different. Excitation of the porphyrin again yields C-^{3}P, which can be detected via its triplet-triplet absorption spectrum. However, the porphyrin triplet state now decays with a time constant of 80 ns, and its spectrum is replaced by that of the carotenoid triplet state with a maximum at about 540 nm, which decays on the μs time scale. Thus, triplet-triplet transfer in solution is nearly as fast as it is in **6**. The explanation for this change in behavior is that in fluid solution, intramolecular motions about the bonds in the flexible linkage allow the molecule to momentarily assume conformations in which the π-electron systems of the two chromophores are in or near van der Waals contact, and thus triplet-triplet transfer via the electron exchange mechanism is rapid. This is analogous to normal collisional quenching between unlinked molecules in solution. In the glassy matrices, however, the molecule is locked in its most stable, extended conformations, and orbital overlap and therefore electron exchange interactions are precluded.

Similar results have been obtained for carotenopyropheophorbide **3**. This motionally mediated triplet-triplet energy transfer can provide a relatively high degree

STRUCTURE 8. Carotenoporphyrin with polymethylene linkage.

of photoprotection. The rate of singlet oxygen bleaching of the dye DPBF following excitation of aerated solutions of **3** was only about 5% that observed in a comparable solution of methyl pyropheophorbide-*a*.[23]

A third route to photoprotection via carotenoid quenching of tetrapyrrole triplet states is through a triplet energy transfer relay. Carotenoid-porphyrin-pyropheophorbide triad **9** illustrates this approach.[24] Excitation of an acetone solution of model pyropheophorbide (Ppd) **10** with a 670-nm laser pulse gives the singlet state, which undergoes intersystem crossing to yield ^{3}Ppd with a quantum yield of ~0.80. In the absence of oxygen, this state decays slowly over a period of 300 μs. However, in the presence of air, singlet oxygen (detected through its luminescence at 1270 nm) is generated with a rate constant of 2.5×10^9 $M^{-1}s^{-1}$. The quantum yield of $^1O_2$ is 0.80, and its lifetime under these conditions is 51 μs. Excitation of the pyropheophorbide moiety of dyad model **11** yields identical results. In aerated solutions, singlet oxygen is produced with a quantum yield of 0.80.

The results for triad **9** are quite different. Excitation of the pyropheophorbide in aerated solutions yields singlet oxygen, but the quantum yield is only 0.36. A clue to the explanation for this reduced quantum yield is provided by the results of laser flash experiments in the absence of oxygen. Excitation of the Ppd moiety of **9** yields C-P-^{3}Ppd, but this state decays rapidly. The decay is coordinated with the rise of the carotenoid triplet state with a rate constant of 2.9×10^6 s^{-1}, which then decays with a rate constant of 1.9×10^5 s^{-1} (typical for carotenoid triplet states). Thus, triplet-triplet energy transfer from C-P-^{3}Ppd to the carotenoid to give ^{3}C-P-Ppd is competing with singlet oxygen sensitization by C-P-^{3}Ppd and reducing the yield of singlet oxygen. The carotenoid is providing photoprotection.

These observations may at first seem puzzling, as the carotenoid moiety of **9** is separated from the pyropheophorbide by the porphyrin moiety, and strong orbital overlap is thereby precluded. However, additional studies demonstrate[24] that the triplet energy transfer is occurring via an intramolecular triplet energy transfer relay. The situation is best understood by reference to FIGURE 1, which shows the energies of the various excited states and their interconversion pathways. Excitation of the pyropheophorbide moiety (either directly by excitation at 670 nm or via singlet-singlet energy transfer from the porphyrin moiety, step 1) yields C-P-^{1}Ppd, which undergoes intersystem crossing to the triplet to give C-P-^{3}Ppd with a quantum yield of 0.80. Decay of this triplet by the usual photophysical processes, step 4, is very slow, but in the presence of air, C-P-^{3}Ppd produces singlet oxygen at the rate discussed above (step 6). However, competing with singlet oxygen sensitization is an endergonic triplet energy transfer to the porphyrin (step 5) to yield C-^{3}P-Ppd, which lies about 0.11 eV higher in energy than C-P-^{3}Ppd. The porphyrin triplet state is quenched very rapidly by the carotenoid (step 7) to yield ^{3}C-P-Ppd. This triplet relay ceases to function at 77 K, as expected from its activated nature.

It is likely that a similar triplet relay operates in the reaction center of the photosynthetic bacterium *Rb. sphaeroides*. The carotenoid in this reaction center is separated from the bacteriochlorophyll special pair by a bacteriochlorophyll monomer. The special pair, the site of triplet formation, has a triplet energy of about 0.94 eV, whereas the adjacent bridging chlorophyll has its triplet state at about 1.02 eV. Thus, thermally activated triplet energy transfer from the special pair to the carotenoid via the intervening bacteriochlorophyll monomer might be expected here as well. In fact, triplet transfer is rapid and efficient at ambient temperatures, but the rate slows significantly below 50 K, and at 10 K transfer is not observed.

STRUCTURES 9–11. (9) Carotenoid-porphyrin-pyropheophorbide triad, (10) model pyropheophorbide, and (11) porphyrin-pyropheophorbide dyad model.

Carotenoid Quenching of Tetrapyrrole Fluorescence

As mentioned above, carotenoids play a role in the quenching of chlorophyll excited singlet states in photosynthetic organisms at high light levels. This quenching may well be a photochemical process, as it is known that chlorophyll fluorescence is quenched by β-carotene in the laboratory.[25] In addition, the carotenoporphyrin species discussed earlier in this paper show some quenching of the porphyrin excited singlet state by the attached carotenoid when the electronic interaction between the moieties is relatively strong.[19] The mechanism of this quenching process is uncertain. When it was first observed by Beddard and co-

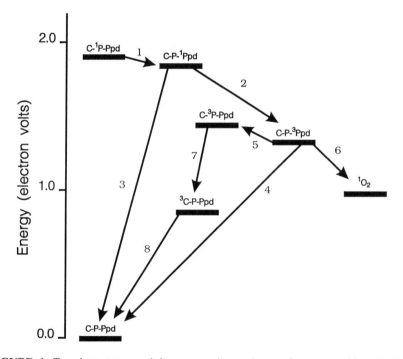

FIGURE 1. Transient states and interconversion pathways for carotenoid-porphyrin-pyropheophorbide **9**.

workers,[25] electron transfer from the carotenoid to the porphyrin first excited singlet state to form $C^{\bullet+}$-$P^{\bullet-}$ was suggested as a possibility. More recently, however, the quenching in a covalently linked carotenoporphyrin molecule was reported to be due to singlet-singlet energy transfer to the low-lying carotenoid S_1 state mentioned earlier.[26] Does this latter observation rule out the electron transfer quenching possibility, or can it be a viable option? Carotenoporphyrin **12** was recently synthesized in order to investigate this question.

Dyad **12** features a porphyrin bearing 15 fluorine atoms, which are strongly electron withdrawing and will stabilize a negative charge on the porphyrin nucleus. Thus, **12** has been designed to favor electron transfer of the type discussed above.[27] Fluorescence decay measurements in *n*-hexane, toluene and butyronitrile revealed quenching of the porphyrin first excited singlet state by the carotenoid with rate constants of 1.3×10^7, 2.1×10^9, and 1.8×10^{10} s^{-1}, respectively. The increase of quenching rate constant with solvent dielectric constant is consistent with electron transfer quenching and solvent stabilization of the resulting charge-separated state. Transient absorption studies were undertaken in order to further investigate this interpretation. Indeed, excitation of the porphyrin moiety of **12** in butyronitrile solution with a 150 fs, 590-nm laser pulse resulted in the observation of the spectrum of a carotenoid radical cation, with an absorption maximum at $\sim$960 nm. This cation was indicative of the formation of C$^{\bullet+}$-P$^{\bullet-}$. Kinetic studies showed that the cation absorption band rises with a time constant of 2.9 ps and decays with a lifetime of 51 ps. Detailed consideration of the transient absorption and emission results indicate that the 51 ps time constant is associated with the formation of C$^{\bullet+}$-P$^{\bullet-}$ from C-^{1}P, whereas the lifetime of C$^{\bullet+}$-P$^{\bullet-}$ is only 2.9 ps. Thus, under favorable conditions, carotenoids can indeed quench tetrapyrrole singlet states via electron transfer. However, the applicability of this mechanism to *in vivo* processes has yet to be determined.

STRUCTURE 12. Carotenoporphyrin.

Carotenoids and Human Health

It is clear from the above examples that carotenoids perform a variety of important functions in the photosynthetic apparatus of plants and other organisms, and that these can be mimicked in the laboratory with properly designed model systems. The model studies in turn help us understand the basic mechanisms of the natural processes. But what is the relevance of these findings for nonphotosynthetic organisms such as human beings? As demonstrated by the carotenoporphyrin results discussed above, the basic photophysics and photochemistry of carotenoids are not peculiar to photosynthesis, and will be present wherever carotenoids are found. Carotenoid polyenes absorb light of certain wavelengths very strongly, and are therefore capable of screening out radiation at these wavelengths in some situations. At the same time, carotenoids are poor singlet energy donors to all pigments, not just chlorophylls, and carotenoids are thus relatively unlikely to serve as sensitizers for the singlet states of other pigments which may be harmful or beneficial to a given organism. Carotenoid singlet states are very short lived, and thus unlikely to carry out photochemistry based on diffusional encounters with substrate molecules. Carotenoid singlet states typically decay to the ground state via internal conversion, and will not produce triplet states by intersystem crossing.

On the other hand, carotenoid triplet states have very low energies (<1.0 eV), and are readily formed by triplet-triplet energy transfer from a host of other pigments, including porphyrins of various types. Under favorable circumstances, carotenoids can quench higher energy, potentially harmful triplet states and thus preclude reaction of those states with other molecules. Unlike the triplet states of many naturally occurring pigments, carotenoid triplets cannot produce singlet oxygen, and indeed carotenoids are excellent quenchers of $^1O_2$. As this quenching is for the most part physical in nature (energy transfer), a single carotenoid molecule can in principle quench many singlet oxygen molecules. All of the above considerations apply *in vivo,* as far as is known.

The photophysical properties of carotenoids discussed above make them suitable for a variety of potential health-related applications. One of these will be illustrated here. It is well known that certain porphyrins localize in some malignant tumor tissues.[28-30] If the porphyrin is illuminated with light of the proper wavelength, powerful oxidizing agents will be produced, and considerable tissue damage will result. Most or all of this tissue damage is thought to result from the porphyrin triplet state, in particular through the sensitized formation of singlet oxygen as discussed in detail above. These effects form the basis of photodynamic therapy of tumors.

Because porphyrins are strongly fluorescent in the visible region of the spectrum, they are also potentially useful agents for detection or visualization of tumor tissue. The porphyrin concentrates in the tumor, and excitation with light results in red fluorescence which can finely delineate the boundary between healthy and diseased tissue. This diagnostic application of tumor-localizing porphyrins is severely limited, however, by the fact that although the porphyrins show a preferential localization in tumor tissue, some of the porphyrins or their degradation products remain in skin and other tissues. Thus, illumination of a patient by natural, environmental or diagnostic light can result in side effects ranging from skin erythema to serious inflammation and necrosis. These problems manifest themselves a few hours after administration of the drug and may persist for as many as six to seven weeks, until the drug is completely eliminated from the skin.

The results for photosynthetic model compounds discussed above suggest a solution to this problem. In properly designed carotenoporphyrins, the carotenoid is a powerful quencher of the triplet state of the attached porphyrin, but has little effect on its singlet-state properties, including fluorescence. Thus, a tumor-localizing carotenoporphyrin could function well as a diagnostic agent, but eliminate photosensitization problems arising from the porphyrin triplet state. In fact, carotenoporphyrin **7** seems to function in just this manner.

As mentioned above, experiments under laboratory conditions show that the carotenoid moiety of **7** quenches the porphyrin triplet state completely within a few ns of excitation. Preliminary *in vivo* experiments with **7** were carried out with mice bearing an infiltrating type of tumor, MS-2 fibrosarcoma. The carotenoporphyrin was injected intravenously in unilamellar liposomes, or as an emulsion (Cremophor EL). At fixed times after injection, various tissues were extracted and the carotenoporphyrin concentration was measured by absorption and fluorescence techniques. Typical results are shown in FIGURE 2. It is clear that by 24 hr after injection, a considerable amount of the carotenoporphyrin has localized in the tumor. Relatively small amounts are present in the surrounding muscle tissue and in the skin. Importantly, experiments with Balb/c mice under visible irradiation have thus far shown no indication of skin sensitization damage. Thus, the agent seems to be functioning as expected. It will be noted from FIGURE 2 that the carotenoporphyrin localizes in the liver and spleen, and that elimination from these tissues is slow. This is possibly an undesirable side effect, which fine-tuning of the carotenoporphyrin structure may reduce or eliminate.

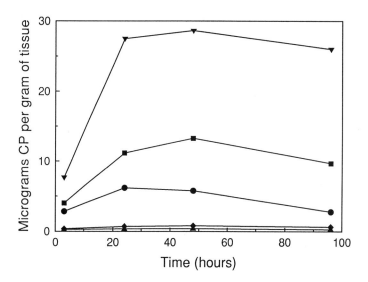

FIGURE 2. Amounts of carotenoporphyrin **7** recovered from selected tissues of mice bearing the MS-2 fibrosarcoma, as a function of time after intravenous administration. The curves represent tumor (●), liver (▼), spleen (■), skin (◆), and muscle (▲) tissue.

CONCLUSIONS

The unique photophysical properties of carotenoids make them eminently suited for a variety of functions in the photosynthetic apparatus of organisms. The study of synthetic model systems has helped elucidate the biological roles of photosynthetic carotenoids, and illustrates how these same photochemical effects can be incorporated into man-made systems. Because carotenoid photophysical and photochemical properties may be expected to remain essentially unchanged in other milieu, the basic photochemistry revealed in natural and artificial photosynthesis may be applied to other systems, including nonphotosynthetic organisms. In fact, direct utilization of the results of photosynthetic model system studies can lead to potentially useful therapeutic agents, as illustrated by the tumor visualization factor discussed above.

REFERENCES

1. SHREVE, A. P., J. K, TRAUTMAN, T. G. OWENS & A. C. ALBRECHT. 1991. Chem. Phys. Lett. **178:** 89–96.
2. TRUSCOTT, T. G. 1990. Photochem. Photobiol/B: Biology **6:** 359–371.
3. KOHLER, B. E. 1991. *In* Conjugated Polymers: The Novel Science and Technology of Conducting and Nonlinear Optically Active Materials. J. L. Bredas & R. Silbey, Eds. 405–434. Dodrecht. Kluwer.
4. WASIELEWSKI, M. A. & L. D. KISPERT. 1986. Chem. Phys. Lett. **128:** 238–243.
5. TRAUTMAN, J. K., A. P. SHREVE, T. G. OWENS & A. C. ALBRECHT. 1990. Chem. Phys. Lett. **166:** 369–374.
6. JONES, P. F., W. J. JONES & B. H. DAVIES. 1992. J. Photochem. Photobiol. A: Chem. **68:** 59–75.
7. BENSASSON, R., E. A. DAWE, D. A. LONG & E. J. LAND. 1977. J. Chem. Soc. Faraday Trans. I **73:** 1319–1325.
8. KIRK, J. T. O. 1983. Light and Photosynthesis in Aquatic Environments. Cambridge University Press. Cambridge.
9. GRIFFITHS, M., W. R. SISTROM, G. COHEN-BAZIRE & R. Y. STANIER. 1955. Nature (London) **176:** 1211–1214.
10. KRINSKY, N. I. 1966. Biochemistry of Chloroplasts. T. W. Goodwin, Ed. Vol. **1:** 423–430. Academic Press. New York.
11. COGDELL, R. J. & H. A. FRANK. 1987. Biochim. Biophys. Acta **895:** 63–79.
12. DEMING-ADAMS, B. 1990. Biochim. Biophys. Acta **1020:** 1–24.
13. FORSTER, T. 1959. Disc. Faraday Soc. **27:** 7–17.
14. DIRKS, G., A. L. MOORE, T. A. MOORE & D. GUST. 1980. Photochem. Photobiol. **32:** 277–280.
15. MOORE, A. L., G. DIRKS, D. GUST & T. A. MOORE. 1980. Photochem. Photobiol. **32:** 691–696.
16. CHACHATY, C., D. GUST, T. A. MOORE, G. A. NEMETH, P. A. LIDDELL & A. L. MOORE. 1984. Org. Magn. Reson. **22:** 39–46.
17. LIDDELL, P. A., D. BARRETT, L. R. MAKINGS, P. J. PESSIKI, D. GUST & T. A. MOORE. 1986. J. Am. Chem. Soc. **108:** 5350–5352.
18. WASIELEWSKI, M. A. & L. D. KISPERT. 1986. Chem. Phys. Lett. **128:** 238–243.
19. GUST, D., T. A. MOORE, A. L. MOORE, C. DEVADOSS, P. A. LIDDELL, R. HERMANT, R. A. NIEMAN, L. J. DEMANCHE, J. M. DEGRAZIANO & I. GOUNI. 1992. J. Am. Chem. Soc. **114:** 3590–3603.
20. SCHENCK, C. C., P. MATHIS, M. LUTZ, D. GUST & T. A. MOORE. 1983. Biophys. J. **41:** 123a.
21. YEATES, T. O., H. KOMIYA, A. CHIRINO, D. C. REES, J. P. ALLEN & G. FEHER. 1988. Proc. Natl. Acad. Sci. USA **85:** 7993–7997.
22. MOORE, A. L., A. JOY, R. TOM, D. GUST, T. A. MOORE, R. V. BENSASSON & E. J. LAND. 1982. Science **216:** 982–984.
23. LIDDELL, P. A., G. A. NEMETH, W. R. LEHMAN, A. M. JOY, A. L. MOORE, R. V. BENSASSON, T. A. MOORE & D. GUST. 1982. Photochem. Photobiol. **36:** 641–645.
24. GUST, D., T. A. MOORE, A. L. MOORE, A. A. KRASNOVSKY, P. A. LIDDELL, D. NICODEM, J. M. DEGRAZIANO, P. KERRIGAN, L. R. MAKINGS & P. J. PESSIKI. 1993. J. Am. Chem. Soc. **115:** 5684–5691.
25. BEDDARD, G. S., R. S. DAVIDSON & K. R. TRETHEWEY. 1977. Nature (London) **267:** 373–374.
26. OSUKA, A., T. NAGATA, K. MARUYAMA, N. MATAGA, T. ASAHI, I. YAMAZAKI & Y. NISHIMURA. 1991. Chem. Phys. Lett. **185:** 88–94.
27. HERMANT, R. M., P. A. LIDDELL, S. LIN, R. G. ALDEN, H. K. KANG, A. L. MOORE, T. A. MOORE & D. GUST. 1993. J. Am. Chem. Soc. **115:** 2080–2081.
28. MOAN, J. & K. BERG. 1992. Photochem. Photobiol. **55:** 931–948.
29. HENDERSON, B. W. & T. J. DOUGHERTY. 1992. Photochem. Photobiol. **55:** 145–157.
30. KESSEL, D. 1990. Photodynamic Therapy of Neoplastic Disease. D. Kessel, Ed. Vol. II: ch. 1. CRC Press. Boca Raton, FL.

Antioxidant Action of Carotenoids *in Vitro* and *in Vivo* and Protection against Oxidation of Human Low-Density Lipoproteins[a,b]

LESTER PACKER

Department of Molecular and Cell Biology
University of California, Berkeley
251 Life Science Addition
Berkeley, California 94720

INTRODUCTION

Carotenoids have aroused considerable interest as antioxidants in the past decade. Epidemiological studies indicate that they may have a protective effect against a variety of chronic degenerative diseases in which reactive oxygen species are thought to play a role.[1] In our laboratory we have taken a multifaceted approach to the study of these compounds as well as retinoids, investigating their antioxidant capacity in a variety of *in vitro* systems, in LDL, and measuring the uptake of carotenoids from dietary sources. These experiments make it clear that the system in which the activity of these compounds is investigated greatly influences their antioxidant capacity, and conclusions about antioxidant potency can only be drawn after studies in a number of *in vitro* systems, as well as *in vivo* experiments, are conducted.

In Vitro *Assessment of Antioxidant Capacity*

In assessing *in vitro* antioxidant activity, several assays should be used. In this way, factors such as solubility or steric hindrance, which may be of overiding importance in one environment but not another, can be varied and the antioxidant capacity of a substance in a variety of milieus may be evaluated. For these reasons, we have used four different types of assays to measure *in vitro* antioxidant activity of retinoids and carotenoids: interaction with the stable free radical 1,1-diphenyl-2-picrylhydrazyl radical (DPPH), interaction with the water-soluble fluorescent reporter molecule phycoerythrin, interaction with the lipid-soluble reporter molecule parinaric acid (in hexane and in liposomes), and chemiluminescence of dioleyl-phosphatidyl choline (DOPC) liposomes.

[a] Vitamin E-deficient LDL sample from Hamburg, Germany. Supported by National Institutes of Health Grant #RO1 CA47597-04, Henkel Corporation, and the Palm Oil Institute of Malaysia (PORIM).

[b] This research was supported by funds provided by the Cigarette and Tobacco Surtax Fund of the State of California through the Tobacco-Related Disease Research Program of the University of California, Grant RT-28, and by funds from the Council for Tobacco Research, Grant 444018.

Retinoids and DPPH Radicals

DPPH is a stable free radical whose signal is easily followed by electron spin resonance (ESR); antioxidants can quench the signal.[2] The concentration dependence of this quenching is the basis for the assay. In the experiments described here, 30 μl of DPPH (200 μM) and 30 μl of sample in ethanol were mixed (30 μl of ethanol only for controls) and 50 μl of this solution was placed in a capillary tube, which was placed in the ESR cavity. Manganese oxide was used as an internal standard; its peak height was assumed to be constant and the peak height of the DPPH control was taken as 100%. TABLE 1 shows the results of this assay for 11 retinoids. Only Ro 22-1318 and Ro 4-3870 (13-*cis*-retinoic acid), at a concentration of 2.5 mM, had any quenching effect on the DPPH signal. For comparison, glutathione, vitamin C and vitamin E completely quenched the signal at this concentration; hence, in this assay the antioxidant action of Ro 4-3870 and Ro 22-1318 are small in comparison to vitamins C and E, and glutathione.

TABLE 1. Effect of Retinoids on the Electron Spin Resonance Signal of 1,1-Diphenyl-2-Picrylhydrazyl (DPPH) Radical[a]

Common Name	Ro Number	Inhibition (% of Control)
Furyl analog of retinoic acid	22-1318	77.3
13-*cis*-Retinoic acid	04-3870	81.7
Acitretin	10-1670	95.6
Etretin	10-9359	97.5
all-*trans*-Retinoic acid	01-5488	99.7
Arotinoid acid	13-7410	100.1
Theinyl analog of retinoic ester	21-6583	101.5
Arotinoid sulfone ester	15-1570	111.7
Motretinide	11-1430	112.3
Termarotene	15-0778	115.1
Arotinoid ester	13-6298	118.8

[a] Retinoids at 2.5 mM were added to a 100 μM (final concentration) solution of DPPH. Each value is the mean of two or three determinations.

Phycoerythrin and Parinaric Acid Assays

Phycoerythrin is a water-soluble fluorescent compound whose fluorescence is quenched upon oxidation. Thus, by measuring the effect of an antioxidant on the rate of decay of fluorescence in the presence of an oxidizer, one may evaluate the antioxidant potency of the substance.[3] In the case of phycoerythrin, sparingly water-soluble substances such as retinoids and carotenoids may be used as long as the concentration is kept below the critical micellar concentration. The antioxidant efficiency of a compound may be evaluated in terms of number of moles of peroxy radical quenched per mole of antioxidant added; FIGURE 1 illustrates the effect of adding Trolox, a water-soluble analog of vitamin E, to a phycoerythrin system in which free radicals were generated by the decay of the temperature-sensitive compound 2,2'-azobis(2-amidino-propane)-HCl (AAPH). In FIGURE 1a the Trolox was added before radical generation was initiated, whereas in FIGURE 1b it was added during the course of the reaction. Trolox is a highly efficient antioxidant, quenching 2 moles of free radicals per

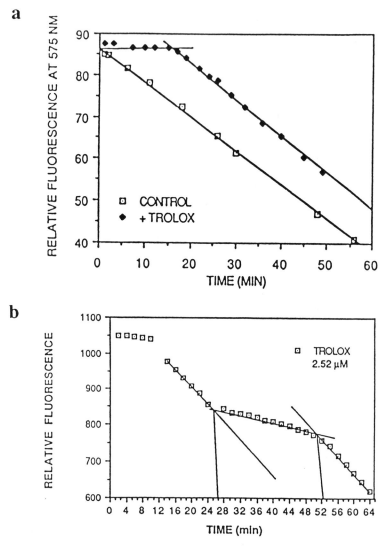

FIGURE 1. Fluorescence decay assay of Trolox (a vitamin E analog) antioxidant activity, with Trolox being added **(a)** before radical generation and **(b)** during the course of the reaction.

mole of Trolox. TABLE 2 shows the antioxidant efficiency for four retinoids and for Trolox as evaluated by this assay. Two retinoids which showed no activity in the DPPH assay (all-*trans*-retinoic acid and acitretin) are quite effective in the phycoerythrin acid assay; in fact, acitretin had the highest efficiency in quenching free radicals of the retinoids tested. By this assay, all four retinoids had high antioxidant efficiency (between 1 and 1.6), though not as great as Trolox (antioxidant efficiency of 2).

TABLE 2. Reaction Stoichiometry of Antioxidants, Using Phycoerythrin
Fluorescence Decay Assay

Substance	Amount Added (μmol)	Reaction Stoichiometry (Mol Peroxy Radicals Consumed/mol)
13-*cis*-Retinoic acid	13.40	1.10
	2.52	1.04
all-*trans*-Retinoic acid	7.92	1.06
	2.52	1.05
Acitretin	2.50	1.60
Furyl analog	2.50	1.52
Trolox	2.52	2.00

The lipid-soluble molecule *cis*-parinaric acid is a fluorescent molecule whose fluorescence is quenched on oxidation, similar to phycoerythrin. Assays of antioxidant efficiency may be carried out in hexane solution, using the lipid-soluble thermo-labile free radical initiator 2,2′-azobis(2,4-dimethylvaleronitrile) (AMVN).[4] In addition, the generation of peroxyl radicals by AMVN and interaction of peroxyl radicals with retinoids and carotenoids in DOPC liposomes may be followed by chemiluminescence produced in the presence of luminol and detected with a luminometer.[4] The antioxidant is incorporated into the liposomes.

In the hexane system, addition of carotenoids but not retinoids delayed the AMVN-induced *cis*-parinaric acid fluorescence decay (FIG. 2). This indicates that the carotenoids have a high scavenging capacity for hydrophobic radicals but

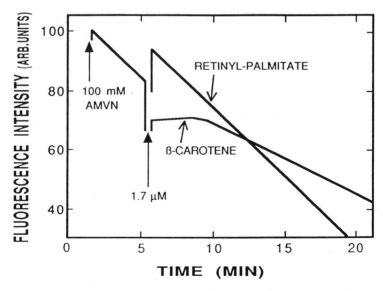

FIGURE 2. Effects of β-carotene and retinyl palmitate in the *cis*-parinaric acid fluorescence decay assay.

retinoids are not as efficient. The values for the number of moles of peroxyl radicals scavenged per mole of antioxidant may be calculated and are shown in TABLE 3 for a number of retinoids, carotenoids, and, for comparison, α-tocopherol and Trolox. Trolox has the same chromanol nucleus as α-tocopherol, with similar antioxidant activity, yet it had no antioxidant activity in this system, owing to its hydrophilic character, compared to an efficiency of 2 for α-tocopherol, as expected. This illustrates the necessity of testing antioxidants in a variety of aqueous and lipid environments to adequately reflect the variety of cellular and extracellular environments in which they may operate. The contrast between the high efficiencies of the carotenoids and the lack of efficiency of the retinoids in this system may be partially explained by the number of conjugated double bonds in the two classes of compounds. Retinoids have 5 conjugated double bonds while carotenoids have 11; thus, carotenoids may compete highly efficiently with cis-parinaric acid (which has only 4 conjugated double bonds) for AMVN-derived peroxyl radicals while retinoids cannot compete so overwhelmingly. Still, there must be some other factor or factors at work to explain the efficiency of 0 for the retinoids. There must also be some other factor at work to explain the extremely high efficiency of the carotenoids, around 30 moles of radical quenched per mole of carotenoid. Possibly, oxidation products of carotenoids may possess enough quenching potential to still compete successfully for peroxyl radicals with cis-parinaric acid. In this system carotenoids were about fifteen times as efficient as α-tocopherol in radical quenching.

In the chemiluminescent DOPC liposome system, retinoids and carotenoids inhibited the chemiluminescence caused by radical formation, as did α-tocopherol. The inhibition was concentration-dependent in all cases (FIG. 3). The concentrations for half-inhibition were 10, 37, 160 and over 200 μM for α-tocopherol, β-carotene, retinyl-palmitate, and retinoic acid, respectively. β-Carotene, which was a stronger scavenger than α-tocopherol in hexane, was weaker in the liposomal system, and retinoids, which had no radical-scavenging activity in the hexane, showed marked activity in the liposomal system. These results indicate that it is not simple chemical reactivity (as measured in the hexane solution) that determines antioxidant capacity in a membrane system; other factors, such as the interaction

TABLE 3. Reaction Stoichiometry of Carotenoids and Retinoids with Peroxyl Radicals in Hexane as Compared to Alpha-Tocopherol

Substance	Reaction Stoichiometry (mol Peroxyl Radicals Consumed/mol, Mean ± SE)	No. of Conjugated Double Bonds
β-Carotene	30.8 ± 0.8	11
Cryptoxanthin	29.4 ± 1.2	11
Lutein	29.6 ± 1.6	11
Canthaxanthin	30.2 ± 0.8	11\
Lycopene	27.2 ± 1.0	11
Zeaxanthin	31.4 ± 0.8	11
Retinyl-palmitate	0.0	5
Retinoic acid	0.0	5
Retinol	0.0	5
α-Tocopherol	2.0 ± 0.0	—
Trolox	0.0	—

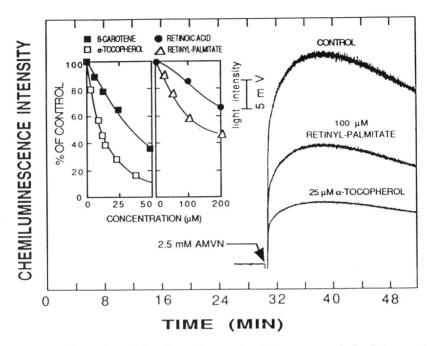

FIGURE 3. Comparison of the effects of α-tocopherol, β-carotene, retinyl-palmitate, and retinoic acid on luminol-amplified chemiluminescence in DOPC liposomes. *Inset* shows the concentration dependence of chemiluminescence quenching by the compounds tested.

of antioxidants with membrane components, are also involved. Mobility of scavenging molecules in membranes is one of the possible factors. Note that carotenoids were still about five times as efficient as retinoids in the membrane system, again indicating that the number of double bonds is involved in the radical-scavenging efficiency of these compounds.

A final lipid system is a hybrid of the hexane-parinaric acid system and the DOPC liposome system. In this model, parinaric acid is incorporated into DOPC liposomes and acts as a reporter molecule in the same way as in the simpler hexane system.[5,6] When the protective effects of α-tocopherol, ubiquinol, and β-carotene were compared in this system, α-tocopherol was clearly superior (FIG. 4), though both β-carotene and ubiquinol possessed antioxidant capability. One can also compare the antioxidant efficiency of liposomes containing α-tocopherol alone to that of liposomes containing α-tocopherol plus one other antioxidant, either in the liposome or in the surrounding medium. If the effects are additive, this indicates little or no interaction between the antioxidants. But if the effects are synergistic, there is probably interaction between the antioxidants. FIGURE 5 illustrates this for ascorbate and β-carotene. The effect of ascorbate is synergistic with that of α-tocopherol, consistent with the well-known ability of ascorbate to regenerate tocopherol from the tocopheroxyl radical.[7,8] On the other hand, the effect of β-carotene appears to be merely additive, indicating little or no interaction between the antioxidants in this system.

Carotenoid Animal Feeding Studies

Little quantitative data are available on the absorption of carotenoids from biological sources. Therefore, we examined the absorption of various carotenoids from Palm Oil Carotene enriched fraction (POC) incorporated into the diet of rats, and also examined the resistance of various tissues to lipid peroxidation in supplemented and unsupplemented animals. The carotenoid content of POC is given in TABLE 4. It was incorporated into the diet of male Sprague-Dawley rats at a concentration of 7.5 g POC/kg diet, and rats were fed this diet for periods up to 10 weeks. Rats were sacrificed at various times, and their tissue concentrations of lycopene, β-carotene, α-carotene, and total carotenoids were measured by HPLC. In addition, lipid peroxidation was induced in liver homogenates by the lipophilic azo-initiator AMVN. Lipid peroxidation products were measured by thiobarbituric acid reactive substances (TBARS) assay.

At no time were carotenoids detectable in adipose tissue or skin. Heart and skeletal muscle initially had no detectable carotenoids, but by 10 weeks levels of β-carotene in these tissues were 17 ± 4 ng/g and 6 ± 1 ng/g wet tissue, respectively.

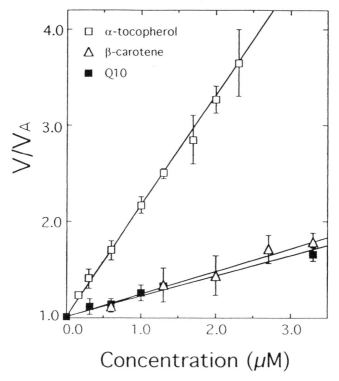

FIGURE 4. Relationship between V/V_A and antioxidant concentration in *cis*-parinaric acid-incorporated liposomes. V = the rate of initial fluorescence decay of *cis*-parinaric acid in the absence of antioxidants; V_A = the rate of initial fluorescence decay of *cis*-parinaric acid in the presence of the antioxidants indicated in the figure.

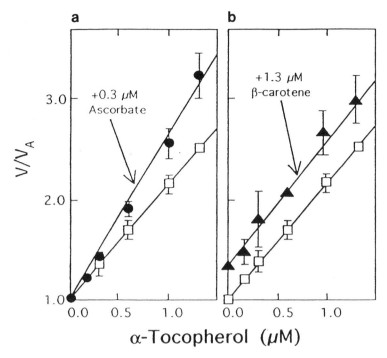

FIGURE 5. Effect of **(a)** ascorbate and **(b)** β-carotene on the plot of V/VA against α-tocopherol concentration.

The greatest increase in β-carotene concentration was in liver, where levels increased from 7.3 to 145 ng/g wet tissue over 10 weeks (FIG. 6). When liver homogenates were exposed to AMVN the correlation between TBARS and carotenoid content was found to be in the order α-carotene > β-carotene > lycopene ($r = 0.673 > 0.487 > 0.401$).

These results indicate that high amounts of not only β-carotene, but also lycopene and α-carotene, can be absorbed by the liver, and can afford significant antioxidant protection to that organ. In agreement with other researchers,[9,10] we confirmed that the rat, unlike humans, does not accumulate carotenoids in adipose tissue.

Carotenoids in LDL

LDL as a Model System—Interactions between Carotenoids and Vitamin E

Low-density lipoproteins (LDL) are an attractive system in which to study the interactions of antioxidants. They contain the major lipid-soluble antioxidants, including vitamin E, carotenoids, and ubiquinols.[11-14] They are easily isolated and represent an important component of the plasma, especially in terms of cardiovascular disease.[15] Many methods have been developed for inducing oxidation in

TABLE 4. The Carotene Composition of Palm Oil Carotene Enriched Fraction (POC)

Carotene	mg/kg POC
phytoene	1200
phytofluene	240
β-carotene	40,000
α-carotene	26,640
ξ-carotene	trace
γ-carotene	trace
δ-carotene	480
neusporene	trace
β-zeacarotene	trace
α-zeacarotene	trace
lycopene	2720
cis-β-carotene	720
cis-α-carotene	4400

LDL and for studying the effects.[16,17] For these reasons we decided to examine the effects of oxidation on carotenoids in LDL.

Carotenoids Are Destroyed by Processes That Directly Destroy Only Vitamin E. When LDL are exposed to UV light of a wavelength around 295 nm, the vitamin E is selectively destroyed. By doing this, one may examine the interaction of other antioxidants with vitamin E, since antioxidants which are depleted under this condition must interact with vitamin E in some way. When this experiment is carried out, one finds that not only is vitamin E destroyed, but β-carotene as

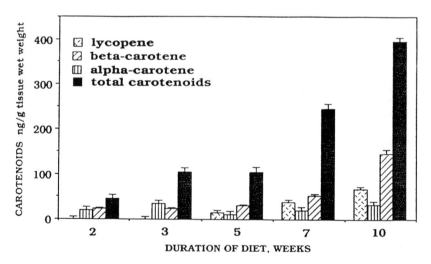

FIGURE 6. Accumulation of carotenoids in liver of animals fed a palm oil carotene enriched fraction. N = 3.

TABLE 5. Effect of UV Irradiation, Dihydrolipoic Acid (DHLA), and Ascorbate on Beta-Carotene Content of Human Low-Density Lipoprotein

Treatment	β-Carotene pmol/mg Protein	% Control	% Spared
Control	320	100.0	—
+UV	80	25.0	0.0
+UV and DHLA	120	37.5	12.5
+UV and ascorbate	175	54.7	29.7
+UV, DHLA, and ascorbate	300	93.75	68.7

well (see TABLE 5). Thus, there must be some interaction between the vitamin E radical formed during UVB radiation and β-carotene in LDL. These results imply that the components of the LDL are arranged in such a way that the two antioxidants can interact, even though some investigators believe that they are located in different parts of the LDL particle. Furthermore, when antioxidants such as dihydrolipoic acid or ascorbate are added to the LDL preparation, they exert some protective effect on the β-carotene, and together they have a synergistic protective effect (TABLE 5). These antioxidants can reduce oxidized compounds and "recycle" antioxidants such as vitamin E,[19] and they exhibit synergism in this recycling. But β-carotene is chemically destroyed when it reacts with radicals, and cannot be regenerated by oxidation-reduction reactions.[19] These compounds thus probably protect β-carotene indirectly, by reducing the vitamin E radical as it is formed, back to vitamin E, and keeping the radical's steady-state concentration low.

Carotenoids Protect Low-Density Lipoprotein (LDL)

In collaboration with Bernard Arrio and Dominique Bonnefont Rousselot, we have used a new technique, laser Doppler electrophoresis (LDE), to measure the changes in mobility in human LDL caused by oxidation. LDE measures the electrophoretic mobility of particles, such as LDL, whose size can range between 0.01 and 30 μm, in liquid suspensions. The particles are analyzed by independent laser Doppler measurements at four different angles simultaneously with 256-channel resolution each. Comparisons of simultaneous laser Doppler spectra from four angles allow the detection of very small particles as well as the separation of effects due to electrophoretic inhomogeneity, thermal diffusion, and flow inhomogeneity.[20,21] For these experiments, the 25.6° angle was used to obtain data for graphs.

In one experiment, LDL from a normolipidemic subject was isolated. The LDL was either left untreated (control) or was supplemented with an extract from *Dunaleiella salina* which initially consists of equal amounts of all-*trans* and 9-*cis* β-carotene (Betatene®, a gift of Henkel Corp., La Grange, IL). It was first dissolved in hexane at 60°C and thereafter diluted in ethanol. LDL suspensions were pretreated with 12.5 μM Betatene 24 hours before inducing oxidation by the addition of 10 μl of appropriate stock solution to 1 ml of the LDL preparation. In all cases control LDL preparations were treated with the same volume of ethanol alone for the same length of time as the β-carotene-treated samples. Incorporation of β-carotene into the LDL was confirmed by scanning the absorption spectrum of the β-carotene-treated samples vs control samples (all samples were scanned after dialysis): the treated samples absorbed strongly at 465 nm (λmax for β-carotene), while the control samples showed only weak absorbance at this wavelength. Both control and β-carotene supplemented samples were then subjected to oxidation by three methods: Cu^+ oxidation, AAPH oxidation, and γ-radiolysis.

In LDL treated with Cu^+, there is a pronounced shift toward a more negative mobility as well as a greater heterogeneity of mobilities. The Betatene-treated LDL has a less pronounced shift toward a negative mobility and displays greater homogeneity of populations; it thus appears, at least by LDE, that β-carotene is protective against oxidative stress in LDL. Biochemical analyses give further

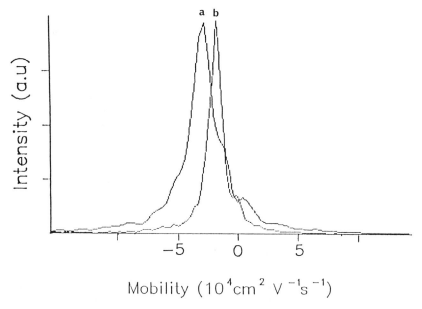

FIGURE 7. LDE spectrum illustrating the protective effect of β-carotene against AAPH oxidation. (a) Vitamin E-deficient LDL; (b) same LDL sample treated with β-carotene. Both samples oxidized by treatment with AAPH.

indication that Betatene pretreatment was protective for LDL in all three different methods of oxidation. In the Betatene-treated LDL, compared to control, there was 1–23% less loss of vitamin E, especially when oxidation was initiated by γ-radiolysis, and 10–50% less lipid peroxidation, as measured by TBARS, the degree of protection depending on the type of oxidation used.

LDL was also obtained from a vitamin E-deficient subject. This LDL contained 15% the vitamin E concentration of LDL from normolipidemic subjects.[22] Using this LDL allowed us to determine whether supplementation with β-carotene could compensate for the loss of vitamin E in this LDL. Control samples and Betatene-treated samples were oxidized by treatment with AAPH and compared by LDE. In this case the population shifts toward a more negative mobility, and heterogeneity appears. FIGURE 7 shows Betatene-pretreated E-deficient LDL oxidized with

AAPH compared to control E-deficient LDL oxidized with AAPH. Betatene prevents some of the shift toward a more negative mobility and there is no loss of homogeneity on oxidation. This indicates that β-carotene can at least partially compensate for loss of vitamin E in LDL.

Although the concentration of carotenoids in normal LDL is far lower than that of vitamin E,[23] these results indicate that β-carotene can play a significant protective role against oxidation in LDL. LDL samples prepared from the vitamin-E-deficient subject, which contained almost undetectable endogenous levels of vitamin E, could be readily oxidized, but could be afforded protection by pretreatment with β-carotene prior to oxidant (AAPH) exposure. Our results are in agreement with β-carotene supplementation of LDL from normolipidemic subjects, both by us in the present studies, and by others, where supplementation was found to prevent increased negative charge changes as measured by agarose gel electrophoresis.[24] Our findings provide direct evidence for the importance of β-carotene in protection of LDL against oxidation, even in the presence of low exogenous vitamin E. Carotenoids and vitamin E may act independently to protect LDL, since β-carotene antioxidant action is not based on redox reactions as is the case with vitamin E. However, it is not yet known if a synergistic protective antioxidant effect is afforded by the presence of both vitamin E and carotenoids in the same LDL particle.

ACKNOWLEDGMENTS

We gratefully acknowledge our collaborators in these studies: Bernard Arrio, Dominique Bonnefont Rouselot, Judith Catudioc, Elena Serbinova, Yuen May Choo, Midori Hiramatsu, and Masahiko Tsuchiya.

REFERENCES

1. GEY, K. F. 1993. Br. Med. Bull. **49.** In press.
2. HIRAMATSU, M., R. PACKER & L. PACKER. 1990. *In* Meth. Enzymol. L. Packer, Ed. Vol. **190:** 273–280. Academic Press. New York, NY.
3. GLAZER, A. N. 1990. *In* Meth. Enzymol. L. Packer & A. N. Glazer, Eds. Vol. **186:** 161–168. Academic Press. New York, NY.
4. TSUCHIYA, M., G. SCITA, D. F. T. THOMPSON, L. PACKER, V. E. KAGAN & M. A. LIVREA. 1993. *In* Retinoids: Progress in Research and Clinical Applications. M. A. Livrea & L. Packer, Eds. 525–536. Marcel Dekker, Inc. New York, NY.
5. TSUCHIYA, M., G. SCITA, H. J. FREISLEBEN, V. E. KAGAN & L. PACKER. 1992. *In* Meth. Enzymol. L. Packer, Ed. Vol. **213:** 460–472. Academic Press. New York, NY.
6. KUYPERS, F. A., J. J. M. VAN DEN BERG, C. SCHALKWIJK, B. ROELOFSEN & J. A. F. OP DEN KAMP. 1987. Biochim. Biophys. Acta **921:** 266.
7. PACKER, J. E., T. R. SLATER & R. L. WILLSON. 1979. Nature **278:** 737–738.
8. NIKI, E. 1987. Chem. Phys. Lipids **44:** 227–253.
9. LAKSHMAN, M., K. ASHER, M. ATTLESEY, S. SATCHITHANANDAM, I. MYCHKOVSKY & P. COUTAKIS. 1989. J. Lipid Res. **30:** 1545–1550.
10. MATHEWS-ROTH, M., S. WELANKIWAR, P. SEHGAL, C. LAUSEN, M. RUSSETT & N. KRINSKY. 1990. J. Nutr. **120:** 1205–1209.
11. ESTERBAUER, H., M. DIEBER-ROTHENEDER, G. WAEG, G. STRIEGL & G. JURGENS. 1990. Chem. Res. Toxicol. **3:** 77–92.
12. ESTERBAUER, H., M. DIEBER-ROTHENEDER, G. WAEG, H. PUHL & F. TATZBER. 1990. Biochem. Soc. Trans. **18:** 1059–1061.

13. DIEBER-ROTHENEDER, M., H. PUHL, G. WAEG, G. STRIEGL & H. ESTERBAUER. 1991.
    J. Lipid Res. **32:** 1325–1332.
14. ESTERBAUER, H., H. PUHL, M. DIEBER-ROTHENEDER, G. WAEG & H. RABL. 1991.
    Ann. Med. **23:** 573–581.
15. GOLDSTEIN, J. L. & M. S. BROWN. 1977. Annu. Rev. Biochem. **46:** 897–930.
16. BONNEFONT-ROUSSELOT, D., M. GARDES-ALBERT, S. LEPAGE, J. DELATTRE &
    C. FERRADINI. 1992. Radiat. Res. **132:** 228–236.
17. STEINBRECHER, V. P. 1987. J. Biol. Chem. **262:** 3603–3608.
18. KAGAN, V. E., E. A. SERBINOVA, T. FORTE, G. SCITA & L. PACKER. 1992. J. Lipid
    Res. **33:** 385–397.
19. PALOZZA, P. & N. I. KRINSKY. 1992. *In* Meth. Enzymol. L. Packer, Ed. Vol. **213:**
    403–420. Academic Press. New York, NY.
20. RIVIERE, M.-E., B. JOHANNIN, D. GAMET, V. MOLITOR, G. A. PESCHEK & B. ARRIO.
    1988. Meth. Enzymol. **167:** 691–700.
21. BLOOMFIELD, V. A. & T. K. LIM. 1978. Meth. Enzymol. **48:** 415–494.
22. KOHLSCHÜTTER, A., C. HUBNER, W. JANSEN & S. G. LINDNER. 1988. J. Inherited
    Metab. Dis. **11**(Suppl. 2): 149–152.
23. ESTERBAUER, H., J. GEBICKI, H. PUHL & G. JÜRGENS. 1992. Free Radical Biol. Med.
    13: 341–390.
24. JIALAL, I., E. P. NORKUS, L. CRISTOL & S. M. GRUNDY. 1991. Biochim. Biophys.
    Acta **1086:** 134–138.

Biological Functions
of Dietary Carotenoids

ADRIANNE BENDICH

Human Nutrition Research
Hoffmann-La Roche Inc.
Nutley, New Jersey 07110

INTRODUCTION

The growing interest in carotenoids has resulted in research to better define the functions of these molecules. In parallel, there have been numerous studies describing the activities of carotenoids in areas of human health including chemoprevention, cardiovascular disease and cataract prevention as well as effects on immune responses. This paper focuses on the last of these topics, reporting recent findings of beneficial effects of beta carotene supplementation on immune function in several populations at risk for immunosuppression.

Biological Functions

Of the 600 carotenoids found in nature, only about 40 are regularly consumed by humans.[1] Few of the carotenoids in human diets have provitamin A activity, the classic biological function attributed to carotenoids. Beta carotene has the highest potential vitamin A activity (one sixth that of retinol); however, all other provitamin A carotenoids are currently assigned one twelfth the activity of vitamin A (retinol). Other than their potential to serve as precursors of vitamin A, there is no nutritional value placed on carotenoids.

Yet we have known for decades that carotenoids with nine or more conjugated double bonds are potent quenchers of singlet oxygen, a biological function which is independent of any provitamin A activity. Likewise, carotenoids have antioxidant potentials which are well above that seen with vitamin A.

New biological functions include the recent finding that certain carotenoids can activate the expression of genes which encode the message for production of a protein, connexin 43, which is an integral component of the gap junctions required for cell-cell communications.[2] Beta carotene, and canthaxanthin, but not vitamin E, have this capacity, suggesting that gene activation is not associated with antioxidant capacity. Retinoic acid can activate the gene, but requires the binding to a retinoid receptor, whereas beta carotene does not bind the retinoid receptor. Thus, the carotenoid effect on gene expression is independent of any provitamin A activity.

A second new function of carotenoids involves their capacity to modulate the enzymatic activities of lipoxygenases.[3] Because the end products of lipoxygenase activity are proinflammatory and immunomodulatory molecules, there can be many biological consequences of carotenoid regulation of the enzyme's activity.

Biological Actions

Investigations concerning the observed actions associated with dietary carotenoids have, for the most part, not examined the specific carotenoid function responsible for the observed activities. Realistically, it may be many decades before we can determine the mechanisms of actions which result in the observed associations. This situation is not unusual in clinical research. Small pox vaccinations were implemented well before we even knew of the existence of lymphocytes or their importance in disease prevention. Thus, the observed activities of carotenoids can provide important insights for improving human health and preventing chronic disease.

Cancer Prevention

Cumulative data from almost 100 separate epidemiological studies have consistently shown that individuals with the highest intakes of carotenoid-rich fruits and vegetables have the lowest risk for many cancers, including those affecting the lung, oral cavity, stomach and esophagus. Serum beta carotene levels are often lowest in the highest risk groups. The most recent studies include analyses of the six major carotenoids in serum (beta carotene, alpha carotene, lutein, lycopene, zeaxanthin and cryptoxanthin); high serum levels of several of these carotenoids are associated with decreased risk of certain cancers, although the link with beta carotene remains the strongest.[4] Even though the intervention trial for the prevention of skin cancer with beta carotene supplementation was positive,[5] several investigators have shown that beta carotene supplementation can decrease the size and recurrence of oral precancerous lesions.[6] Intervention trials may have greater potential for success in individuals with precancerous conditions than in those with preexisting disease.

Cardiovascular Disease Prevention

Preliminary evidence that beta carotene supplementation significantly reduced the progression of cardiovascular disease in physicians with preexisting disease[7] has spurred investigation into the role of beta carotene and other carotenoids in cardiovascular function. Beta carotene administered orally to subjects does not appear to protect their isolated LDL from subsequent *in vitro* oxidation; however, there are findings that indicate that beta carotene can alter the oxidative modification of lipoprotein (a).[8]

Carotenoids have been shown to alter macrophage function (reviewed in Ref. 9).[10] Macrophages are transformed into foam cells which are an integral component of the atherosclerotic plaque. Macrophages also produce reactive oxygen species and control many actions of other immune cells. Other possible mechanisms of carotenoid cardioprotection could include elevation of HDL concentrations and/or alterations in platelet function and fibrin formation.

Cataract Prevention

Several studies have recently found a significant association between high intakes of carotenoid-rich diets and lowered risk of cataracts.[11] Two carotenoids found in the eye, lutein and zeaxanthin, can quench singlet oxygen and may reduce the oxidative stress on lens proteins.

Photosensitivity Prevention

Beta carotene and other carotenoids lacking vitamin A activity can quench singlet oxygen and have been shown to protect laboratory animals from UV-induced inflammation and certain cancers. Clinically, beta carotene supplementation has been used successfully in the treatment of inherited light sensitivity disorders.[12]

Immune Functions

Laboratory animal studies have shown that carotenoids enhance a number of indices of immune function independent of any provitamin A effect (reviewed in Ref. 9). Research on the effects of carotenoids on human immune responses, however, has been limited to beta carotene. Watson et al.[13] have published the majority of the studies examining the effects of beta carotene supplementation on human immune responses. They reported that supplementation of healthy older adults (av. 56 years) with either 30, 45 or 60 mg/day of beta carotene for two months significantly enhanced the percentage in peripheral blood of white blood cells (leukocytes) with cell receptors indicative of natural killer (NK) cells, and of lymphocytes with interleukin 2 (IL 2) and transferrin receptors. NK cells can kill tumor cells and virally infected cells. IL 2 receptors are present on activated T helper lymphocytes, and transferrin receptors are also markers for activated lymphocytes. Immune responses often decline with age, and there is a greater risk of cancer and infection in the elderly. This short-term intervention trial suggests that beta carotene enhances immune parameters which may prevent immune-mediated morbidity in the elderly.

In addition to the elderly, cigarette smokers are also at risk for immune suppression, infections and cancer. Beta carotene supplementation (30 mg/day/2 months) reduced the progression of oral precancerous lesions in the mouths of 70% of smokers in the trial, while at the same time enhancing NK cell receptors and in vitro killing of tumor cells by NK cells.[14,15] As discussed above, several other groups have seen that beta carotene supplementation significantly prevents the progression of oral leukoplakia; however, this is the only group that has linked the clinical response with immunological parameters.

Exposure to UV light has been shown to depress human immune responses and also to increase the risk of skin cancer. Specifically, UV exposure caused a significant reduction in circulating total lymphocytes and helper T lymphocytes, resulting in an inversion of the helper/suppressor T cell ratio from 1.5 to 0.8.[16] UV light also decreases antioxidant enzyme levels in the skin while increasing lipid peroxide levels. White et al.[17] reported a significant decrease in circulating plasma carotenoids following exposure to UV light. In a placebo-controlled trial, beta carotene supplementation (30 mg/day/7 wk) blocked the UV-induced depression in overall immune responses, as determined by delayed type hypersensitivity (DTH) skin tests.[18] The number of DTH responses was significantly decreased, but returned to baseline by the end of the study. In contrast, the vigor of the

TABLE 1. Beta Carotene Supplementation and DTH Induration in UV-Exposed Subjects[a]

	DTH Induration (mm)	
	Beta Carotene (30 mg/day)	Placebo
Baseline	24.5 ± 2.4	23.5 ± 2.2
Pre-UV	25.3 ± 4.3	30.3 ± 3.1
Post-UV	20.3 ± 3.9	11.8 ± 1.5*
Final	25.0 ± 4.3	18.7 ± 2.0*

* $p < 0.05$ compared to baseline, pre-UV and final values.
[a] Data derived from Fuller et al.[18]

response, as measured by the induration diameter, was still significantly reduced in the placebo group at the end of the study (TABLE 1).

UV light, either from lamps or sunlight, activated human HIV gene expression in transgenic mice.[19] The immune system of HIV-infected patients is severely compromised, because the virus attacks helper T lymphocytes. Exposure to UV could adversely affect HIV-infected patients in two ways: by activating the viral genetic material and by further reducing immune responses.

Coodley et al.[20] have recently completed a placebo-controlled, double-blind crossover study of the effects of high-dose beta carotene supplementation on the peripheral leukocyte population in HIV-infected patients. Supplementation with 180 mg/day for one month caused a significant increase in total white blood cells, and the percent change in helper T lymphocytes, resulting in a significant improvement in the helper/suppressor ratio (FIG. 1). Total lymphocyte and B lymphocyte levels were also positively affected. The majority of the patients

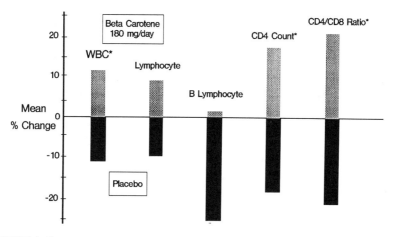

FIGURE 1. Beta carotene supplementation enhances HIV patient's immune profile. * $p < 0.02$. Data derived from Coodley et al.[20]

TABLE 2. Effect of Beta Carotene Supplementation on Individual CD4 Counts in HIV-Infected Patients[a]

	Beta Carotene (180 mg/day) (n = 14)	Placebo (n = 13)
Improved	8	1
Stayed the same	2	4
Worsened	4	8

[a] Data derived from Coodley et al.[20]

showed improvement during beta carotene supplementation, while most of the patients given the placebo worsened (TABLE 2). Garewal et al.[21] supplemented HIV-infected patients with 60 mg/day of beta carotene for 3 months and did not see an improvement in helper T lymphocyte number, but did see an increase in NK cells and increases in other markers of lymphocyte activation. The difference between these two studies may reflect the decreased intestinal absorption of many micronutrients found in HIV infection.[22] HIV-infected patients may require more than 60 mg/day of beta carotene to raise helper T lymphocyte levels.

Of importance is the recent finding by Ward et al.[23] that HIV-infected patients from the United States had significantly decreased serum vitamin A levels, which could be increased with supplementation. Vitamin A supplementation significantly increased the helper T lymphocyte levels in vitamin A-deficient children in Indonesia and increased the helper/suppressor ratio from 0.97 to 1.32.[24] Low serum vitamin A levels were associated with low helper T lymphocyte levels and increased risk of mortality in IV-drug using, HIV-infected U.S. adults.[25] It is possible, therefore, that the beta carotene supplementation increased vitamin A levels as well as beta carotene levels, and that the resulting immune cell changes seen in the Coodley et al.[20] and Garewal et al.[21] studies were due to vitamin A. On the other hand, Loya et al.[26] showed that a carotenoid could block the HIV reverse transcriptase enzyme without affecting human cells. Beta carotene was not reported to have been tested in this system; however, the ability to reduce viral replication may not be limited to only one carotenoid. Thus, even though the mechanisms of action of beta carotene on immune parameters in HIV-infected patients is yet to be elucidated, the findings are sufficiently promising to warrant further research.

CONCLUSIONS

The research focussing on the activities of carotenoids indicates that these molecules have diverse biological functions, not all of which are present in each carotenoid, i.e., not all carotenoids have provitamin A activity. Moreover, the diverse carotenoids are not functionally equipotent.

With regard to immune parameters, recent intervention studies show that beta carotene can protect against UV-induced immunosuppression. Preliminary reports suggest that beta carotene supplementation enhanced certain immune markers in HIV-infected patients and in other population groups at risk for immunosuppression. The biological functions responsible for immunoenhancement are yet to be fully determined.

REFERENCES

1. BEECHER, G. Personal communication.
2. BERTRAM, J. S. 1993. This volume.
3. CANFIELD, L. M. & J. G. VALENZUELA. 1993. This volume.
4. ZIEGLER, R. G. 1993. This volume.
5. GREENBERG, E. R. 1993. This volume.
6. GAREWAL, H. S. 1993. This volume.
7. HENNEKENS, C. H. 1993. This volume.
8. NARUSZEWICZ, M. E., E. SELINGER & J. DAVIGNON. 1992. Oxidative modification of lipoprotein (a) and the effect of β-carotene. Metabolism **41:** 1215–1224.
9. BENDICH, A. 1991. Beta-carotene and the immune response. Proc. Nutr. Soc. **50:** 263–274.
10. BACHMANN, H., R. NEMZEK & J. W. COFFEY. 1993. This volume.
11. KNEKT, P., M. HELIOVAARA, A. RISSANEN, A. AROMAA & R-K. AARAN. 1992. Serum antioxidant vitamins and risk of cataract. Br. Med. J. **305:** 1392–1394.
12. MATTHEWS-ROTH, M. M. 1993. This volume.
13. WATSON, R. R., R. H. PRABHALA, P. M. PLEZIA & D. S. ALBERTS. 1991. Effect of β-carotene on lymphocyte subpopulations in elderly humans: evidence for a dose-response relationship. Am. J. Clin. Nutr. **53:** 90–94.
14. GAREWAL, H. & G. J. SHAMDAS. 1991. Intervention trials with beta-carotene in precancerous conditions of the upper aerodigestive tract. *In* Micronutrients in Health and in Disease Prevention. A. Bendich & C. E. Butterworth, Jr., Eds. 127–140. Marcel Dekker, Inc. New York, NY.
15. PRABHALA, R. H., H. S. GAREWAL, M. J. HICKS, R. W. STAMPLINER & R. R. WATSON. 1991. The effects of 13-cis retinoic acid and beta-carotene on cellular immunity in humans. Cancer **67:** 1556–1560.
16. HERSEY, P., G. HARAN, E. HASIC & A. EDWARDS. 1983. Alteration of T cell subsets and induction of suppressor T cell activity in normal subjects after exposure to sunlight. J. Immunol. **31:** 171–174.
17. WHITE, W. S., C. KIM, H. J. KALKWARF, P. BUSTOS & D. ROE. 1988. Ultraviolet light-induced reductions in plasma carotenoid levels. Am. J. Clin. Nutr. **47:** 879–883.
18. FULLER, C. J., H. FAULKNER, A. BENDICH, R. S. PARKER & D. ROE. 1992. Effect of beta-carotene supplementation on photosuppression of delayed-type hypersensitivity in normal young men. Am. J. Clin. Nutr. **56:** 684–690.
19. MORREY, J. D., S. M. BOURN, T. D. BUNCH, R. W. SIDELL & C. A. ROSEN. 1992. HIV-1 LTR activation model: evaluation of various agents in skin of transgenic men. J. Acquir. Immun. Def. Synd. **5:** 1–9.
20. COODLEY, G. O., H. D. NELSON, M. O. LOVELESS & C. FOLK. 1993. Beta carotene in HIV infection. J. Acquir. Immun. Def. Synd. In press.
21. GAREWAL, H. S., N. M. AMPEL, R. R. WATSON, R. H. PRABHALA & C. L. DOLS. 1992. A preliminary trial of beta-carotene in subjects infected with the human immunodeficiency virus. J. Nutr. **122:** 728–732.
22. COODLEY, G. & D. E. GIRARD. 1991. Vitamins and minerals in HIV infection. J. Gen. Intern. Med. **6:** 472–479.
23. WARD, B. J., J. H. HUMPHREY, L. CLEMENT & R. E. CHAISSON. 1993. Vitamin A status in HIV infection. Nutr. Res. **13:** 157–166.
24. SEMBA, R. D., MUHILAL, B. J. WARD, D. E. GRIFFIN, A. L. SCOTT, G. NATADISASTRA, K. P. WEST & A. SOMMER. 1993. Abnormal T-cell subset proportions in vitamin-A-deficient children. Lancet **341:** 5–8.
25. SEMBA, R. D., N. M. H. GRAHAM, J. PALENICEK, W. T. CAIAFFA, A. L. SCOTT, L. CLEMENT, A. SAAH & D. VLAHOV. 1993. Increased mortality associated with

vitamin A deficiency during HIV-1 infection. Brief summary of poster presentation for IVACG 1993.

26. LOYA, S. Y. KASHMAN & A. HIZI. 1992. The carotenoid halocynthiaxanthin: a novel inhibitor of the reverse transcriptases of human immunodeficiency virus type 1 and type 2. Arch. Biochem. Biophys. **293:** 208–212.

Assessment of Carotenoid Intakes in Humans[a]

JEAN H. HANKIN,[b] LOÏC LE MARCHAND,

LAURENCE N. KOLONEL, AND LYNNE R. WILKENS

Cancer Research Center of Hawaii
University of Hawaii
Honolulu, Hawaii 96813

Inverse associations of vegetable and fruit consumption with cancer risk have been demonstrated by several epidemiologic studies using a diet history or food frequency questionnaire.[1-3] Investigators have also reported an inverse relationship between cancer and a β-carotene index derived from the vitamin A content of selected food items.[1-5] The recent availability of food composition data on the five main carotenoids found in serum (α-carotene, β-carotene, lycopene, lutein, and β-cryptoxanthin)[6] has enhanced our ability to assess the intake of these potential inhibitors of cancer risk.

In this paper, we shall discuss the use and importance of these carotenoid values in epidemiologic studies, the appropriate dietary methodologies for assessing carotenoid intakes, and the selection of relevant food items for diet history or food frequency questionnaires.

Use of Carotenoid Food Composition Values in Epidemiologic Studies

The daily intake of carotenoids is generally more variable than the intake of protein, fat, and carbohydrate. Although most persons may vary their choice of meats and starches (potatoes, rice, pasta) from day to day, the daily intake of these nutrients is usually relatively stable. In contrast, depending on the particular yellow or green vegetables or yellow fruits a person consumes, there are likely to be large daily fluctuations in carotenoid intakes. For example, 100-gram servings of cooked mustard greens, spinach and broccoli provide very different amounts of carotenoids, as shown in TABLE 1.[6] Equally variable composition patterns are seen among yellow vegetables, such as carrots, corn and acorn squash, and yellow fruits, such as mangoes, papayas and cantaloupe (TABLE 1). These differences have relevance in the development of appropriate questionnaires for dietary assessment of carotenoids.

We recently had an opportunity to utilize the new food composition carotenoid values in reanalyzing dietary data from a case-control study of lung cancer that was conducted among the multiethnic population of Hawaii in 1983–1985.[1] In this study, we initially assessed the intake of β-carotene according to a procedure adopted by the FAO/WHO Expert Group on Vitamin A Requirements.[7] This Group recommended that the vitamin A content of foods be divided into retinol,

[a] This research was supported by National Cancer Institute Grant PO1 CA33619.

[b] Correspondence to: Dr. Jean H. Hankin, Epidemiology Program, Cancer Research Center of Hawaii, University of Hawaii, 1236 Lauhala Street, Honolulu, HI 96813.

β-carotene, and other carotenoids with vitamin A activity according to specified percentages for different food groups. As shown in TABLE 2, we found a dose-dependent inverse association between β-carotene intake and lung cancer risk in both males and females. Even stronger inverse associations were demonstrated for tomatoes, dark green vegetables, cruciferous vegetables, and all vegetables, suggesting that other constituents of vegetables might also be protective against this cancer. We found no association with fruits, retinol, vitamin C, folic acid, iron, or dietary fiber in this analysis.

With the new quantitative values of the five major carotenoids in vegetables and fruits from Mangels *et al.*,[6] we reanalyzed these data to assess more directly the association of these nutrients with lung cancer risk.[8] Although the two methods for assessing β-carotene intake were not identical, the correlation between the intakes based on the calculated index and the new food composition values for our study subjects was 0.9, confirming our early published results concerning β-carotene intake and lung cancer risk.[1] Using the new carotenoid values, there

TABLE 1. Carotenoid Content of Selected Vegetables and Fruits[a]

Food Item	β-Carotene μg/100 g	α-Carotene μg/100 g	Lutein[b] μg/100 g	β-Cryptoxanthin μg/100 g
Mustard greens, ckd[c]	2,700	0[d]	9,900	0[d]
Spinach, ckd	5,500	0[d]	12,600	0[d]
Broccoli, ckd	1,300	1[d]	1,800	0[d]
Carrots, ckd	9,800	3,700	260[d]	0[d]
Corn, yellow, ckd	51	50	780	0[d]
Acorn (winter) squash, ckd	2,400	110	1,300	0[d]
Mangoes, raw	1,300	0	0	54
Papaya, raw	99	0	0[d]	470
Cantaloupe, raw	3,000	35	0	0

[a] From Mangels *et al.*[6] (Reprinted by permission from the *Journal of the American Dietetic Association*.)
[b] Lutein + zeaxanthin.
[c] ckd = cooked.
[d] Imputed value (see ref. 6).

were strong inverse associations with lung cancer risk for β-carotene, α-carotene, and lutein (TABLE 3).[8] No association was found for lycopene or β-cryptoxanthin. However, the protective relationship with total carotenoid intake or with the sum of β-carotene, lutein, and α-carotene (data not shown) was still not so high as with the total vegetable intake, suggesting that other components in these foods may also have cancer-inhibiting properties.

Appropriate Methodologies for Assessing Carotenoid Intakes

Measured food records and 24-hour recalls are useful for validating diet histories, for dietary counseling of patients, and for monitoring subjects participating in intervention trials. For example, in a recent feasibility trial to determine whether we could motivate cancer patients to increase their vegetable and fruit intake to eight servings a day, dietitians utilized unannounced 24-hour recalls to monitor

TABLE 2. Odds Ratios[a] for Lung Cancer by Intake Level of β-Carotene and Selected Vegetables by Sex, Hawaii, 1983–1985[b]

	Males (230 Cases, 597 Controls)					Females (102 Cases, 268 Controls)				
β-Carotene/Vegetables	Q_4 (High)	Q_3	Q_2	Q_1 (Low)	p for Trend[c]	Q_4 (High)	Q_3	Q_2	Q_1 (Low)	p for Trend
β-Carotene[d]	1.0	1.5	2.4	1.9	0.001	1.0	1.9	2.4	2.7	0.01
Tomatoes	1.0	2.5	1.8	2.3	0.002	1.0	1.5	3.1	3.7	<0.001
Dark green vegetables	1.0	1.4	1.9	2.0	0.003	1.0	3.7	3.4	3.9	0.001
Cruciferous vegetables	1.0	1.4	2.3	2.2	0.001	1.0	3.2	4.6	4.7	<0.001
All vegetables	1.0	1.9	2.3	2.7	<0.001	1.0	3.2	3.0	7.0	<0.001

[a] Adjusted by logistic regression for age, ethnicity, smoking status, pack-years of cigarette smoking, and cholesterol intake (for males only).
[b] From Le Marchand et al.[1]
[c] Test of significance for trend variable assigned the median value of the quartile.
[d] Computed as a percentage of vitamin A as recommended by FAO/WHO.[7]

TABLE 3. Odds Ratios[a] for Lung Cancer by Intake Level of Carotenoid Intake and Sex, Hawaii, 1983–1985[b]

Carotenoid	Males (230 Cases, 597 Controls)					Females (102 Cases, 268 Controls)				
	Q_4 (High)	Q_3	Q_2	Q_1 (Low)	*p* for Trend[c]	Q_4 (High)	Q_3	Q_2	Q_1 (Low)	*p* for Trend
β-Carotene[d]	1.0	1.8	2.5	2.1	0.001	1.0	2.1	2.2	3.8	0.003
α-Carotene	1.0	2.2	2.1	2.3	0.001	1.0	1.7	2.4	2.2	0.02
Lutein	1.0	1.5	1.5	1.8	0.04	1.0	0.9	2.3	3.6	0.002
Lycopene	1.0	1.4	1.6	1.5	0.07	1.0	0.6	0.7	1.3	0.83
β-Cryptoxanthin	1.0	1.3	0.9	1.1	0.81	1.0	1.1	0.9	1.1	0.99

[a] Adjusted by logistic regression for age, ethnicity, smoking status, pack-years of cigarette smoking, and cholesterol intake (for males only).
[b] From Le Marchand *et al.*[8] (Reprinted by permission from *Cancer Epidemiology, Biomarkers & Prevention*.)
[c] Test of significance for trend variable assigned the median value of the quartile.
[d] Computed from analytical data.[6]

fruit and vegetable dietary intakes, and used food records to assess quantitative changes in carotenoid intakes during a three-month interval. The food records appeared to adequately measure changes in intake since, for most carotenoids, good correlations were found between changes in intake and in plasma levels during the intervention.[9] Spearman correlation coefficients were as follows: lycopene 0.66, lutein 0.50, β-cryptoxanthin 0.49, β-carotene 0.34, α-carotene 0.23, and total carotenoids 0.67.

On the other hand, for research concerning the etiology of diseases, such as cancer and heart disease, investigators seek information on the usual diet consumed during a considerable period of time. This has led to the development of quantitative diet histories for estimating the usual intakes of particular foods and food groups among participants in epidemiologic studies.[10–12] Thus, this would be the method of choice for assessing the usual intakes of carotenoids as well. Using this method, respondents are asked to recall food consumption covering a one-year period. For carotenoid assessment, a one-year period would be the minimal acceptable time span, particularly, since seasonal fruits and vegetables must be adequately covered. To simplify and reduce bias in data collection for these studies, most researchers have designed structured diet history questionnaires that include lists of food items representative of the eating patterns of the study population. This method is more objective than the open-ended interviews that were utilized in early research concerning diet and child growth[13,14] and diet and heart disease.[15,16]

Some questionnaires of this type, such as that of Willett's,[17] are semiquantitative, in that subjects are asked to mark the correct frequency of consumption for a specified quantity of each food item. Although not stated, it is assumed that respondents will adjust the frequency if their serving size differs from the stated amount. Other questionnaires, such as the instrument developed by Block,[18] obtain frequencies and ask the participant to indicate the serving size (small, medium, or large) according to the defined medium portion of each listed food.

For studies in Hawaii, we developed a diet history method over many years that was suitable for a multiethnic population in which both frequencies and portion sizes are recorded. In a recent extension of this work, we developed two optically scannable versions to reduce the workload of processing the dietary information. The first questionnaire was designed to be administered by trained interviewers in case-control studies. Both frequencies and portion sizes are recorded. Based on a review of interviews in which open-ended consumption frequencies were obtained, we developed an appropriate series of frequency intervals. The following categorization (similar to that used by Willett and Block) was selected: never or hardly ever, once a month, 2 to 3 times a month, once a week, 2 to 3 times a week, 4 to 6 times a week, once a day, and 2 or more times a day. We use the same intervals for seasonal items, but with the frame of reference restricted to the period of a usual season. For example, since mangoes are available for about three months a year in Hawaii, subjects are asked about their frequency during the three-month period.

We designed the second instrument for self-administration in a multiethnic cohort study in Hawaii and Los Angeles. Participants receive the questionnaire by mail and are asked to complete the frequencies and quantities of each food item, along with additional questions on their eating habits, their other lifestyle practices, and their health and ethnic background, and to return the completed questionnaire in the self-addressed envelope. This diet history utilizes the same frequency intervals as the first instrument, but differs from the first questionnaire in a few ways. First, we added a few items frequently consumed by the Hispanic and Black populations of Los Angeles. Second, to reduce the length of the questionnaire, we combined some of the individual foods into groups of items with similar nutrient values. Each of the listed food groups includes suggestions of appropriate items. For example, the item "sausage" appears as: **Sausage** (such as pork, beef, chorizo, Polish, Vienna, Portuguese, hot links).

We have found that estimating amounts usually consumed is easier if people are provided with suitable visual aids, such as food models or photographs, showing usual portion sizes. For our case-control studies in which interviews are generally conducted in the participants' homes, color photographs are utilized for those items with variable serving sizes. Participants choose small, medium, or large portions, multiple servings of a particular portion, or combinations of two or more portion sizes to best reflect their consumption patterns. We recently validated this diet history method among a representative sample of 60 to 65 persons from each of the five major ethnic groups (Japanese, Caucasian, Hawaiian, Filipino, and Chinese).[19] We compared the questionnaire with four one-week food records that were obtained at three-month intervals during a one-year period. The correlation of β-carotene intake estimated by these two methods was 0.6. It seems likely that the results would be similar for the other carotenoids.

For the self-administered questionnaire used in our cohort study, we printed black and white photographs showing three typical portion sizes of meat items, meat and vegetable mixed dishes, cooked vegetables, and lettuce or salads. Respondents are asked to select their usual portion size from the photographs or from the listed household measurement. For example, the choices for "Broccoli" are as follows: Photo A (¼ cup or less) **OR** Photo B (about ½ cup) **OR** Photo C (1 cup or more).

Selection of Food Items for Assessing Carotenoids in Diet Histories

The particular food items included in a diet history questionnaire for assessing carotenoid intakes should be those that are consumed by a sizable number of persons in the population to be studied, that vary in frequency and quantity consumed among the members of the population, and that together account for a significant proportion of the intake of the five major carotenoids in the diet.

Investigators have utilized various methods to select food items for diet history questionnaires. For a study among a large cohort of nurses, Willett *et al.*[17] started with an extensive list of foods, which, after several pretests, was reduced by stepwise regression analysis. Block *et al.*[20,21] analyzed 24-hour recalls of adults in the NHANES II survey. They selected food items for their questionnaire that contributed >90% of the total population intake of energy and 17 nutrients, including "vitamin A or provitamin A." A number of other investigators have utilized the Willett and Block questionnaires, which permit the addition or substitution of a few items.

For Hawaii, we derived our basic diet history[22,23] from three-day measured food records of a random sample of the population. The foods were selected to contribute >85% of the intakes of energy, macronutrients, micronutrients, and dietary fiber of each ethnic group. Actually, the foods in the questionnaire contribute more than 85% of most nutrients, since a food that is a major contributor to a particular nutrient, such as β-carotene, but not to protein, is still included in the protein calculation.

For the Hawaii–Los Angeles cohort study, we obtained additional three-day food records from members of the Black and Hispanic populations in Los Angeles.

We then utilized the food record data from Hawaii and Los Angeles to select appropriate items for the self-administered questionnaire. As noted above, some items that are similar in nutrient value and are used interchangeably in the diet have been combined into food groups. On the other hand, since one of our objectives is to test the association of carotenoids and other antioxidants with cancer risk, we separated frequently consumed green and yellow-orange vegetables and yellow and citrus fruits into discrete items in the diet history. A preliminary validation of the questionnaire suggests that the selected items and food groups are appropriate for assessing carotenoid intakes in this cohort.

SUMMARY

The availability of new food composition carotenoid values for fruits and vegetables increases our ability to test hypotheses concerning the role of antioxidant nutrients and cancer risk. To estimate the usual carotenoid intakes, a quantitative diet history covering a one-year period is recommended for epidemiologic studies on diet and cancer. The particular food items in the diet history questionnaire should be representative of the eating patterns of the study population, should contribute more than 85% of the individual carotenoid intakes, and should distinguish between the high and low consumers of particular carotenoids.

REFERENCES

1. LE MARCHAND, L., C. N. YOSHIZAWA, L. N. KOLONEL, J. H. HANKIN & M. T. GOODMAN. 1989. Vegetable consumption and lung cancer risk: a population-based case-control study in Hawaii. J. Natl. Cancer Inst. **81:** 1158–1164.
2. STEINMETZ, K. & J. D. POTTER. 1991. Vegetables, fruits, and cancer. II. Mechanisms. Cancer Causes and Control. **2:** 427–442.
3. BLOCK, G., B. PATTERSON & A. SUBAR. 1992. Fruit, vegetables, and cancer prevention: a review of the epidemiologic evidence. Nutr. & Cancer. **18:** 1–29.
4. HINDS, M. W., L. N. KOLONEL, J. H. HANKIN & J. LEE. 1984. Dietary vitamin A, carotene, vitamin C and risk of lung cancer in Hawaii. Am. J. Epidemiol. **119:** 27–237.
5. COLDITZ, G. A., M. J. STAMPFER & W. C. WILLETT. 1987. Diet and lung cancer: a review of the epidemiologic evidence in humans. Arch. Intern. Med. **147:** 157–160.
6. MANGELS, A. R., J. M. HOLDEN, G. R. BEECHER, M. FORMAN & E. LANZA. 1993. The carotenoid content of fruits and vegetables: an evaluation of analytical data. J. Am. Dietet. Assoc. **93:** 284–296.
7. WU LEUNG, W. T., R. R. BUTRUM & F. H. CHANG. 1972. Food Composition Table for Use in East Asia. Food & Agriculture Organization. Rome, Italy.
8. LE MARCHAND, L., J. H. HANKIN, L. N. KOLONEL, G. R. BEECHER, L. R. WILKENS & L. P. ZHAO. Intake of specific carotenoids and lung cancer risk. Cancer Epidemiol. Biomarkers Prev. In press.
9. LE MARCHAND, L., J. H. HANKIN, F. S. CARTER, C. ESSLING, D. LUFFEY, A. A. FRANKE, L. R. WILKENS, R. V. COONEY & L. N. KOLONEL. Plasma carotenoids and ascorbic acid as markers of compliance to a high fruit and vegetable dietary intervention. J. Natl. Cancer Inst. Submitted for publication.
10. WILLETT, W. C. 1990. Nutritional Epidemiology. Oxford University Press. New York.
11. HANKIN, J. H. 1991. Dietary intake methodology. *In* Research: Successful Approaches. E. R. Monsen, Ed. 173–194. American Dietetic Association. Chicago.
12. BLOCK, G., F. E. THOMPSON, A. M. HARTMAN, F. A. LARKIN & K. E. GUIRE. 1992.

Comparison of two dietary questionnaires validated against multiple dietary records collected during a 1-year period. J. Am. Diet. Assoc. **92:** 686–693.

13. REED, R. B. & B. S. BURKE. 1954. Collection and analysis of dietary intake data. Am. J. Public Health **44:** 1015–1026.

14. BEAL, V. A. 1967. The nutritional history in longitudinal research. J. Am. Diet. Assoc. **51:** 426–432.

15. MANN, G. V., G. PEARSON, T. GORDON, T. R. DAWBER, L. LYELL & D. SHURTLEFF. 1962. Diet and cardiovascular disease in the Framingham study. I. Measurement of dietary intake. Am. J. Clin. Nutr. **11:** 200–225.

16. PAUL, O., M. H. LEPPER, W. H. PHELAN et al. 1963. A longitudinal study of coronary heart disease. Circulation **28:** 20–31.

17. WILLETT, W. C., L. SAMPSON, M. J. STAMPFER et al. 1985. Reproducibility and validity of a semiquantitative food frequency questionnaire. Am. J. Epidemiol. **122:** 51–65.

18. BLOCK, G., A. M. HARTMAN, C. M. DRESSER, M. D. CARROLL, J. GANNON & L. GARDNER. 1986. A data-based approach to diet questionnaire design and testing. Am. J. Epidemiol. **124:** 453–469.

19. HANKIN, J. H., L. R. WILKENS, L. N. KOLONEL & C. N. YOSHIZAWA. 1991. Validation of a quantitative diet history in Hawaii. Am. J. Epidemiol. **133:** 616–628.

20. BLOCK, G., C. M. DRESSER, A. M. HARTMAN & M. D. CARROLL. 1985. Nutrient sources in the American diet: quantitative data from the NHANES II survey. I. Vitamins and minerals. Am. J. Epidemiol. **122:** 13–26.

21. BLOCK, G., C. M. DRESSER, A. M. HARTMAN & M. D. CARROLL. 1985. Nutrient sources in the American diet: quantitative data from the NHANES II survey. II. Macronutrients and fats. Am. J. Epidemiol. **122:** 27–40.

22. HANKIN, J. H. 1986. A diet history method for research, clinical, and community use. J. Am. Diet. Assoc. **86:** 868–875.

23. HANKIN, J. H. 1989. Development of a diet history questionnaire for studies of older persons. Am. J. Epidemiol. **50:** 1121–1127.

Absorption and Transport
of Carotenoids

JOHN W. ERDMAN, JR., TIFFANY L. BIERER,
AND ERIC T. GUGGER

Division of Nutritional Sciences
451 Bevier Hall
University of Illinois
905 South Goodwin Avenue
Urbana, Illinois 61801

The absorption and transport processes of carotenoids are quite complex and to a large degree not well understood.[1-5] In his 1957 book on Vitamin A, Thomas Moore[1] wrote, "There are many complicating factors, both chemical and physiological, which will make it difficult to give an account of the absorption of vitamin A, and its provitamins, which is both clear and reasonably comprehensive." In this review, the authors summarize the current knowledge of both the absorption and transport of carotenoids, but Moore's words still hold true today. There is some information available on human absorption of β-carotene and a few select carotenoids, but only under defined dietary conditions. This information is generally limited to plasma appearance curves following a meal or is indirect in nature via measurement of fecal excretion of unabsorbed carotenoids.

People most often consume carotenoids as components of foods. Various food matrix effects add a level of complexity that does not readily allow for an accurate prediction of carotenoid absorption or vitamin A values from foods or from meals.[4] Nevertheless, we review here the major factors of both dietary and nondietary origin that affect uptake and metabolism.

Absorption of Carotenoids

Absorption is defined as movement of dietary carotenoids, or metabolites of carotenoids, to the lymphatic or portal circulation. Uptake by mucosal cells in itself is not sufficient for absorption as mucosal cells have short half lives and are sloughed off into the lumen of the gastrointestinal tract along with their contents. Moreover, carotenoids may or may not be metabolized or transported within these cells.

Several processes are necessary for optimal absorption to occur: 1) sufficient digestion of the food matrix to release carotenoids, 2) formation of lipid micelles in the small intestine, 3) uptake of carotenoids by intestinal mucosal cells, and 4) transport of carotenoids or their metabolic products to the lymphatic and/or portal circulation. Each process is briefly reviewed below.

FIGURES 1 and 2 depict the events that are thought to take place during the absorption of β-carotene. Numerous dietary and nondietary factors affect carotenoid absorption and utilization as shown in TABLE 1.

Digestion of the Food Matrix

β-Carotene absorption from oil solutions, aqueous dispersions, or antioxidant-protected commercial beadlets can be quite high, perhaps up to 50%.[2,6,7] However,

76

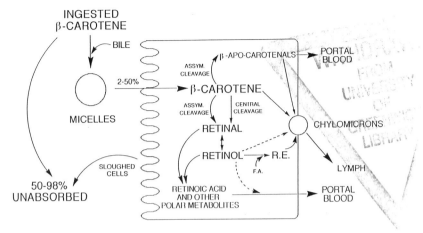

FIGURE 1. Uptake of β-carotene from lipid micelles into intestinal mucosal cells, possible metabolic events within the cell, and movement of β-carotene and/or its metabolic products to lymph and portal blood.

absorption can be very low, *i.e.*, as low as 1–2% from raw, uncooked vegetables such as the carrot.[2] Stahl and Sies,[8] for example, found no plasma appearance peak of lycopene from tomato juice unless the juice was heated first. Particle size of uncooked foods is particularly important; pureed or finely chopped vegetables yield considerably higher β-carotene absorption compared to whole or sliced raw vegetables.[2,3]

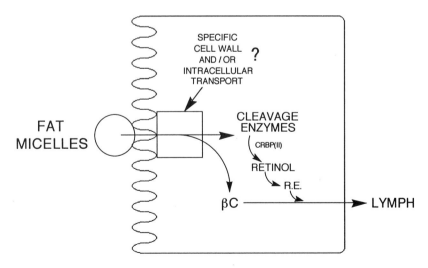

FIGURE 2. Intramucosal cell transport of β-carotene. The possible existence of specific cell wall and/or intracellular transport systems is raised.

In nature, carotenoids in a wide variety of plants, animals and microorganisms are found in protein complexes. These complexes, called carotenoproteins, exist in various forms. We have suggested[9-11] that carotenoproteins may have an inhibitory effect upon carotenoid digestion and absorption. Mild heating, such as steaming, appears to improve the extractability of β-carotene from vegetables and also β-carotene bioavailability.

In green, photosynthetic plant tissue, carotenoids are localized in the thylakoid membranes of chloroplasts, while in nonphotosynthetic tissues carotenoids are primarily found in chromoplasts.[12] In chloroplasts, carotenoids are found symbiotically with the chlorophylls in the multicomponent pigment-protein complexes of photosystems I and II.[13] Detergent isolation of these pigment-protein complexes

TABLE 1. Dietary and Nondietary Factors Affecting the Absorption and Utilization of Carotenoids

Dietary factors
Digestibility of food matrix
Particle size of food
Fat level—bile acid secretion
Antioxidant level, especially vitamin E
Dietary fiber level and type
Level of carotene in meal
Interactions with other carotenoids
Protein level and status
Iron, zinc status
Vitamin A level and status
Others?
Nondietary factors
Intestinal malabsorption diseases
Intestinal parasites
Hormone status
Thyroid
Others?
Drug Interactions
Ethanol & other P_{450} inducers
Cholestyramine
Others?
Liver or kidney disease

generally results in improved carotenoid release as the treatment becomes increasingly harsh or denaturing. It would therefore appear necessary to denature these pigment-protein complexes, with, for example, mild heating, for efficient utilization of carotenoids from photosynthetic tissue.

In chromoplasts, carotenoids can be found in a variety of substructures which determine chromoplast type.[14] There are four main types of chromoplasts, and one or more different types may be found in the same plant tissue. The most common type of chromoplast is the globulous, which contains carotenoid in lipid droplets with only traces of associated protein. Tubulous chromoplasts contain tubules consisting of a carotenoid nematic liquid crystal core stabilized by phospholipids and a 30-kD protein, which represents 28% of the tubule dry weight. Membranous chromoplasts contain lipid and carotenoid-rich concentric membrane structures which are associated with a variety of proteins. These proteins represent 22% of the membrane dry weight. Crystalline chromoplasts contain crystals of pure carotenoid surrounded by a layer of thickened membrane sheets. In the carrot, these membranes contain a major protein of 18 kD (unpublished results from the authors' laboratory). The specific role of these chromoplast substructures and their protein components has yet to be determined with respect to carotenoid bioavailability.

While mild heating of vegetables leads to improved bioavailability, additional heating can cause isomerization of the naturally-occurring all-trans double bonds of carotenoids to cis configurations which reduces the biological value of the carotenes. For example, canning of sweet potatoes and carrots results in the conversion of 75% of all-trans β-carotene to 13- or 9-cis isomers.[15] Further heating in the presence of oxygen can result in oxidation of the carotenes with a subsequent loss of vitamin A activity. Antioxidants such as vitamin E and BHT provide protection from oxidation during heating or storage of foods.

Formation of Lipid Micelles

Dietary fat stimulates bile flow from the gall bladder which facilitates the emulsification of fat and fat-soluble vitamins into lipid micelles within the small intestine. Without micelle formation, carotenoids are poorly absorbed. Several researchers have shown that the absence of dietary fat or very low levels of fat in the diet substantially reduces human carotene absorption.[4–5,16–18] For example, Roels *et al.*[17] showed that in boys with vitamin A deficiency in an African village, supplementation of their carotene-sufficient but low-fat diets (about 7% of calories) with 18 gm/day of olive oil substantially improved carotene absorption (from less than 5% to 25%).

In the same regard, disruption of lipid micelle formation with bile acid sequesterant drugs such as cholestyramine reduces carotenoid absorption. Some forms of dietary fiber may also inhibit carotenoid utilization, perhaps by reducing lipid micelle formation.[19,20] Rock and Swendseid[20] recently found that when 12 grams of citrus pectin was added to a control meal containing 25 mg β-carotene, the plasma β-carotene response in female subjects was significantly reduced.

Gastrointestinal malabsorption problems will severely limit carotenoid absorption. Intestinal parasites are particularly damaging. Steatorrhea, or fat malabsorption syndromes caused by pancreatic or gall bladder disorders are similarly troublesome.

Uptake of Carotenoids by Mucosal Cells

Carotene absorption is thought to be a passive process. The assumption is that carotenoids within lipid micelles come in contact with the intestinal epithelial cell membranes and that transport from micelles to the plasma membrane and/or cytosol of the cell occurs in concert with the transport of fatty acids, monoglycerides and other partially hydrolyzed lipids from within the lipid micelle. It is easier to visualize the more polar carotenoids moving in this manner than the nonpolar hydrocarbon carotenes. Nevertheless, β-carotene appears simultaneously in lymph with the newly absorbed fat from a meal, and thus it is assumed that these lipids move together across the plasma membrane and within the mucosal cell.

The possibility exists that there are specific cell wall and/or intracellular transport mechanisms for carotenoid transport (see FIG. 2), although none have been found. Because many of the hundreds of carotenoids in foods differ only slightly in structure, it is also possible that there is competition between carotenoids for uptake into mucosal cells and for absorption. We[21] have studied the effects of concurrent feeding of canthaxanthin or lycopene with β-carotene using the ferret model and found that canthaxanthin was particularly antagonistic to β-carotene uptake into blood plasma and tissues. The diketo carotenoid, canthaxanthin, may be a competitor for uptake at the mucosal cell wall and/or may compete within the mucosal cell with β-carotene for intracellular transport, processing or enzymatic action.

Because mature intestinal mucosal cells have short half-lives, carotenoids that were taken up by these cells that are neither metabolized nor absorbed will be returned to the intestinal lumen when the cells are sloughed off. Re-uptake by mucosal cells further along the gastrointestinal tract is possible, but has not been studied.

Transport of Carotenoids and/or Their Metabolic Products to the Lymph or Portal Circulation

Humans are somewhat unique in that they can cleave provitamin A active carotenoids to vitamin A within the intestinal mucosal cells or they can absorb a whole variety of carotenoids intact. Most species do not absorb carotenoids intact. The ferret and the preruminant calf absorb carotenoids intact and are appropriate animal models to study transport and metabolism of carotenoids.[22,23]

FIGURE 1 depicts a number of cleavage products of one carotenoid, β-carotene. (Enzymatic cleavage of carotenoids is discussed elsewhere in this book and will not be covered here.) A variety of forms of vitamin A and a series of apocarotenoids can be formed. Depending upon their polarity, these products move to the lymph or directly to portal blood.

The control mechanisms regarding mucosal cell uptake, cleavage pathways, and transport to portal blood and lymph are poorly understood. It is clear from studies with numerous animal species that as dietary carotene levels increase, the efficiency of their conversion to vitamin A is substantially decreased. This suggests that regulatory mechanism(s) are in place to limit mucosal cell uptake and/or transport and/or conversion of vitamin A when dietary carotenes are high and/or when vitamin A status is adequate.

The Recommended Dietary Allowances (RDA) for preformed vitamin A and the provitamin A active carotenoids have been established assuming that carotenoids are less well absorbed than vitamin A and are inefficiently converted to vitamin A.[24] Sauberlich and co-workers[25] found that with synthetic forms of β-carotene and all-trans retinyl acetate that 2 μg of β-carotene was equivalent to 1 μg of retinol in its ability to cure vitamin A deficiency in humans. Thus with highly absorbed forms of β-carotene, we would assume a 2 to 1 weight for weight conversion efficiency. The RDA, however, uses conversion factors of 6 to 1 and 12 to 1 for β-carotene and other provitamin A active carotenoids, respectively, recognizing that compared to more purified forms, dietary carotenes are much more poorly absorbed.

In FIGURE 2, we suggest that specific cell wall and/or intracellular transport mechanisms may exist in mucosal cells. If present, the transport systems could help direct (or metabolically channel) carotenoids a) to cleavage enzymes, b) to chylomicrons, or c) to neither. Option (c) would result in their loss to the intestinal lumen following normal cell turnover.

Ong and co-workers have intensively investigated preformed vitamin A absorption. They have demonstrated the important role of cellular retinol-binding protein type two, CRBP (II), in directing vitamin A metabolism during vitamin A absorption through the epithelial cell layer of intestinal mucosa. It is not known whether CRBP (II) interacts with carotenoid cleavage enzymes or transport systems. However, Ong[26] hypothesizes that "carotene cleavage might logically be regulated by requiring apo CRBP (II) for release of product inhibition, thus preventing

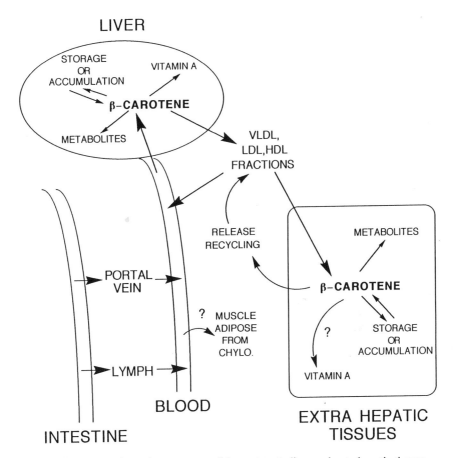

FIGURE 3. Postabsorption transport of β-carotene to liver and extrahepatic tissues.

oversynthesis of vitamin A from carotenes." As essential as CRBP (II) is to vitamin A absorption, it seems logical that this binding protein will play an important role in carotene absorption and/or conversion as well.

Transport of Carotenoids

The postabsorptive movement of carotenoids and/or their metabolic products is depicted in FIGURES 3 and 4. The metabolism of absorbed carotenoids has not been extensively studied and is not well understood. Most assumptions are derived from studies of plasma appearance and disappearance of carotenoids and limited amounts of human surgical and autopsy tissue carotenoid analyses.

It is clear that humans transport carotenoids in blood plasma exclusively via lipoproteins. Krinsky et al.[27] followed by other workers[28–31] reported that under fasting conditions, up to 75% of plasma hydrocarbon carotenoids are found in the LDL fractions. Most of the remaining carotenoids are associated with HDL and to a lesser degree with VLDL. The polar carotenoids are found more equally distributed between LDL and HDL fractions. Carotenoids appear initially in blood

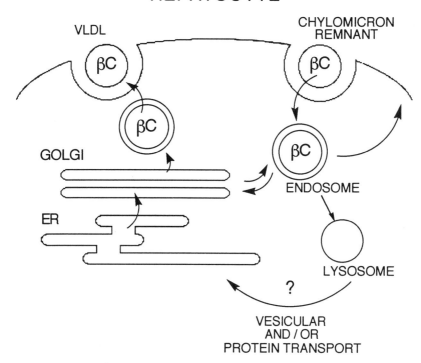

FIGURE 4. Uptake of a chylomicron remnant containing β-carotene by a hepatocyte and the repackaging of β-carotene into VLDL. *Arrows* depict movement of lipid, and possibly β-carotene, within the cell.

chylomicron and VLDL fractions followed sequentially by appearance in LDL and then HDL fractions.[28–31] Generally, the appearance of β-carotene in lipoprotein fractions follows the same time-course as newly absorbed triglycerides from the same meal.

Some people are classified as nonresponders. For example, Johnson and Russell[29] found that only 4 of 11 subjects administered an oral dose of 120 mg β-carotene demonstrated a plasma response. Of interest with the 4 responders was that surges of chylomicron β-carotene occurred every few days following the single β-carotene dose, suggesting delayed release of β-carotene from mucosal cells. It is possible that these surges were the result of re-uptake of β-carotene from the intestinal lumen following sloughing off of the epithelial cells. Elsewhere in this book,[32] we report that after an earlier β-carotene-containing meal, a small surge of β-carotene in chylomicrons was seen in a preruminant calf after a second carotene-free meal.

Kowalewski et al.,[33] in 1951, reported direct absorption of carotenoids from the small intestine into the portal vein of dogs. Portal vein absorption occurred following both water- and oil-soluble carotenoid administration. A small amount of lymphatic absorption was also observed with the oil solution, but this represented only a minor amount. Portal absorption of carotenoids has also been suggested by others.[29] Our laboratory[32] did not detect significant portal absorption of a water soluble β-carotene dose in the preruminant calf while lymphatic absorption predominated.

In humans, chylomicrons (CM) and VLDL, composed mainly of triglycerides, are packaged in the intestine and transported through the lymphatic system to the thoracic duct. This then empties into the subclavian vein and enters the main circulation. Lipoprotein lipase acts on the CM by hydrolyzing core triglycerides, resulting in the formation of a CM remnant. The CM remnants are then taken up by the liver where the internalized carotenoids are utilized to produce vitamin A, and/or are stored or repackaged and released with VLDL particles (FIG. 4). In humans, CM and VLDL β-carotene levels peak early (4–8 hours) following a β-carotene dose due to excretion from the intestine. As these are cleared by the liver, LDL β-carotene levels start to rise with a peak level at 24–48 hours post dosing, while HDL levels peak at 16–48 hours.[28] Carotenoids, especially the carotenes, are believed to be transported in the nonpolar core of lipoproteins.[33]

It is unclear whether there is transfer of carotenoids from CM to extrahepatic tissues prior to uptake of CM remnants by the liver. Nor is it known what factors come into play regarding uptake of carotenoids by tissues or their recycling from tissues back to plasma (FIG. 3). Carotenoid concentrations vary substantially from tissue to tissue.[34–36] Adrenal and reproductive tissues have particularly high carotenoid concentrations, especially in β-carotene. One plausible explanation is that tissues, such as human adrenal, testes and liver, which have a larger number of LDL receptors and the highest rate of lipoprotein uptake accumulate carotenoids passively with the uptake of large amounts of LDL.[34,35] The variable concentrations and forms of carotenoids in different tissues[34–38] suggest that other factors come into play. For example, the macular pigment of the eye contains primarily lutein and zeaxanthin[37,38] and the bovine pineal gland is very high in β-carotene[39] suggesting specific functions and/or uptake mechanisms must be in place.

As depicted in FIGURE 3, carotenoids accumulate and/or are stored in tissues. The term "storage" implies that a specific storage mechanism and/or function(s) exist in tissues for carotenoids. It is assumed that, at least in the liver, β-carotene and other provitamin A active carotenoids would be available for conversion to vitamin A. Carotenes may then be stored there for that purpose. Bovine corpus luteum has a very high β-carotene concentration[40] and the question arises as to a role of β-carotene in reproductive performance.

CONCLUSION

Numerous complex events influence the absorption and transport of carotenoids. Although much has been accomplished since 1957, when Moore[1] warned us of the complexity of these processes, we are not much closer to being able to predict the actual absorbability of carotenoids from a meal or the ability of a carotene-containing food to provide vitamin A activity. A variety of factors known to influence carotenoid absorption and utilization were noted in this review. Much more research is needed, however, to refine our knowledge base. Additional work will have significance regarding maintenance of vitamin A status of populations as well as on nonvitamin A roles of carotenoids in health promotion.

REFERENCES

1. MOORE, T. 1957. Vitamin A. 151. Elsevier Publ. Corp. Amsterdam.
2. RODRIQUEZ, M. S. & M. I. IRWIN. 1972. A conspectus of research on vitamin A requirements of man. J. Nutr. **102:** 909–968.
3. HUME, E. M. & H. A. KREBS. 1949. Vitamin A requirement of human adults. Medical Research Council Special Report Series #264 (London). 1–145. His Majesty's Stationery Office. Great Britain.
4. ERDMAN, J. W., JR. 1988. The physiologic chemistry of carotenes in man. Clin. Nutr. **7:** 101–106.
5. OLSON, J. A. 1991. Vitamin A. *In* Handbook of Vitamins, 2nd ed. L. J. Machlin, Ed. 1–57. Marcel Dekker, Inc. New York.
6. GOODMAN, D-W. S., R. BLOMSTRAND, B. WERNER, H. S. HUANG & T. SHIRATORI. 1966. The intestinal absorption and metabolism of vitamin A and β-carotene in man. J. Clin. Invest. **45:** 1615–1623.
7. BLOMSTRAND, R. & B. WERNER. 1967. Studies on the intestinal absorption of radioactive β-carotene and vitamin A in man. Scand. J. Clin. Lab. Invest. **19:** 337–345.
8. STAHL, W. & H. SIES. 1992. Uptake of lycopene and its geometric isomers is greater from heat-processed than from unprocessed tomato juice in humans. J. Nutr. **112:** 2161–2166.
9. DIETZ, J. M., S. SRI KANTHA & J. W. ERDMAN, JR. 1988. Reverse phase HPLC analysis of α & β-carotene from selected raw and cooked vegetables. Plant Foods Hum. Nutr. **38:** 333–341.
10. BRYANT, J. D., J. D. McCORD, L. K. UNLU & J. W. ERDMAN, JR. 1992. The isolation and partial characterization of α & β-carotene carotenoprotein(s) from carrot (*Daucus carota L*) root chromoplasts. J. Ag. Food Chem. **40:** 545–549.
11. POOR, C. L., T. L. BIERER, N. R. MERCHEN, G. C. FAHEY, JR. & J. W. ERDMAN, JR. 1993. The accumulation of alpha- and beta-carotene in serum and tissues of preruminant calves fed raw and steamed carrot slurries. J. Nutr. In press.
12. KIRK, J. T. O. & R. A. E. TILNEY-BASSETT. 1978. The Plastids: Their Chemistry, Structure, Growth and Inheritance. Elsevier/North-Holland Biomedical Press. New York.
13. THORNBER, J. P. 1986. Biochemical characterization and structure of pigment-proteins of photosynthetic organism. *In* L. A. Staehelin & C. J. Arntzen, Eds. Encyclopedia of Plant Physiology, Vol. 19: 98–142. Springer-Verlag. Berlin.
14. SITTE, P., H. FALK & B. LIEDVOGEL. 1980. Chromoplasts. *In* Pigments in Plants, 2nd edit. F.-Ch. Czygan, Ed. 117–148. Gustav Fisher. Stuttgart.
15. CHANDLER, L. A. & S. J. SCHWARTZ. 1987. HPLC separation of cis-trans carotene isomers in fresh and processed fruits and vegetables. J. Food Sci. **52:** 669–672.
16. DIMITROV, N. V., C. MEYER, D. E. ULLREY, W. CHENOWETH, A. MICHELAKIS, W. MALONE, C. BOONE & G. FINK. 1988. Bioavailability of β-carotene in humans. Am. J. Clin. Nutr. **48:** 298–304.
17. ROELS, O. A., M. E. TROUT & R. DUJAQUIER. 1958. Carotene balances in boys in Ruanda where vitamin A deficiency is prevalent. J. Nutr. **65:** 115–127.
18. PRINCE, M. R. & J. K. FRISOLI. 1993. Beta-carotene accumulation in serum and skin. Am. J. Clin. Nutr. **57:** 175–181.
19. ERDMAN, J. W., JR., G. C. FAHEY & C. B. WHITE. 1986. Effects of purified dietary fiber sources on beta-carotene utilization in chicks. J. Nutr. **116:** 2415–2423.
20. ROCK, C. L. & M. E. SWENDSEID. 1992. Plasma β-carotene response in humans after meals supplemented with dietary pectin. Am. J. Clin. Nutr. **55:** 96–99.

21. WHITE, W. S., K. M. PECK, T. L. BIERER, E. T. GUGGER & J. W. ERDMAN, JR. 1993. Interactive effects of oral β-carotene and canthaxanthin in ferrets. J. Nutr. In press.

22. GUGGER, E. T., T. L. BIERER, T. M. HENZE, W. S. WHITE & J. W. ERDMAN, JR. 1992. β-carotene uptake and tissue distribution in the ferret (*mustela putorius furo*). J. Nutr. **122:** 115–119.

23. POOR, C. L., T. L. BIERER, N. R. MERCHEN, G. C. FAHEY, JR., M. R. MURPHY & J. W. ERDMAN, JR. 1992. Evaluation of the preruminant calf as a model for study of human carotenoid metabolism. J. Nutr. **122:** 262–268.

24. ANON. 1989. Recommended Dietary Allowances, 10th edit. Food & Nutrition Board, National Academy of Sciences. 80–87. NAS Press. Washington, DC.

25. SAUBERLICH, H. E., H. E. HODGES, D. L. WALLACE, H. KOLDER, J. E. CANHAN, J. HOOD, N. RAICA, JR. & L. K. LOWRY. 1974. Vitamin A metabolism and requirements in humans studied with the use of labelled retinol. Vitam. Horm. **32:** 251–275.

26. ONG, D. E. 1993. Retinoid metabolism during intestinal absorption. J. Nutr. **123:** 351–355.

27. KRINSKY, N. I., D. G. CORNWELL & J. L. ONCLEY. 1958. The transport of vitamin A and carotenoids in human plasma. Arch. Biochem. Biophys. **73:** 233–246.

28. CORNWELL, D. G., F. A. KRUGER & H. B. ROBINSON. 1962. Studies on the absorption of beta-carotene and the distribution of total carotenoid in human serum lipoproteins after oral administration. J. Lipid Res. **3:** 65–70.

29. JOHNSON, E. J. & R. M. RUSSELL. 1992. Distribution of orally administered β-carotene among lipoproteins in healthy men. Am. J. Clin. Nutr. **56:** 128–135.

30. REDDY, P. P., B. A. CLEVIDENCE, E. BERLIN, P. R. TAYLOR, J. G. BIERI & J. C. SMITH. 1989. Plasma carotenoid and vitamin E profile of lipoprotein fractions of men fed a controlled typical US diet. FASEB J. **3**(4): A955 (Abstract #4235).

31. BJORNSON, L. K., H. J. KAYDEN, E. MILLER & A. N. MOSHELL. 1976. The transport of α-tocophorol and β-carotene in human blood. J. Lipid Res. **17:** 343–352.

32. BIERER, T. L., N. R. MERCHEN, D. R. NELSON & J. W. ERDMAN, JR. 1993. Transport of newly-absorbed beta-carotene by the preruminant calf. *In* Carotenoids in Human Health. L. M. Canfield, N. I. Krinsky & J. A. Olson, Eds. This volume.

33. KOWALEWSKI, K., E. HENROTIN & J. VANGEERTRUYDEN. 1951. Role of portal and lymphatic circulation in the transport of orally administered carotene. Acta Gastro-Enterol. Belg. **14:** 7–15.

34. KAPLAN, L. A., J. M. LAU & E. A. STEIN. 1990. Carotenoid composition, concentrations and relationships in various human organs. Clin. Physiol. Biochem. **8:** 1–10.

35. SCHMITZ, H. H., C. L. POOR, R. B. WELLMAN & J. W. ERDMAN, JR. 1991. Concentrations of selected carotenoids and vitamin A in human liver, kidney and lung tissue. J. Nutr. **121:** 1613–1621.

36. STAHL, W., W. SCHWARZ, A. R. SUNDRIST & H. SIES. 1992. Cis-trans isomers of lycopene and β-carotene in human serum and tissues. Arch. Biochem. Biophys. **294:** 173–177.

37. BONE, R. A., J. T. LANDRUM & S. L. TARSIS. 1985. Preliminary identification of the human macular pigment. Vision Res. **25:** 1531–1535.

38. HANDELMAN, G. J., E. A. DRATZ, C. C. REAY & F. J. G. M. VAN KUIJK. 1988. Carotenoids in the human macular and whole retina. Invest. Ophthalmol. Visual Sci. **29:** 850–855.

39. SHI, H., H. C. FURR & J. A. OLSON. 1991. Retinoids and carotenoids in bovine pineal gland. Brain Res. Bull. **26:** 235–239.

40. CHEW, B. P., D. M. HOLPUCH & J. V. O'FALLON. 1984. Vitamin A & β-carotene in bovine and porcine plasma, liver, corpora lutea and follicular fluid. J. Dairy Sci. **67:** 1316–1322.

Study of β-Carotene Metabolism in Humans Using ^{13}C-β-Carotene and High Precision Isotope Ratio Mass Spectrometry

ROBERT S. PARKER,[a] JOY E. SWANSON,
BONNIE MARMOR, KEITH J. GOODMAN,
AMY B. SPIELMAN, J. THOMAS BRENNA,
SHARON M. VIERECK, AND WESLEY K. CANFIELD

Division of Nutritional Sciences
Cornell University
Savage Hall
Ithaca, New York 14853-6301

INTRODUCTION

β-Carotene is a nutrient of growing importance in the biomedical community, but its metabolism in humans is poorly understood. The following are examples of fundamental aspects of β-carotene metabolism essentially unknown in the human: (a) range of absorption efficiency between individuals; (b) range of efficiency of intestinal conversion to vitamin A, and the extent to which conversion is regulated; (c) physiological, behavioral, or dietary factors affecting absorption or metabolism, including effects on the pattern of metabolites produced from β-carotene; (d) rates of turnover of plasma β-carotene or retinol pools in healthy or diseased states. The two major factors contributing to this knowledge deficit have been the lack of characterized animal models which resemble the human with respect to β-carotene physiology and metabolism, and the lack of appropriate methodological tools with which to study β-carotene metabolism in humans at levels typical of daily dietary intake.

While stable isotopes have been used to examine various aspects of retinol metabolism in humans, particularly estimation of liver vitamin A stores by isotope dilution,[1] there are no reports of application of stable isotope methodology in the study of β-carotene metabolism in humans. Previous approaches have involved the use of either (a) pharmacological doses of β-carotene sufficient to elevate plasma β-carotene levels, or (b) radioactive forms of β-carotene. β-Carotene labeled with either ^{14}C or ^{3}H was employed in two earlier studies of β-carotene absorption and intestinal metabolism in a small number of surgical patients with catheterized thoracic lymph ducts.[2,3] These studies have indicated that β-carotene absorption efficiency is probably low to moderate, and highly variable between subjects.

A stable isotope tracer method is needed for human studies of β-carotene since (a) most individuals possess sizable endogenous pools of β-carotene and its vitamin

---

[a] To whom correspondence should be addressed.

A metabolites, (b) blood levels of β-carotene do not change appreciably following single doses less than 15 milligrams, so that blood β-carotene levels cannot be used to estimate absorption efficiency; (c) blood levels of retinol are regulated and do not vary significantly over time in well-nourished individuals, so that blood retinol levels cannot be used to study conversion of β-carotene to retinol; and (d) radioactive forms of β-carotene pose unacceptable risks. We report here a stable isotope tracer method which we have developed and applied to the area of β-carotene metabolism in human subjects, and which we have successfully employed in preliminary studies at oral doses as low as 0.5 milligrams.[4]

METHODS

Unicellular green algae were grown with ^{13}C as the sole carbon source by Martek, Inc., Columbia, MD, and a crude hexane extract of algal biomass was supplied to our laboratory. Perlabeled ^{13}C-β-carotene (>95% ^{13}C) was purified by repeated crystallization from petroleum ether. The preparation used for the experiment described below contained about 5% α-carotene and about 1% cis-β-carotene isomers. One milligram of this material was dissolved in 20 g tricaprylin, a C-8 triglyceride (Sigma, St. Louis, MO), and emulsified with 70 ml skim milk and 30 grams of fresh banana (for taste and emulsion stability).

A 41-year old male, in good health, was placed on a low carotenoid diet for 48 hours prior to the ^{13}C-β-carotene dose. On the morning of the dose, the subject was fitted with an indwelling catheter with three-way stopcock in a forearm vein. A baseline blood sample was taken, and the subject then consumed the ^{13}C-β-carotene emulsion and a light breakfast (one-half bagel) containing no additional fat. The dose was taken with an additional 100 ml skim milk to rinse the dose container and mouth. Subsequent blood samples were taken at the times shown below. The low carotenoid diet was continued through 24 hours after the dose. A light, low fat lunch was consumed three hours after the dose, and an evening meal nine hours after the dose.

At each time point, 2.2 gram plasma aliquots were deproteinized with one volume ethanol and lipids extracted twice with three volumes hexane. Lipid extracts were subjected to semipreparative high pressure liquid chromatography (HPLC) using a Vydac TP201 column (Separations Group, Hesperia, CA) and methanol-dichloromethane (86 : 14), and fractions corresponding to retinol, all-trans β-carotene, and retinyl ester were collected. Peak areas of each of these three analytes were integrated for calculation of plasma concentration, corrected for recovery. At each time point, one-half of the collected retinol was combined with the retinyl ester fraction and saponified in ethanol with saturated aqueous potassium hydroxide at 40°C for 25 minutes. All retinol fractions (unesterified, or combined retinol plus retinyl ester-retinol after saponification) were further purified by analytical reverse-phase HPLC in acetonitrile-water (80 : 20). Retinyl ester-retinol could not be analyzed independently since the low mass of this plasma fraction (two orders of magnitude below that of retinol) yielded imprecise isotope ratios. All-trans β-carotene fractions were further purified by saponification followed by analytical reverse-phase HPLC on a Vydac TP201 column using methanol-dichloromethane (97 : 3) then hydrogenated to the thermally stable perhydro-β-carotene analog using platinum oxide under hydrogen gas overnight at 65°C.

Isotope ratios of unesterified retinol, combined retinol-plus-retinyl ester-retinol, and perhydro-β-carotene were determined using gas chromatography-combustion-gas isotope ratio mass spectrometry (GCC-IRMS). This technique was recently described and reviewed by Goodman and Brenna.[5] A Finnigan MAT (Bremen, Germany) 252 high precision GIRMS instrument interfaced to a Varian 3400 GC via a ceramic combustion furnace was employed. A 30-meter DB-1 column (J&W Scientific, Folsom, CA) was used for retinol analysis, and a nine-meter Ultra-1 (Hewlett-Packard, Palo Alto, CA) column used for perhydro-β-carotene analysis. A calibrated external CO_2 standard was obtained from Oztech, Fremont, CA. Masses corresponding to 44 (^{12}C-CO_2) and 45 (^{13}C-CO_2) were continuously monitored, and $^{13}C/^{12}C$ isotope ratios calculated relative to the calibrated standard. The atom percent ^{13}C in each fraction at each time point was calculated, and the atom percent excess ^{13}C obtained by subtracting the atom percent ^{13}C at baseline from that of all subsequent time points. The concentration (nM) of ^{13}C-labeled analyte present in plasma at each time point was then calculated by multiplying the atom percent excess ^{13}C by the total plasma concentration of that analyte (labeled plus unlabeled, as determined by HPLC). The concentration of labeled retinyl ester was obtained by subtracting the appropriate concentration of ^{13}C-retinol from the combined ^{13}C-retinol plus ^{13}C-retinyl ester-retinol concentration. Since the GCC-IRMS method was used only to measure isotope ratio and not analyte concentration, recovery of analyte during the HPLC purification and/ or hydrogenation steps was not important.

Duplicate plasma samples from each time point were prepared and analyzed independently as described above. Retinol standards were prepared by hydrolysis of retinyl acetate (Sigma Chemical, St. Louis, MO) with potassium hydroxide. β-Carotene was purchased from Fluka Chemical Corp., Ronkonkoma, NY.

RESULTS

Resolution of plasma retinol, all-trans β-carotene, and retinyl esters by semi-preparative HPLC is illustrated in FIGURE 1. Plots of plasma concentration of total (labeled plus unlabeled) retinol, all-trans β-carotene, and retinyl esters over the 24-hour period after the dose of ^{13}C-β-carotene calculated from this HPLC data revealed that only the retinyl ester fraction showed a peak which may be attributed to newly absorbed vitamin A, while the other two fractions showed no such peaks (data not shown). Total retinyl esters showed two peaks, one at 5 hours and a second at 11–14 hours. The first peak likely reflected absorption of the retinyl palmitate in the skim milk taken with the dose, and the second peak retinyl palmitate in the commercial frozen entree consumed as the evening meal. Plasma retinol concentration averaged 2794 nM over the first 22 hours after the dose, and β-carotene concentration averaged 258 nM.

GCC-IRMS chromatograms of the mass 44 signal and the corresponding delta values are shown for a plasma retinol fraction prepared as described in Methods (FIG. 2). The term "delta" is a unit of the $^{13}C/^{12}C$ ratio expressed in parts per thousand relative to an international carbon standard (PeeDee Belemnite), where higher delta values reflect greater enrichment with ^{13}C. The plasma retinol was collected from plasma taken 22 hours after the ^{13}C-β-carotene dose, and shows significant enrichment in ^{13}C, as illustrated by the elevated delta values associated with the retinol peak, as compared with a retinol standard (standard delta, −27). FIGURE 3 shows traces of masses 44 and 45 at the time of elution of the perhydro-β-carotene peak (22 hours after dose), also showing enrichment in ^{13}C as illustrated by the stronger mass 45 signal relative to the mass 44 signal.

FIGURE 4 illustrates the kinetics of concentration of ^{13}C-retinol, ^{13}C-retinyl ester, and [13]C-*β*-carotene in plasma over the first five hours following the dose. All three labeled analytes had appeared by three hours with retinyl ester the predominant labeled species, with lower concentrations of unesterified retinol and *β*-carotene. At five hours, the molar ratio of the labeled species of retinyl ester : retinol : *β*-carotene was 4.5 : 1.5 : 1. Plots of concentrations of the three labeled analytes through 22 hours after the dose are shown in FIGURE 5. Two concentration peaks for plasma retinyl ester were observed, a broad doublet peak

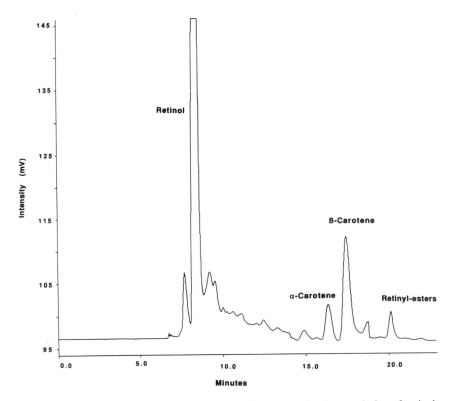

FIGURE 1. HPLC chromatogram of plasma lipid extract, showing resolution of retinol, all-trans *β*-carotene, and retinyl esters. Eluant was monitored at 325 nm from 0 to 13 minutes, 460 nm from 13 to 18 minutes, and 325 nm from 18 to 24 minutes. Column, 10 mm × 25 cm Vydac TP201; mobile phase, methanol-dichloromethane, 86 : 14, 1.7 ml/minute.

at 5–9 hours, and a second, sharper peak at 13 hours. Three peaks were observed for *β*-carotene, at 7, 13, and 16 hours. A single broad peak was observed for ^{13}C-retinol at about 12 to 14 hours. Excellent reproducibility of the concentration of the labeled species was generally obtained for all three analytes, as at many time points the error bars were within the figure symbols.

At all time points the labeled species represented only a small proportion of the total concentration (labeled plus unlabeled) of each analyte. At the times corresponding to the maximum concentration of each ^{13}C-labeled analyte during the 22-hour period, the proportion of total analyte existing in the plasma as the labeled species was approximately 1.2% for β-carotene, 0.8% for retinol, and 9.2% for retinyl ester. The higher proportion for retinyl ester reflects both the fact that retinyl esters were the primary metabolites of ^{13}C-β-carotene and the low pool size of retinyl esters in the plasma.

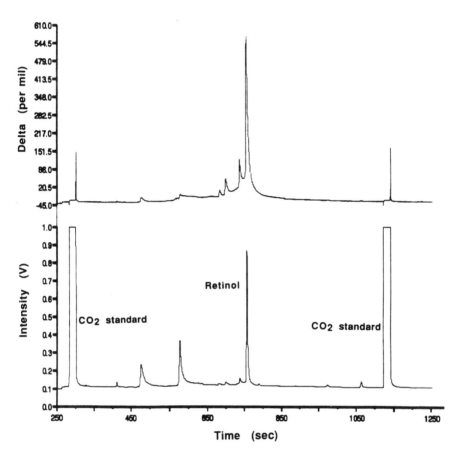

FIGURE 2. GCC-IRMS chromatogram of a retinol fraction prepared from plasma collected 22 hours after an oral dose of 1.0 mg ^{13}C-β-carotene (*bottom*). The *bottom trace* represents the mass 44 signal, and the *top trace* the corresponding delta trace, which is an expression of the ^{13}C/^{12}C ratio expressed in parts per thousand relative to an international carbonate standard. The peak corresponding to the retention time of standard retinol is indicated; for comparison, the delta value for the standard (synthetic) retinol was -27.

DISCUSSION

Our development of a method based on the use of per-labeled ^{13}C-β-carotene and a new generation of high precision gas isotope ratio mass spectrometers now permits the study of metabolism of small doses of β-carotene typical of daily

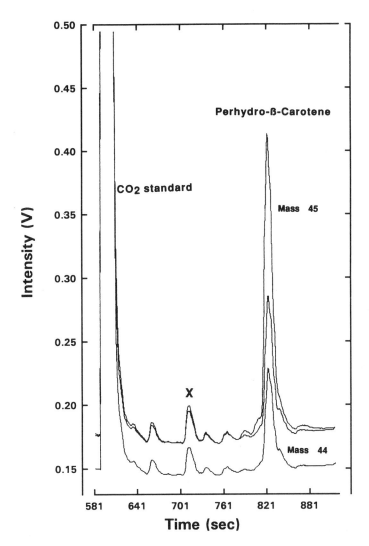

FIGURE 3. GCC-IRMS plot of mass 44 and mass 45 signals vs time for a plasma β-carotene fraction, from plasma collected 22 hours after an oral dose of ^{13}C-β-carotene. The *third trace* is mass 46, which is used to make a minor correction in isotope ratio due to ^{17}O. This computer-generated post-run plot represents data collected from 580 sec to 900 sec of the chromatogram. The peak corresponding to the retention time of standard perhydro-β-caro-tene is indicated. Amplifier gains are matched so as to produce comparable signals at natural abundance for the three traces. The greater elevation in mass 45 relative to mass 44 reflects ^{13}C enrichment in the perhydro-β-carotene peak, compared to other unidentified peaks (X) in the chromatogram which show no such enrichment.

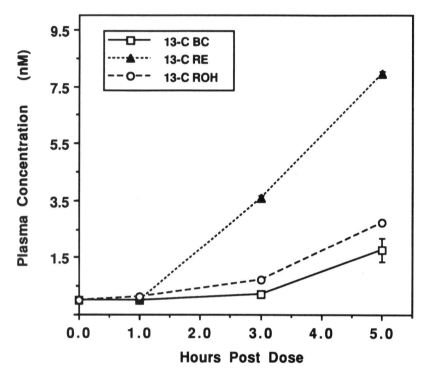

FIGURE 4. Plot of plasma concentration of ^{13}C-β-carotene, ^{13}C-retinyl esters, and ^{13}C-retinol from 0 to 5 hours following an oral dose of 1.0 mg ^{13}C-β-carotene. Concentrations of the labeled analytes were determined as described in Methods.

dietary intake. Here we show that ^{13}C from a 1.0-mg dose of ^{13}C-β-carotene can be traced into plasma β-carotene, retinyl ester and retinol pools, and the biokinetics of each pool followed throughout the absorption period. Furthermore, the reproducibility of data obtained from two independent plasma analyses from the same points is generally excellent, particularly at lower levels of ^{13}C enrichment. Issues of precision of isotope ratio measurement as a function of ^{13}C enrichment have been discussed in detail by Goodman and Brenna.[5]

Both ^{13}C-labeled retinyl ester and β-carotene plasma concentration curves showed multiple peaks during the first 24 hours following the dose. This may have resulted from incomplete absorption of ^{13}C-β-carotene during the initial few hours, followed by a stimulation of further absorptive episodes by consumption of the midday and evening meals. ^{13}C-Retinol showed only one peak, but these data are complicated by the fact that after the initial few hours, retinol probably existed in two plasma pools: retinol associated with chylomicrons (and chylomicron remnants), and retinol associated with retinol binding protein. We are currently studying the distribution of labeled retinol between these two pools at various times after the ^{13}C-β-carotene dose to determine how quickly labeled retinol is secreted by the liver following the uptake of labeled retinyl ester or retinol associated with chylomicrons.

This is the first tracer study to report appearance and disappearance of labeled β-carotene and its primary metabolites in human plasma. Earlier, Goodman *et al.*[2] and Blomstrand and Werner[3] used radioactivity-labeled β-carotene to follow the appearance of β-carotene and its metabolites in human lymph following a single oral dose, using surgical patients with cannulated thoracic ducts. These two studies found that only 8–17% of the administered radioactivity was recoverable in lymph, and that retinyl esters accounted for 61–90% of absorbed radioactivity. Retinol accounted for 2–9% and β-carotene 2–28% of absorbed label. These early studies have provided most of what we know of the metabolism of β-carotene in humans. However, because of issues of risk associated with radioactivity and the invasive procedure necessary for cannulation of the thoracic duct, this model cannot be used routinely.

Our approach involves the use of plasma, in which the vitamin A and β-carotene pools are in a much more dynamic state than is the case with lymph. Consequently,

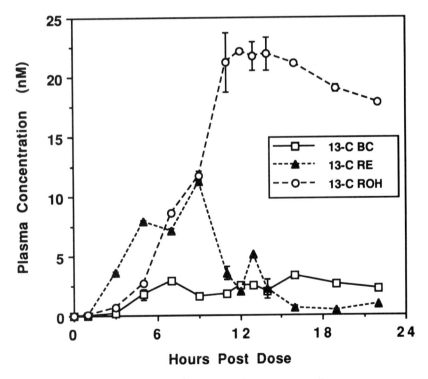

FIGURE 5. Plots of plasma concentration of ^{13}C-β-carotene, ^{13}C-retinyl esters, and ^{13}C-retinol from 0 to 22 hours following an oral dose of 1.0 mg ^{13}C-β-carotene. Concentrations of the labeled analytes were determined as described in Methods.

we shall need to rely on pharmacokinetic approaches to make inferences about the extent of absorption of β-carotene. We have not yet attempted such an analysis with this data set. However, it is apparent that in the study reported here, most of the absorbed dose was converted to vitamin A, with retinyl esters predominating. If it is assumed that all three analytes at this time point were removed from the plasma at the same rate (e.g., via chylomicron remnant clearance by the liver), then on a molar basis about 64% of absorbed ^{13}C from ^{13}C-β-carotene entered the plasma as retinyl esters, 21% as retinol, and 14% as intact β-carotene. These values are within the ranges reported by the two lymph radioactivity studies cited above. While our data show that labeled retinol peaked at a higher concentration than either retinyl ester or β-carotene, this may reflect liver output of protein-bound retinol, which likely turns over at a much slower rate than β-carotene or vitamin A associated with chylomicrons. Thus plasma ^{13}C-retinol may be reflective of intestinal production of retinol from β-carotene only early in the absorptive process. We are currently continuing these studies, including extending the plasma data collection to later time points. Other preliminary data from our laboratory[4] has indicated that changes in plasma concentration of ^{13}C-labeled retinol and β-carotene can be observed as long as three weeks after an oral dose of one milligram ^{13}C-β-carotene.

Several large scale intervention studies involving regular consumption of 40- to 50-mg doses of β-carotene are currently under way to determine if β-carotene supplements of this magnitude reduce risk of cancer or cardiovascular disease. Unfortunately, essentially nothing is known of the effect in humans of prior β-carotene intake on the metabolism of subsequent doses, or whether β-carotene is metabolized differently at high vs low doses. The data of Dimitrov et al.[6,7] show that in several subjects receiving 15 or 45 mg β-carotene per day for several weeks, plasma β-carotene levels peaked as early as 10 days, then declined steadily even though dosing continued. Assuming that lack of compliance is not responsible for these findings, one may speculate that (a) absorption efficiency was impaired, (b) there was induced metabolism of β-carotene to vitamin A or other products, or (c) there was enhanced plasma clearance of β-carotene.

These issues and other fundamental aspects of β-carotene metabolism are best investigated using a tracer method such as that reported here, in which plasma input (and clearance) of both labeled β-carotene and its intestinal retinoid metabolites can be measured. Interpretation of results of intervention studies with β-carotene supplements, whether for prevention of chronic disease or vitamin A deficiency, will be more difficult in the absence of a more complete understanding of β-carotene metabolism in the human.

REFERENCES

1. FURR, H. C., O. AMEDEE-MANESME, A. J. CLIFFORD, H. R. BERGEN, III, A. J. JONES, D. P. ANDERSON & J. A. OLSON. 1989. Vitamin A concentrations in liver determined by isotope dilution assay with tetradeuterated vitamin A and by biopsy in generally healthy adult humans. Am. J. Clin. Nutr. 49: 713–716.
2. GOODMAN, D. S., R. BLOMSTRAND, B. WERNER, H. S. HUANG & T. SHIRATORI. 1966. The intestinal absorption and metabolism of vitamin A and β-carotene in man. J. Clin. Invest 45(10): 1615–1623.
3. BLOMSTRAND, R. & B. WERNER. 1967. Studies on the intestinal absorption of radioactive β-carotene and vitamin A in man. Conversion of β-carotene into vitamin A. Scand. J. Clin. Lab. Invest. 19: 339–345.
4. PARKER, R. S., J. E. SWANSON, S. M. VIERECK, A. B. SPIELMAN, J. T. BRENNA &

K. J. GOODMAN. 1992. Metabolism and biokinetics of ^{13}C-*β*-carotene in humans following a small oral dose. FASEB J. **6**(5): A1645.

5. GOODMAN, K. J. & J. T. BRENNA. 1992. High sensitivity tracer detection using high precision isotope ratio monitoring gas chromatography and highly enriched [U-^{13}C]-labeled precursors. Anal. Chem. **64**(1): 1088–1095.

6. DIMITROV, N. V., C. W. BOONE, M. B. HAY *et al.* 1987. Plasma beta-carotene levels kinetic patterns during administration of various doses of beta-carotene. Nutr. Growth Cancer **3**: 227–238.

7. DIMITROV, N. V., C. MEYER, D. E. ULLREY, W. CHENOWETH, A. MICHELAKIS, W. MALONE, C. BOONE & G. FINK. 1988. Bioavailability of *β*-carotene in humans. Am. J. Clin. Nutr. **48**: 298–304.

Effects of Nutritional Status on Carotene Uptake and Bioconversion[a]

NOEL W. SOLOMONS AND JESUS BULUX

Center for Studies of Sensory Impairment,
Aging and Metabolism (CeSSIAM)
Research Branch for the
National Committee for the Blind and Deaf of Guatemala
"Dr. Rodolfo Robles V." Eye and Ear Hospital
Diagonal 21 y 19 Calle, Zona 11
Guatemala City, Guatemala 01011

INTRODUCTION

Retinoids, specifically vitamin A, are essential nutrients in metabolism of vertebrates. It is obvious from a casual look at natural history that it is not necessary to ingest preformed vitamin A in the diet, as strict herbivorous species can produce all the vitamin A necessary for adequate nutriture from the precursor carotenoids in foods of plant origin. As is reviewed in a number of contributions to this volume, the intestine is the site for the hydrolysis of provitamin A carotenes and the liberation of retinoids with vitamin A activity. When it comes to human populations, one does not have the luxury of focusing exclusively on the metabolism of a single nutrient, as the *interaction* among nutrients is a complex—but fundamental—reality. Moreover, although the strategies, tactics, logistics and ethics for studying, in this instance, carotene metabolism, are limited and fraught with pitfalls in human subjects, *the best model for human physiology is man and woman*. The present paper will attempt to discuss and critique the experimental approaches of utility in detecting and quantifying carotene uptake and biological conversion to vitamin A in *human* investigation and to review its interaction with the underlying nutritional status of the host and with the preformance of the intestinal mechanisms for absorption and bioconversion of dietary carotenoids. We shall include a review of the literature and reports on recent experience in Guatemala from the CeSSIAM in collaboration with the University of Arizona.

Bioavailability and Bioconversion of Carotenes

Operational concepts and specific definitions are important for the discussion that follows. *Bioavailability* is used here in the sense and connotation originated in pharmacology, namely, that which relates to the intestinal uptake and passage

[a] We would like to acknowledge the financial assistance of the Thrasher Research Fund, AkPharma Inc., and the U.S. Agency for International Development in the research cited from Guatemala and in the writing of this paper.

of a compound into the systemic circulation. We have left moot any more elaborate issues of the subsequent participation in biological functions in the host. In fact, as other contributions to this volume have documented, not all of the biological functions of intact carotenoids or indices for their measurement have been elucidated.

Carotenoids can be classified as "provitamin A" and "nonprovitamin A" with respect to their capacity to yield retinal upon central or eccentric enzymatic cleavage.[1] The term *bioconversion* is used to refer to the cleavage of a provitamin A compound to yield a molecular precursor of vitamin A (retinal) which is documented by its detection in the systemic circulation or as part of a new contribution to hepatic vitamin A stores. We recognize that other retinoids may be derived from intestinal cleavage of carotenoids,[2,3] but the literature on this phenomenon in humans is sparse, and is totally devoid of instances of interaction with host nutritional status.

Nutritional Status and Intestinal Function

Although, as we shall discuss below, "nutritional status" becomes an elusive concept in its practical application to human individuals and populations, we can identify two conceptual domains for interactions of nutriture and intestinal function. The first relates to some nutritional "insult" (or tissue damage or dysfunction from nutritional deficiency {or excess}) that would change the normal response of the digestive and absorptive mechanisms of the alimentary tract to a meal. The second relates to the reality of *homeostatic* regulation of the body which, in the case of nutrients, tends to "optimize" the content of stores and concentrations of tissues. Too little of a nutrient can damage morphology and function, but, at the same time too much of the same substance may be toxic. By implication, then, the body perceives nutritional status as something to be regulated, and intestinal function becomes "responsive" to the need of the body either to admit or exclude a specific nutrient.

In general terms, we have both animal and human models for the paradigm of nutritional damage to intestinal function. Protein-energy malnutrition (PEM) is defined both in terms of deficits in anthropometric status in relation to a reference population[4] and as the overt, clinical syndromes of marasmus and kwashiorkor.[5] The latter syndrome, protein deficiency associated with edema, has been associated with transient maldigestion of lipids, protein, and disaccharides and malabsorption of fatty acids, vitamin A, and vitamin B_{12}.[6] Lesions in pancreatic secretion and in the turnover of mucosal cells can be implicated in the digestive and absorptive dysfunctions in severe, edematous PEM. Alternatively, the regulation of iron absorption and metabolism in kwashiorkor remains intact.[7] Deficiencies of various micronutrients are also associated with intestinal lesion that could interfere with absorption of other micronutrients. The deficiency syndromes associated with malabsorption include folic acid deficiency,[8] pellagra,[9] and zinc deficiency.[10] Clinical diarrhea is a prominent feature of each of the aforementioned micronutrient deficiencies.

With regard to homeostasis, often termed "the wisdom of the body," our inquiry would be focussed on the "wisdom of the *gut*," that is, on the capacity of mechanisms of enhancement or inhibition (upregulation or downregulation) to bring a nutrient supply into harmony with the body's need to have enough, but not too much. Control by the intestine can operate not only at the level of uptake but also at the level of excretion.

The mammalian intestine's handling of *iron* is the classical example and model for homeostatic regulation of absorption.[11,12] Iron is poorly soluble and precipitates readily with other chemicals in the diet, yet it is the third most abundant element in the earth's crust and an excessive accumulation in the body is toxic. Thus, the gut has a bidirectional system to enhance iron absorption when stores are low but to restrict its uptake when stores are sufficient.

Several nutrients have organic precursors or provitamin forms, which require some form of digestion or chemical transformation to become the active vitamin. The *intestine* is the site of only one such conversion of a provitamin to a vitamin, that of provitamin A carotenoids to vitamin A. However, we can examine analogies with respect to the hepatic decision to convert the amino acid, *tryptophan,* to the vitamin, *niacin,* and the process in the dermis of the skin that converts *7-dehydrocholesterol* into *vitamin D*. The tryptophan-niacin story is illustrative of a capacity for *up*regulation. When individuals are consuming niacin-deficient diets, the amount of tryptophan converted to the vitamin is increased.[13] The dermal biosynthesis of vitamin D is illustrative of a capacity for *down*regulation. Although one can become intoxicated and damaged by excessive amounts of vitamin D taken orally, the solar activated synthesis in the skin is self-limited and one cannot become vitamin D toxic from sun exposure.[14]

With respect to carotene and the gut, it has been postulated that there is a bidirectional control, not of uptake, but of its bioconversion to active vitamin A. What is well demonstrated is the downregulation with high intakes;[15] one cannot become vitamin A toxic consuming carotenoids. Animal studies[16] suggest that rates of bioconversion are higher in vitamin A deficiency states, but this demonstration in humans is currently under study (see below).

Methodological Considerations in Human Research

Nutritional Status Assessment

One would think that nutritional science would have developed a consensus on the meaning of a term as basic as "nutritional status." Such, however, is not the case. This term can refer to the total-body content of a specific nutrient as indicated by a measure of internal reserves or stores of the compound. Or, it can refer to its presence, in the *activated* form, in the target tissues, as indicated by biopsies of peripheral tissues. Or, it can refer to the integration of the active nutrient in the metabolism of the host, as indicated by tests of physiological function (functional assessment).[17] In experimental animals, one has the luxury not only of assessing nutritional status at each and all of the aforementioned levels but also of starting with genetically defined and uniform organisms and controlling and manipulating their dietary intake of all nutrients.

In human and clinical nutrition, such is not the case. Precisely where our interest in nutrition and carotene metabolism is most relevant—in *man* and *woman*—the circumstances of human existence and genetic variation, including variability in diet, different rates of disease, parasitoses of different intensities, and diverse ethnicities with more or less interbreeding, confound one's ambition to study and compare homogeneous population samples. Also, bioethics govern one's attitude to induce impaired nutritional status or to maintain individuals in states of nutritional deficiency once diagnosed. When moving from the cell culture well through the laboratory metabolic cage to free-living populations, the degree of experimental freedom for invasive collection procedures and the homogeneity of populations are drastically diminished.

Assessment of nutritional status with respect to vitamin A and of what might be called "carotene status" provides a critical variable in the hypotheses regarding interaction of nutritional status and carotene handling, but diagnosis of status is not unequivocal.

Vitamin A Status. Since the liver is the primary site of vitamin A storage, hepatic biopsy would be the most direct manner to establish nutritional status. It is obviously too invasive for routine use. Stable isotope technology[18] holds the promise of assessing the total-body pool by a dilution approach, but the cost is prohibitive and the time is protracted. In fact, circulating retinol levels are the most commonly used index of status. This indicator has serious limitations as a surrogate for hepatic reserves[19] as it does not change in proportion to liver stores.

The standard of functional tests for vitamin A status, and perhaps for functional tests in general, is the dark adaptation test.[20] In recent years, a series of functional approaches to assessing vitamin A status included the Relative Dose Response, Modified Relative Dose Response, and Conjunctival Impression Cytology.

It would be by means of these indices that one would ask the question about vitamin A status in relation to intestinal metabolism of carotenes.

Carotene Status. Since carotenoids are not classified as nutrients, talking about their "status" is not semantically pure. However, we can use it here in the sense of quantifying the body deposits of this compound. This is most often indexed using circulating levels of β-carotenes or total carotenes. Subcutaneous fat needle biopsies are not overly invasive, and have been used to gauge carotene status. Most recently rectal mucosal biopsy[21] and buccal mucosal scrapings[22] have been employed.

Quantification of Carotene Uptake from the Diet

The kinds of variables that one would want to associate with nutritional status variables are those of quantifying the uptake of carotene from diet or enteral doses. There are two basic formats: that of a formal absorption test and that related to accumulation in the body over time with continuous feeding. The former involves a single test dosing; the latter requires multiple dosing over a finite period of time.

A commonly used single-dose absorption test in gastroenterology and pharmacology is the "tolerance test" which involves the feeding of a large dose of β-carotene and making serial samples at predetermined intervals postdosing. FIGURE 1 is a schematic illustration of three possible plasma concentration responses to an oral, challenge dose of β-carotene administered either as a food or supplement. As illustrated in TABLE 1, a number of authors have employed this "tolerance test" approach to evaluate plasma appearance of carotenes after a single dose. Interestingly, the literature differs as to whether 8, 24 or 48 h is the point of apogee in concentration. What is clear, in practice, however, is that the rise and fall of carotene is much more prolonged than that seen with other nutrients. Plasma appearance methods have interpretive caveats and pitfalls. Although no logic can deny that if one sees a new appearance of a substance after oral administration of the same compound, it is likely to be the result of its recent absorption. If one does not see a plasma rise, however, that does not mean that there was no absorption. Also, the proportionality among the peak-heights of the curves or the areas under the curves of plasma change cannot necessarily be assumed to reflect the relative magnitude of uptake. Issues of rates of clearance impinge on these latter two assumptions.

The other format is multiple dosing (usually daily administration) of β-carotene supplements or a food-source and following the change in circulating carotene levels at a fixed interval. FIGURE 2 represents schematically this approach to assessing carotene bioavailability. A series of pitfalls are inherent in the differential interpretation of magnitude of increment in concentration. As shown in FIGURE 3, a "ceiling effect" may operate, in which the accumulation of carotene in the plasma is limited due to point of saturation of binding capacity (or some adaptation in plasma clearance). Over the years, this approach has been used by many authors (TABLE 1), including dosing subjects to the point of clinically apparent carotenodermia (yellow discoloration of the skin). The same interpretive assumptions about the meaning of new appearance of circulating carotenes and of their nonappearance obtain for the multiple-dose format, as for the single-dose challenge.

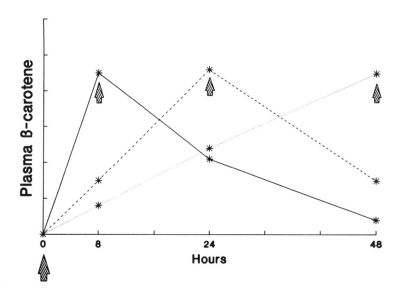

FIGURE 1. Single dose. This is the schematic examination of the conventional paradigm for evaluation of β-carotene bioavailability as a change in plasma (or serum) concentration after a single oral dose of a provitamin A carotene. As depicted, a dose (15 to 50 mg) of β-carotene is given at time zero (*arrow*). Blood samples are taken at 8, 24 and 48 hours. As in other analogous "tolerance tests," the increment in plasma concentration or the area under the curve is interpreted as an index of uptake. Of note is the difference in the time-course of plasma appearance and disappearance for carotene, as compared with other nutrients which peak at 4 to 6 h. The literature differs with some authors finding each of the various time-intervals as the expected time for maximal rise.

TABLE 1. Publications in Which the Rise in Circulating β-Carotene Levels Have Been Used as an Index of Bioavailability or as a Response to Long-Term Supplementation

Short-term monitoring of a single oral dose
    Urbach, C. *et al.* 1952. Exp. Med. Surg. **12:** 7–20.
    Ralli, E. P. *et al.* 1935. J. Lab. Clin. Med. **20:** 1266–1275.
    Murril, W. A. *et al.* 1942. J. Clin. Invest. **20:** 395–400.
    Fujita, A. *et al.* 1957. J. Vitaminol. **3:** 223–234.
    Cornwell, D. G. *et al.* 1962. J. Lipid Res. **3:** 65–70.
    Dimitrov, N. V. *et al.* 1987. J. Nutr. Growth Cancer **3:** 227–238.
    Brown, E. D. *et al.* 1989. Am. J. Clin. Nutr. **49:** 1258–1266.
    Brown, E. D. *et al.* 1989. Clin. Chem. **35:** 310–312.
    Henderson, C. T. *et al.* 1989. J. Am. Coll. Nutr. **8:** 625–635.
    Maiani, G. *et al.* 1989. Eur. J. Clin. Nutr. **43:** 749–461.
    Canfield, L. M. *et al.* 1991. Am. J. Clin. Nutr. **54:** 539–541.
Long-term monitoring of multiple oral doses
    Urbach, C. *et al.* 1952. Exp. Med. Surg. **12:** 7–20.
    Mathews-Roth, M. M. *et al.* 1974. Eur. J. Clin. Nutr. **43:** 175–186.
    Corbett, M. F. *et al.* 1977. Br. J. Dermatol. **97:** 655–662.
    Devadas, P. R. *et al.* 1978. World Rev. Nutr. Diet. **31:** 159–161.
    Jayarahan, P. *et al.* 1980. Indian J. Med. **71:** 53–65.
    Willett, W. C. *et al.* 1983. Am. J. Clin. Nutr. **38:** 559–566.
    Willett, W. C. *et al.* 1983. Am. J. Clin. Nutr. **38:** 631–639.
    Meyer, J. C. *et al.* 1985. J. Am. Med. Assoc. **228:** 1004–1008.
    Jensen, C. D. *et al.* 1986. Nutr. Rep. Int. **33:** 117–123.
    Dimitrov, N. V. *et al.* 1987. J. Nutr. Growth Cancer **3:** 227–238.
    Constantino, J. P. *et al.* 1988. Am. J. Clin. Nutr. **48:** 1277–1283.
    Dimitrov, N. V. *et al.* 1988. Am. J. Clin. Nutr. **48:** 298–304.
    Kim, H. J. *et al.* 1988. Nutr. Res. **8:** 1119–1127.
    Greenberg, E. R. *et al.* 1989. Controlled Clin. Trials **10:** 153–166.
    Hussein, L. & El-Tohamy 1989. Int. J. Vitam. Nutr. Res. **59:** 229–233.
    Hussein, L. & El-Tohamy 1990. Int. J. Vitam. Nutr. Res. **60:** 229–235.
    Albanes, D. *et al.* 1992. Eur. J. Clin. Nutr. **46:** 15–24.
    Micozzi, M. S. *et al.* 1982. Am. J. Clin. Nutr. **55:** 1120–1125.

Quantification of Bioconversion of Carotenes to Retinoids

The other paradigm is measuring the conversion of provitamin A carotenoids to active vitamin A. In theory, as above, the options are to focus on either the intestinal process or the change in body content/nutritional status that resulted. With respect to the former, the fate of a single challenge dose could be followed. In a sophisticated, high-technology setting this could involve the labelling of the carotene molecule with stable[18] (or radioactive) isotopes. The use of the latter would generally be restricted to older adult populations. Alternatively, one could introduce inert side chains, *e.g.*, hydroxyl groups, at known sites on the central chain. The amount of *labeled* or *modified* active vitamin A appearing in the circulation would be a marker for the degree of postdose bioconversion. The former would be determined using gas-chromatographic mass-spectrophotometry (G-C Mass-Spec)[23] and the latter by high precision liquid chromatography (HPLC).[24]

A *low*-technology, less expensive approach derives from the fact that vitamin A released from the gut cells enters the circulation in the form of retinyl esters bound to lipoproteins in chylomicra. If one provided carotene and measured retinyl esters in the early postprandial circulation, this can only be of provitamin A origin.[25] Current methods permit detection of low concentrations of circulating esters. FIGURE 4 schematically illustrates the expected changes in plasma retinyl esters and β-carotene after administration of a large oral dose of the compound.

With the multiple-dose feeding of a provitamin A source, what one would evaluate would be the change in nutritional status of vitamin A. Changes in retinol

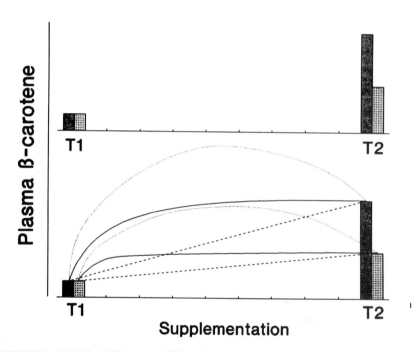

FIGURE 2. Multiple (daily) doses. This is the schematic examination of the conventional paradigm for evaluating β-carotene bioavailability as a change in plasma (or serum) concentration after prolonged, multiple-dose supplementation, T_1 represents some presupplementation sampling and T_2 represents some time after an interval of oral supplementation with a carotene source(s). The *bars* represent two trial populations with different status or treatment, *i.e.*, different source, different dose, different state of intestinal health. The *upper panel* shows the usual evaluation, as the interval differential increase in circulating concentration. The *lower panel* represents various assumptions about the manner that plasma accumulates. One assumption (as represented by the *dashed lines*) is a linear increase with time. Another assumption is that a proportion of the circulating level is cleared daily (as represented by the *solid curves*); when the amount absorbed is equal to the amount cleared, the levels reach a plateau. The final assumption is that the clearance adapts to the amount accumulating, such that an increasing proportion of the circulating level is cleared as levels get higher (as represented by the *dotted curves*). Only if the linear accumulation is correct, can the relative differences in bioavailability be reflected in the changes in β-carotene levels.

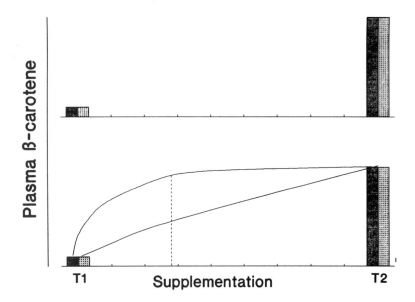

FIGURE 3. "Ceiling effect." The graphic terms of reference that obtain in FIGURE 2 are the same. Another confounder of the interpretation of the accumulation of β-carotene in plasma as a differential index of its bioavailability is the "ceiling" phenomenon. The levels of the compound are identical at the termination of the supplementation trial (*upper panel*), and could be erroneously misconstrued as representing equivalent uptake. In this case, however, there is a limited carrying capacity in the circulation and the two peaks were arrived at with quite distinct dynamics (*lower panel*). Only before the binding capacity is saturated can one appreciate the relative differences in bioavailability.

levels have been used,[26,27] but in theory, improvement in a functional index such as conjunctival morphology/metabolism or dark adaptation in a marginally malnourished population would also be potentially useful.

Malnutrition, Carotene Uptake, and Bioconversion

Preformed Vitamin A Absorption in Severe Malnutrition

Over 20 years ago, in the golden age of interest in clinical malnutrition syndromes, Arroyave[29] reviewed the accumulated experience in animals and humans with regard to the effect of protein and protein-energy deficiency on the metabolism of vitamin A, both at the gut uptake level and in its circulatory transport and hepatic storage. Studies in rats had demonstrated impaired uptake of vitamin A from the diet,[30] as well as impairment of its transport.[30,31] Children with clinical edematous malnutrition (kwashiorkor) manifested attenuated plasma responses (flat tolerance curves) to an oral dose of 75,000 retinol equivalents (RE) of vitamin A as retinyl palmitate.[32] This can be attributed in part to defective intraluminal events due to the effect of severe PEM on biliary and pancreatic function, in part to nutritional mucosal damage, and possibly to impaired lipoprotein synthesis in the protein-deficient gut. It has also been shown that children with severe PEM have difficulty mobilizing injected vitamin A from an intramuscular site to the liver.[33]

Carotene Bioavailability and Bioconversion

Malnutrition of a mild to moderate degree also can be assessed by anthropometric standards aimed at detecting growth failure. Canfield *et al.*[34] performed complex statistical regression analyses to determine whether nutritional status, as assessed

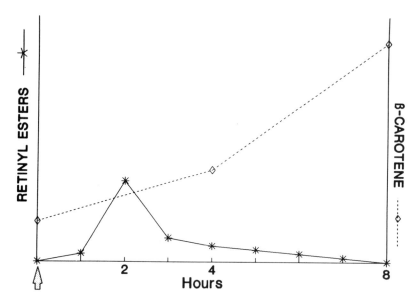

FIGURE 4. This is a schematic representation of the single-dose paradigm for assessing bioconversion as the postprandial appearance of retinyl esters in the circulation. An oral dose of β-carotene (or other carotenoid with provitamin A activity) is given at zero-time (*arrow*). Blood samples are taken at 2, 4, and 8 hours. The course of retinyl esters is shown by the *solid line,* with a peak at 2 h, at a time before clearance of the chylomicra. The *dashed line* represents the expected rise in β-carotene levels. The assumption is that the magnitude of increase is proportional to the extent of carotene to retinal conversion during passage of the meal through the gut.

by anthropometry, had any influence on plasma excursion after a standard oral dose of β-carotene. In this study, performed in collaboration with our group in Guatemala,[34] we used the paradigm shown schematically in FIGURE 1. We found no association between the rise in plasma β-carotene after a 15- or 30-mg oral dose and weight-for-age, height-for-age, or weight-for-height, among children with a high prevalence of deficits in the former two indices.

Studies of β-carotene bioconversion efficiency in severe PEM have yet to be reported. One would *assume* that, at least, the impaired mechanisms that apply to preformed retinol (above) would apply, but a prior, additional derangement of the carotene cleavage in the mucosa may also occur. With respect to mild to moderate malnutrition, defined anthropometrically, Bulux et al.[35] failed to find any association between the retinyl ester response to oral β-carotene and the subjects' anthropometric indices.

Carotene Status and Carotene Bioavailability

There are two alternative hypotheses of a relationship between carotene status and its bioavailability: a negative association, or a positive one. If one has reduced absorption of β-carotene with a greater apparent body reserve, one can input a *retro*regulation which implies causality of the former effect by the latter. If one finds greater absorption of β-carotene in those with an initially greater status, one may assume that a stable, intersubject variability in absorption efficiency is at work.

The simplest way to examine the hypothesis of a relationship between carotene status and carotene absorption would be to perform statistical regressions of the two variables from a *cross-sectional* format. Operationally, this could be done using prevailing circulating carotene levels as the index of "status" and the plasma (or serum) postdose excursion of carotene after a single dose of the test compound (FIG. 1).

Canfield et al.[34] in Guatemala, in a collaboration between our center and the University of Arizona, used a single, oral dose of 15 mg or 30 mg of oral β-carotene as a challenge dose, with the peak postdose rise as the index of carotene bioavailability. Regression analyses failed to find any association between initial plasma β-carotene levels and the postchallenge excursion of that analyte in the bloodstream.

Albanes et al.[36] performed a double-blind controlled trial in 220 Finnish men aged 30 to 69 (average: 50 y). Of these, 111 completed a phase of 60 days of daily supplementation with 20 mg β-carotene capsules and 109 took placebos. The baseline intake of dietary β-carotene was 2.1 mg daily. For the supplemented group, there was an average 10-fold rise from 26.84 ± 19.33 μg/dl (0.50 ± 0.36 μmol/L) to 267.89 ± 132.60 μg/dl (4.99 ± 2.97 μmol/L) with a consistently large coefficient of variation. With both simple and multiple regression analyses, one of the strongest predictors of the peak serum carotene level in the supplemented men was their baseline circulating β-carotene level. The rank ordering was positively correlated ($r = 0.64$).

In Guatemala, we performed a study in school children from a suburb of the capital city. A total of 65 children were divided in four groups to receive 20 days of supplementation with one of four treatments: 1) placebo, 2) 1000 RE of retinyl palmitate, 3) 6 mg of β-carotene, and 4) 50 g of cooked carrots containing 6 mg of β-carotene.[37] Of greatest importance to this discussion is the regression of initial β-carotene levels and the increase in these levels in the β-carotene-supplemented group. No relationship was found (J. Bulux: unpublished finding).

An experimental design that, to our knowledge, has not yet been reported would be to perform some formal, single-dose β-carotene absorption test, before and after a protracted period of oral supplementation. If a negative feedback by carotene status were in operation, one would expect the supplemented group to have a lesser uptake of β-carotene than an unsupplemented group. Unfortunately, the potential of a "ceiling effect" as illustrated in FIGURE 3 intercedes. It is possible that an initial high plasma β-carotene level, close to some saturation point, may impede the further entry of the compound into the circulation even if it has been efficiently absorbed. For the proposed study, an isotope-*labeled* or *modified* oral carotene tracer would be required.

Several studies have shown that it is possible to reduce circulating levels of carotenoids by feeding volunteers a low-carotene diet.[36,39] Something, similar to the converse of the aforementioned design has indeed been performed by Jensen *et al.*[38] with a prospective carotene *depletion* and *repletion* format. In subjects who were fed a low-carotene (fruit- and vegetable-free) diet for 10 days with a consequent decline in carotene levels, it was possible to demonstrate rapid rises in circulating levels after only a few days of feeding a plant source of carotenoids, carrots, in amounts of one or three units daily.

Finally, one could use single-dose challenges as the index of absorption and a prospective carotene-feeding format as the longitudinal and differential challenge. That would mean performing β-carotene tolerance tests before and after a period of carotene supplementation with appropriate placebo controls. To our knowledge, such a design has not been reported in the literature.

Vitamin A Status and Carotene Bioconversion

It is well recognized by clinical experience with carotene supplementers and carotenodermia, that an adequate vitamin A status effectively blocks further bioconversion. The alternate question, also presumably controlled by feedback regulation, is whether the bioconversion of provitamin A to the active vitamin is enhanced in a marginal or deficient vitamin A status. This is suggested in animals,[16] but there is only limited data available in humans.

We, in Guatemala, in collaboration with the University of Arizona[37] have employed the experimental model for human bioconversion discussed in FIGURE 4, namely, monitoring the immediate, postprandial retinyl ester excursions,[25] to explore the interaction of vitamin A status and the extent of intestinal conversion of carotenoids to the active vitamin. In this study, we had a range of retinol concentrations in our rural schoolchildren, ranging from 0.33 to 1.41 μmol/L. The 2-h increment in retinyl ester levels ranged from 0 to 0.24 μmol/L. There was a *trend* toward an inverse association between plasma retinyl ester response and retinol levels ($r = 0.29$), which did not reach significance with the sample size of 20 children. Possibly, a population with even more profound depression of levels would provide a better forum for this inquiry.

In most of the studies of multiple-dose supplementation trials, retinol levels have remained unchanged; this has been expected as the majority of the populations were European or North American adults. Using the rise in circulating retinol levels with prolonged feeding as an index of bioconversion, and feeding, variously, carrots, carrot juice and spinach to Egyptian children with low retinol levels, Hussein and El-Tohamy[27] have produced evidence suggestive of enhanced intestinal β-carotene bioconversion with poor vitamin A status. In these studies, 13 Egyptian schoolchildren with average circulating retinol levels of 0.6 to 0.7 μmol/L (17 to 20 μg/dl) were given three supplementation formats. Seven received the 200,000 IU capsule (60,000 RE), four received a cumulative dose of 25,000 RE as spinach over 40 days and 2 received a cumulative dose of 16,000 RE over the same period as cooked carrots. Retinol levels doubled in all three groups, and total carotene levels remained basically stable. This truly is suggestive of the fact of bioconversion of the dietary carotene. In a related study, in adult volunteers, in which subjects were assigned to 14 days of a vitamin A-free diet (no vitamin from either animal or plant sources), these same Egyptian authors[28] showed that protracted feeding with grated carrots, carrot juice and spinach could stabilize the retinol levels of the subject.

FUTURE CONSIDERATIONS

It would be fair to conclude that our appraisal of the topic of the nutritional status focused more on the limitations in our knowledge, our ability to interpret data, and our capability to generate useful new knowledge when the issue of human investigation is concerned. The simple and accessible (perhaps simplistic) approaches of dosing human subjects with provitamin A sources and following the changes in circulating levels of carotenoids and/or retinoids (retinol; retinyl esters) have dominated the scant literature on carotene bioavailability and bioconversion. These efforts, however, may have taken us as far as we can go within the interpretive limitations. Greatly increased cost and analytical complexity would be needed to begin to apply tracer experiments, with isotope-labeled or modified carotenoid compounds. This will require the mobilization of financial resources and collaborative goodwill. Third World countries have the widespread prevalences of hypovitaminosis A and of other nutritional deficiencies; First World nations have the sophisticated synthetic and analytical chemistry needed in tracer research. This coalition will be needed to refine and extend our knowledge about the feedback homeostatic control of carotene bioavailability and its bioconversion.

We must also admit that certain questions of interaction of nutritional status have not even occurred to nutritional scientists. This points out the need for even wider collaborations, to embrace experts on issues of protein malnutrition and micronutrient deficiencies, notably those of iron, zinc and folic acid in which there would be reasonable hypotheses about an interference with the intestinal handling of dietary carotenes in their uptake and/or bioconversion.

The majority of the world's population lives in poor, developing countries. For every industrial-nation adult at some risk of a chemopreventable chronic disease, there are manifold children in developing countries in search of ways to satisfy their vitamin A requirements, and probably an equal number of adults whose life-styles or exposures also make them candidates for any health benefits that intact carotenes exercise in the diet and in the body.

ACKNOWLEDGMENTS

We appreciate the collaboration of Prof. Louise M. Canfield and her colleagues at the University of Arizona: Prof. Gail Harrison, Laura Kettel, Ann F. Lima, Anna Giuliano, Veronica Ortiz, Jesus Valenzuela, Brian Kelley, Suzanne Worley, and Carol Margolis.

We also express our gratitude to those who have participated in Guatemala: the children of Carchá, Alta Verapaz; Antigua Guatemala; Guajitos and Belén in Guatemala City; and their parents for their willingness to participate in the studies. Thanks to our colleagues at CeSSIAM: Julieta Quan de Serrano, Rosalba Perez, Aura M. Guerrero, Carmen Y. Lopez, Marjorie Haskell, Carlos Rivera, and Carlos Valdez, for their cooperation.

REFERENCES

1. OLSON, J. A. 1990. *In* Present Knowledge in Nutrition. M. L. Brown, Ed. 6th edit. 96–107. ISLI-Nutrition Foundation. Washington DC.
2. OLSON, J. A. 1989. J. Nutr. **119:** 105–108.

3. WANG, X-D., N. I. KRINSKY, G. TANG & R. M. RUSSELL. 1992. Arch Biochem. Biophys. **293:** 298–304.
4. WATERLOW, J. 1973. Lancet **2:** 87–89.
5. Wellcome Trust Working Party. 1970. Lancet **2:** 302–303.
6. SOLOMONS, N. W., J. BULUX & S. MOLINA. 1989. *In* Textbook of Gastroenterology and Nutrition in Infancy. E. Lebenthal, Ed. 2nd edit. 517–533. Raven Press. New York.
7. CABALLERO, B., N. W. SOLOMONS, R. BATRES & B. TORUN. 1985. J. Pediatr. Gastroenterol. Nutr. **4:** 97–102.
8. HERBERT, V. & N. COLEMAN. 1988. *In* Modern Nutrition in Health and Disease. M. G. Shills & V. R. Young, Eds. 7th edit. 388–416. Lea & Febiger. Philadelphia.
9. JACOB, R. A. & M. E. SWENSEID. 1990. *In* Present Knowledge in Nutrition. M. L. Brown, Ed. 6th edit. 163–169. ISLI-Nutrition Foundation. Washington, DC.
10. MOYNAHAN, E. J. 1974. Lancet **2:** 399.
11. GREEN, R., R. W. CHARLTON, H. SEFTEL, T. BOTHWELL, F. MAYET, B. ADAMS, C. FINCH & M. LAYRISSE. 1968. Am. J. Med. **45:** 336–353.
12. LYNCH, S. R. 1984. *In* Absorption and Malabsorption of Mineral Nutrient. N. W. Solomons & I. H. Rosenberg, Eds. 89–124. Alan R. Liss, Inc. New York.
13. NAKAGAWA, I., T. TAKAHASHI, T. SUZUKI & Y. MASANA. 1969. J. Nutr. **99:** 325–330.
14. HOLICK, M. F. 1985. Ann. N.Y. Acad. Sci. **453:** 1–13.
15. MICOZZI, M. S., E. D. BROWN, P. R. TAYLOR & E. WOLFE. 1988. Am. J. Clin. Nutr. **48:** 1061–1064.
16. ERDMAN, J. W. JR., M. A. GRUMMER, & S. D. MILLER. 1984. Fed. Proc. **43:** A3375 (abst.).
17. SOLOMONS, N. W. & L. H. ALLEN. 1983. Nutr. Rev. **41:** 33–50.
18. FURR, H. C., O. AMEDEE-MANESME, A. J. CLIFFORD, H. R. BERGEN, III, A. D. JONES, D. P. ANDERSON & J. A. OLSON. 1989. Am. J. Clin. Nutr. **49:** 713–716.
19. OLSON, J. A. 1984. J. Natl. Cancer Inst. **73:** 1439–1444.
20. CARNEY, E. A. & R. M. RUSSELL. 1980. Am. J. Clin. Nutr. **110:** 552–557.
21. GRANDE, A., S. MOBARHAN, A. KESHAVARIAN, P. BOWEN, M. STACEWIVZ-SPAPUNT-ZAKIS, K. GHAZANFARI, F. KONICEK, A. OLIVERA, A. SHIAU & C. FORD. 1992. FASEB J. **6:** A4169.
22. GILBERT, A. M., H. F. STICH, M. P. ROSIN & A. J. DAVIDSON. 1990. Int. J. Cancer **45:** 855–859.
23. CLIFFORD, A. J., A. D. JONES, Y. TONDEUR, H. C. FURR, H. R. BERGEN & J. A. OLSON. 1986. Proc. Mass. Spectrom. Allied Top. **34:** 327–328.
24. TANUMIHARDJO, S. A., H. C. FURR, J. W. ERDMAN, JR. & J. A. OLSON. 1990. Eur. J. Clin. Nutr. **44:** 219–224.
25. MAIANI, G., S. MOBARHAN, M. CECCANTI, L. RANALDI, S. GETTNER, P. BOWEN, H. FRIEDMAN, A. DELORENZO & A. FERRO-LUZZI. 1989. Eur. J. Clin. Nutr. **43:** 749–761.
26. JALAL, F., M. C. NESHEIM, D. SANJUR & J. P. HABICHT. 1990. FASEB J. **4:** A1373 (abst.).
27. HUSSEIN, L. & M. EL-TOHAMY. 1989. Int. J. Vit. Nutr. Res. **59:** 229–233.
28. HUSSEIN, L. & M. EL-TOHAMY. 1990. Int. J. Vit. Nutr. Res. **60:** 229–235.
29. ARROYAVE, G. 1969. Am. J. Clin. Nutr. **22:** 1119–1128.
30. JAGANNATHAN, S. N. & V. N. PATWARDHAN. 1960. Indian J. Med. Res. **48:** 775.
31. MATHEWS, J. & G. H. BEATON. 1963. Can. J. Biochem. Physiol. **41:** 543–549.
32. ARROYAVE, G., F. VITERI, M. BEHAR & N. S. SCRIMSHAW. 1959. Am. J. Clin. Nutr. **7:** 185–190.
33. PEREIRA, S. M., A. BEGUM, T. ISAAC & M. E. DUMM. 1967. Am. J. Clin. Nutr. **20:** 297–304.
34. CANFIELD, L. M., J. BULUX, J. QUAN DE SERRANO, C. RIVERA, A. F. LIMA, C. Y. LOPEZ, R. PEREZ, L. KETTEL-KHAN, G. HARRISON & N. W. SOLOMONS. 1991. Am. J. Clin. Nutr. **54:** 539–541.
35. BULUX, J., J. QUAN DE SERRANO, C. RIVERA, C. Y. LOPEZ, R. PEREZ, A. F. LIMA, V. ORTIZ, N. W. SOLOMONS & L. M. CANFIELD. 1990. FASEB J. **4:** A924 (abst.).
36. ALBANES, D., J. VIRTAMO, J. RAUTALAHTI, J. HAUKKA, J. PALMGREN, C-G. GREF & O. P. HEINONEN. 1992. Eur. J. Clin. Nutr. **46:** 15–24.

37. BULUX, J., J. QUAN DE SERRANO, R. PEREZ, C. Y. LOPEZ, C. RIVERA, V. ORTIZ, N. W. SOLOMONS & L. M. CANFIELD. 1991. FASEB J. **5:** A1074 (abst.).
38. JENSEN, C. D., G. A. SPILLER, T. S. PATTISON, J. H. WHITTAM & J. SCALA. 1986. Nutr. Rep. Int. **33:** 117–123.
39. ROCK, C. L., M. E. SWENDSEID, R. A. JACOB & R. W. MCKEE. 1992. J. Nutr. **122:** 96–100.

Carotenoids, Cancer, and Clinical Trials

REGINA G. ZIEGLER

Nutritional Epidemiology Section
Environmental Epidemiology Branch
Epidemiology and Biostatistics Program
Division of Cancer Etiology
National Cancer Institute
Executive Plaza North 443
Bethesda, Maryland 20892

In the early 1980s β-carotene was proposed to reduce the risk of cancer. Epidemiologic support for this hypothesis has come from three types of studies: prospective studies of dietary intake and cancer, prospective studies of blood β-carotene levels and cancer, and retrospective studies of dietary intake and cancer.[1,2] In the prospective studies, dietary information and/or blood samples are collected from a group of nondiseased people; and the cohort is followed over time. When a sufficient number of cancer diagnoses or deaths have occurred, the data collected earlier are compared for the cases and either all the noncases in the cohort or a subset of the cohort matched to the cancer cases. In a retrospective study patients with a particular cancer are identified, and comparable control subjects selected. Then information about usual diet prior to symptoms of disease is collected and compared for the cases and controls.

An example of a prospective study involving dietary assessment is the 19-year follow-up of approximately 2000 middle-aged Western Electric Company employees living in Chicago.[3] In the 33 men that subsequently developed lung cancer, provitamin A carotenoids were the only nutrient of those evaluated significantly associated with reduced risk (TABLE 1). The risk of lung cancer was seven times higher in men in the lowest quartile of carotenoid intake than in men in the highest quartile. Other common cancers were not significantly associated with intake of provitamin A carotenoids although carotenoid intake was lower than average in men who subsequently developed head and neck cancers.

An example of a prospective study involving direct measurement of β-carotene in blood is the 10-year follow-up of approximately 7000 Hawaiian Japanese men participating in the Honolulu Heart Program.[4] In a case-cohort analysis of 74 incident lung cancers, age- and smoking-adjusted relative risks of lung cancer increased with serum β-carotene levels; the test for trend was statistically significant (TABLE 2). Men in the lowest quintile of serum β-carotene levels had twice the risk of men in the highest quintile. No significant associations were noted for colon, stomach, rectal, or bladder cancer although β-carotene levels were somewhat lower in the men who subsequently developed colon and stomach cancers than in the controls. There was no association of either serum vitamin A or serum vitamin E with any of the cancers.

Lung has been the cancer site most frequently studied in retrospective studies of carotenoid intake and cancer. In one of the earliest studies to distinguish between carotenoid and vitamin A intake, a population-based case-control study of lung cancer in white men in six high-risk areas of New Jersey,[5] men in the lowest quartile of carotenoid intake had a smoking-adjusted relative risk of 1.7,

TABLE 1. Dietary Intake in Men Who Subsequently Developed Lung Cancer and Those Who Did Not During 19 Years of Follow-up of Western Electric Workers in Chicago[a]

Nutrient	p for Difference between Means*
Carotene index	<0.001
Retinol index	0.38
Energy intake	0.27
Animal protein (%cal)	0.93
Vegetable protein (%cal)	0.10
Animal fat	0.84
Vegetable fat	0.78
Carbohydrate	0.07
Calcium	0.11
Phosphorous	0.26
Iron	0.18
Thiamin	0.19
Riboflavin	0.27
Niacin	0.10
Vitmain C	0.20
Vitamin D	0.85
Cholesterol	0.59

* Based on Student t test.
[a] Derived from Shekelle et al.[3]

relative to men in the highest quartile; but no increase in risk was associated with low retinol (preformed vitamin A) intake (TABLE 3). The protective effect was limited to current and recent smokers. Intakes of vegetables, dark green vegetables, and dark yellow-orange vegetables showed stronger associations than the carotenoid index. The smoking-adjusted relative risks of those in the lowest quartiles of consumption of these food groups were 1.8–2.2, compared to those in the highest quartiles. Two explanations were proposed. Dark green and dark yellow-orange vegetable consumption might be better measures of β-carotene intake than an approximate estimate of provitamin A carotenoids. Alternatively, there might be protective entities in vegetables and fruits in addition to the carotenoids.

TABLE 2. Relative Risks of Lung Cancer in Hawaiian Japanese Men by Quintiles of Serum β-Carotene Concentration[a]

			Relative Risks	
	Cases	Controls	Unadjusted	Adjusted for Age, Smoking
β-Carotene concentration (μg/dl)				
57.1–311.5	7	60	1.0	1.0
34.6–57.0	12	60	1.7	1.5
25.1–34.5	10	59	1.5	1.2
15.1–25.0	21	62	2.9	2.4
0–15.0	24	61	3.4	2.2
p for trend			0.004	0.04

[a] Derived from Nomura et al.[4]

TABLE 3. Smoking-Adjusted Relative Risks of Lung Cancer by Nutrient and Food Group Intake in New Jersey White Male Current and Recent Cigarette Smokers[a,b]

	Level of Consumption			
Nutrient or Food Group	Upper 25%	Middle 50%	Lower 25%	p for Trend
Retinol	1.0	1.1	1.0	0.48
Carotenoids	1.0	1.5	1.7	0.02
Vitamin A	1.0	1.2	1.2	0.26
Dairy products	1.0	0.8	0.9	0.26
Vegetables and fruit	1.0	1.7	1.8	0.005
Fruit	1.0	1.4	1.2	0.28
Vegetables	1.0	1.3	1.7	0.004
Dark green vegetables	1.0	1.4	1.8	0.002
Yellow-orange vegetables	1.0	1.6	2.2	<0.001

[a] Included are 524 cases and 354 controls.
[b] Derived from Ziegler et al.[5]

In these and many other epidemiologic studies, low intake of carotenoids, vegetables, and fruits is consistently associated with increased risk of lung cancer—in both prospective and retrospective studies. Low levels of β-carotene in serum or plasma are consistently associated with the subsequent development of lung cancer. The simplest explanation is that β-carotene is protective. Since retinol is not related in a similar manner to lung cancer risk, β-carotene appears to function through a mechanism that does not require its conversion into vitamin A. Prospective and retrospective studies also suggest that vegetable and fruit intake may reduce the risk of many other cancers; specifically, cancers of the digestive (mouth, pharynx, esophagus, stomach, pancreas, colon, rectum), respiratory (larynx), and urinary tracts (bladder). Whether vegetable and fruit intake influences hormone-related cancers is unclear. Weaker protective effects have been noted for breast cancer than for many other cancers and are not consistently seen. Pertinent data for ovarian and endometrial cancer are limited. Results for prostate cancer are not consistent. Little relevant research exists for a number of cancer sites, such as the lymphatic and hematopoietic cancers. In addition, evidence of reduced risk with high vegetable and fruit intake does not necessarily imply that the dietary etiology is the same as that observed with lung cancer. For example, β-carotene does not seem to explain the reduced risk of esophageal and stomach cancer associated with increased vegetable and fruit intake.

In a population-based case-control study of esophageal cancer in black men in Washington, DC,[6] low vegetable and fruit consumption was significantly associated with an increased risk of esophageal cancer, but so also were low dairy product and egg consumption and low fresh or frozen meat and fish consumption (TABLE 4). Low intake of vitamin C, riboflavin, and vitamin A, as well as of carotenoids, were all associated with elevated risk. These results suggested that generally poor nutrition, characterized by inadequate intake of the basic food groups, was the dominant dietary risk factor. Multiple micronutrient deficiencies might be involved. This explanation is consistent with the geographic pattern of this cancer. Internationally it is endemic in regions with limited diets and

TABLE 4. Ethanol-Adjusted Relative Risks of Esophageal Cancer by Food Group and Nutrient Intake in Washington, DC Black Males[a,b]

Nutrient or Food Group	Level of Consumption		
	Upper 33%	Middle 33%	Lower 33%
Meat and fish	1.0	1.3	0.9
Dairy and eggs	1.0	1.6	2.0[++]
Vegetables and fruits	1.0	2.1	2.4[+++]
Vegetables	1.0	1.7	1.8[++]
Green vegetables	1.0	1.2	1.5[+]
Yellow vegetables	1.0	1.0	1.2
Fruits	1.0	2.8	2.4[+++]
Carbohydrates	1.0	1.1	1.2
Fresh or frozen meat and fish	1.0	1.5	2.1[++]
Precooked or processed meat and fish	1.0	0.9	0.8
Vitamin A	1.0	1.4	1.5
Carotenoids	1.0	1.4	1.6[+]
Vitamin C	1.0	1.3	2.1[+++]
Thiamin	1.0	1.2	1.1
Riboflavin	1.0	1.1	1.6[+]

[a] Included are 120 cases and 250 controls. Statistical significance of trends: [+] $p < 0.10$, [++] $p < 0.05$, [+++] $p < 0.01$.
[b] Derived from Ziegler et al.[6]

impoverished agriculture; within a country it is associated with low socioeconomic status.

In a population-based case-control study of stomach cancer conducted in high- and low-risk areas of Italy,[7] intake of not only β-carotene but also of vitamin C were inversely associated with risk (TABLE 5). However, the associations with β-carotene were weakened in multivariate analyses adjusting for other nutrients. A number of other epidemiologic studies have demonstrated an increased risk of stomach cancer with decreased intake of vitamin C, and it is frequently postulated that vitamin C inhibits the endogenous formation of potentially carcinogenic N-nitroso compounds by preventing the nitrosation of secondary and tertiary amines. Nonetheless in this study, raw vegetables, citrus fruit, and other fresh fruit were at least as protective as vitamin C, suggesting that other constituents in vegetables and fruits might also be important.

Numerous epidemiologic studies, from 75 to 200 depending on the criteria, have demonstrated associations between increased intake of vegetables and fruits and reduced risk of cancer at many, though not all, sites.[1,2,10–12] Indeed many epidemiologists believe that of all the dietary factors postulated to be related to cancer, including fat and calories, the epidemiologic evidence is the most consistent for vegetables and fruits. The public health implications are impressive. In many studies cancer risk among individuals in the highest one-fifth to one-third of vegetable and fruit intake is 50–80% the risk among those in the lowest one-fifth to one-third of intake. This association, if causal, when translated into attributable risk,[13] implies that 10–33% of potential cancers would be prevented were all in the population to adopt the levels of vegetable and fruit intake characteristic of the highest quantile. The lowest two-thirds to four-fifths of the population, lowest in terms of vegetable and fruit intake, stand to benefit. Multiple opportunities for change can be envisioned: first and foremost, increasing vegetable and fruit intake, and once the etiologic important constituents of vegetables and fruits are identified, incorporating them into dietary supplements, fortified foods, and genetically engineered crops.

However, there are alternative explanations for the reduction in cancer risk associated with intake of carotenoids, vegetables, and fruits. β-carotene may be the simplest, but not the only, answer. First, avoidance of smoking, limited drinking, regular physical activity, and judicious utilization of medical care often accompany increased vegetable and fruit intake, and probably explain part of the apparent reduction in risk. Second, other beneficial dietary patterns, such as reduced intake of fat and calories and reduced percent of calories from fat, may be related to increased vegetable and fruit consumption. Third, nutrients other than β-carotene that are concentrated in vegetables and fruits, such as vitamin C and dietary fiber; other carotenoids; and constituents of vegetables and fruits that are not nutrients may play important roles.

To evaluate the possibility that correlated dietary patterns explain the impact of vegetable and fruit intake, we used two nationally representative dietary surveys to identify the nutrients, food groups, and food preparation practices strongly correlated with high vegetable and fruit intake. We used the 115-item food frequency interview administered to 10,000 adults in the 1982–84 Epidemiologic Follow-up (EFS) of the First National Health and Nutrition Examination Study (NHANES I)[9] and the 60-item food frequency interview administered to 20,000 adults in the 1987 National Health Interview Survey.[14] Results from the two data sets were similar. Percentage of calories from fat was inversely correlated with vegetable and fruit intake ($r = -0.25$), although absolute intake of saturated fatty acids, polyunsaturated fatty acids, and cholesterol seemed unrelated. However, since the correlation with percent of calories from fat was only moderate, its

TABLE 5. Adjusted Relative Risks of Stomach Cancer by Food Group and Nutrient Intake in Low- and High-Risk Areas of Italy[a,b]

	Level of Consumption			
	Lower 33%	Middle 33%	Upper 33%	p for Trend
Food groups				
Raw vegetables	1.0	0.8	0.6	<0.001
Cooked vegetables	1.0	0.9	1.1	0.58
Beans	1.0	0.8	0.8	0.10
Onions and garlic	1.0	1.0	0.8	0.04
Citrus fruit	1.0	0.7	0.6	<0.001
Other fresh fruit	1.0	0.6	0.4	<0.001
Dried and preserved fruit	1.0	0.8	1.0	0.87
Bread and pasta	1.0	1.1	1.0	0.99
Milk and dairy products	1.0	1.0	1.1	0.49
	Lower 20%	Middle 20%	Upper 20%	
Nutrients				
Vitamin C	1.0	0.6	0.5	
β-carotene	1.0	0.6	0.6	

[a] Included are 1016 cases and 1159 controls.
[b] Derived from Buiatti et al.[7,8]

TABLE 6. Categorization of 1982–84 NHANES I EFS Participants by Vegetable and Fruit Intake and Percent of Calories from Fat

| | Vegetables and Fruits | | | |
Percent Calories from Fat	Lowest Quartile	Quartile 2	Quartile 3	Highest Quartile
Highest quartile	9.8%	7.3%	5.1%	2.9%
Quartile 3	6.2%	7.0%	6.4%	5.4%
Quartile 2	4.8%	6.0%	6.8%	7.4%
Lowest quartile	4.3%	4.7%	6.7%	9.3%

effects should be separable from that of vegetables and fruits in a sufficiently large epidemiologic study. As demonstrated in TABLE 6, only 33% of the population was ranked in the equivalent quartiles for both exposures (Q1/Q1 + Q2/Q2 + Q3/Q3 + Q4/Q4; 25% would be expected if the exposures were statistically independent); and almost as many, 27%, differed by more than one quartile (Q1/Q3 + Q1/Q4 + Q2/Q4 + Q3/Q1 + Q4/Q1 + Q4/Q2).

A second line of research focuses on whether β-carotene is uniquely protective, or whether high β-carotene blood levels may simply be an indicator of increased intake of all carotenoids and of vegetables and fruits in general. As we began to evaluate liquid chromatography (LC) methods for separating and quantifying the major individual carotenoids in human serum and plasma, it became apparent that there was little published information on recovery of individual and total carotenoids. One reason was the lack of availability of pure reference materials for carotenoids other than β-carotene. Another was that cancer research was narrowly focused on β-carotene. Poor recovery during measurement of a carotenoid can lead to an imprecise estimate of exposure and thus obscure an association. In addition, spurious associations can be generated by differential recovery between cases and controls.

In collaboration with the National Institute of Standards and Technolgoy, we decided to develop a LC method for measuring individual carotenoids in human serum and plasma that would optimize resolution and recovery. In addition, the method had to be reproducible and practical so that it could be used by a variety of laboratories on the large numbers of samples collected in epidemiologic studies. Percentage recoveries of the common serum carotenoids (lutein, zeaxanthin, β-cryptoxanthin, lycopene, α-carotene, and β-carotene) with the NIST-NCI method[15,16] and with three accepted LC methods that have been used in epidemiologic studies are presented in TABLE 7. Recovery was measured by flow injection analysis. The NIST-NCI method gives 93–99% recovery of each of the six carot-

TABLE 7. Percent Recovery of Individual Carotenoids with Different LC Methods

Method	Lutein[a]	Zeaxanthin[a]	β-Cryptoxanthin	Lycopene	α-Carotene	β-Carotene
NIST-NCI	95	94	93	97	99	99
A	80	75	82	68	89	91
B	99	98	85	70	77	84
C	99	91	96	101	94	91

[a] Lutein and zeaxanthin coelute in all methods except NIST-NCI.

enoids. Recovery drops to 70% or less for lycopene and to 80% or less for at least one additional carotenoid with methods A and B. Method C gives quite good recovery of all six carotenoids, but its resolution of individual carotenoids is limited. Of the four methods, only the NIST-NCI method can resolve the structural isomers lutein and zeaxanthin.

The ability of the NIST-NCI method to separate individual serum carotenoids is demonstrated in FIGURE 1. Not only are structural isomers that frequently coelute (α-cryptoxanthin and β-cryptoxanthin, and lutein and zeaxanthin) resolved but geometric isomers are also separated. The two small peaks trailing the all-

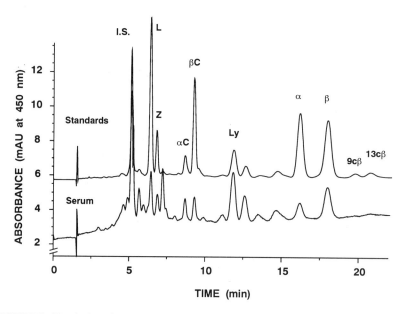

FIGURE 1. Resolution of serum carotenoids with the NIST-NCI LC method. *Upper tracing*: mixture of the six most common serum carotenoids: lutein (L), zeaxanthin (Z), β-cryptoxanthin (βC), lycopene (Ly), α-carotene (α) and β-carotene (β); also seen are α-cryptoxanthin (αC), several unlabeled geometric isomers of lycopene, 9-cis-β-carotene ($9c\beta$), and 13-cis-β-carotene ($13c\beta$). *Lower tracing*: extract of human serum. The internal standard (I.S.) is β-apo-8′-carotenal.

trans β-carotene peak are the 9-*cis* and 13-*cis* isomers, which together comprise approximately 10% of total serum β-carotene. The two peaks after all-*trans* lycopene and the peak before it contain its geometric isomers.

Several projects are now underway that utilize the NIST-NCI method for measuring individual carotenoids. With stored serum from the Japanese men in the Honolulu Heart Program cohort,[4] we are investigating the relationships of individual and total carotenoids in serum to subsequent incidence of lung, oral, pharyngeal, and esophageal cancer. With serum collected from community controls in a large case-control study of cervical cancer,[17] we are analyzing the distribution and demographic, socioeconomic, and lifestyle determinants of individual and total carotenoids in five areas of the United States. Finally, we are comparing in the laboratory the resolution, recovery, and reproducibility of the LC methods commonly used in epidemiologic studies of carotenoids, and quantitatively evaluating how the methods limit epidemiologic analysis and interpretation.

Other carotenoids are not the only constituents of vegetables and fruits that merit further investigation from the perspective of cancer etiology. Vitamin C, like β-carotene found primarily in vegetables and fruits, is a promising candidate.[18] Vegetables and fruits also contribute to the intake of dietary fiber, folate, and vitamin E, each of which may be protective. Other compounds in vegetables and fruits which are not nutrients, such as the dithiolthiones, flavonoids, glucosinolates and indoles, isothiocyanates, phenols, phytoestrogens, sterols, protease inhibitors, and allium compounds, may be important.[11] Although these compounds may not be essential for health or growth, they may play a role in reducing the risk of chronic disease. It is quite likely that at least several protective factors exist in vegetables and fruits and that mechanisms differ for the various cancers. Because the protective factors have not yet been conclusively identified, NCI currently advocates, through its "Five A Day for Better Health" program, consuming at least five servings of vegetables and fruits a day.

Chemoprevention trials will soon begin to answer to what extent β-carotene can explain the reduction in cancer risk consistently associated with increased vegetable and fruit consumption. Data from two of these trials, conducted in Linxian, China[19,20] and in Finland,[21] are now being analyzed, and will be published in 1993 or 1994. Linxian was selected as the site for two randomized placebo-controlled intervention trials of multiple vitamin and mineral supplementation because of its extraordinarily high rates of esophageal and gastric cancer, both of which are associated with low vegetable and fruit intake. Food availability and variety in Linxian have historically been limited, and subclinical deficiencies of several micronutrients have been demonstrated. In the dysplasia trial 3318 subjects, aged 40–69, with cytologically diagnosed dysplasia of the upper gastrointestinal tract were assigned to receive a daily supplement containing 14 vitamins, 12 minerals, and 15 mg of β-carotene or a placebo.[19] Doses were typically 2–3 times the U.S. Recommended Daily Allowances. During the six years of the trial, 462 cancers accrued: 262 of the esophagus and 179 of the stomach, primarily in the cardia region. In the general population trial, 29,584 volunteers, aged 40–69, were randomly assigned to intervention groups according to a one-half replicate of a 2^4 factorial experimental design.[20] The design enabled testing for the effects of four combinations of nutrients: retinol and zinc; riboflavin and niacin; vitamin C and molybdenum; and β-carotene (15 mg), α-tocopherol, and selenium. Micronutrient levels were typically at 1–2 times the U.S. Recommended Daily Allowances. In the 5.25 years of the trial 1307 cancers accrued: 639 esophageal and 546 gastric, primarily in the cardia region.

In the U.S.-Finland lung cancer prevention trial, as in the Linxian trials, a high-risk population in an area of low vegetable and fruit consumption is being investigated. In the past decade Finland has experienced lung cancer incidence rates among the highest in the world, due mainly to the high proportion of smoking males. In a randomized, placebo-controlled trial 29,246 males in Finland, aged 50–69, who smoked 5 or more cigarettes a day were assigned to receive a daily supplement of 20 mg of β-carotene, 50 mg of α-tocopherol, both micronutrients, or neither.[21] During the 5–8 years of the trial approximately 800 cases of lung cancer have accrued, as well as sufficient numbers of prostate, colorectal, and bladder cancer for analysis.

If definitive or marginal protection for one or several cancers is demonstrated in any of these chemoprevention trials, then the results will provide direction for further research and for public health policy. However, negative trials with no evidence of reduced cancer risk will not conclusively rule out a role for micronutrients. The micronutrient levels might have been too low; pharmacologic dosages might have been necessary. Supplements might have been taken for too short a period of time, or too late for a crucial period in carcinogenesis. Other cancer sites or other populations with different exposures might have been more responsive. Other combinations of micronutrients or broader changes in diet might have been more effective. Nonetheless, the results of these early micronutrient supplementation trials will hopefully contribute significantly to our understanding of the role of β-carotene in cancer etiology.

REFERENCES

1. ZIEGLER, R. G. 1989. A review of epidemiologic evidence that carotenoids reduce the risk of cancer. J. Nutr. **119:** 116–122.
2. ZIEGLER, R. G. 1991. Vegetables, fruits, and carotenoids and the risk of cancer. Am. J. Clin. Nutr. **53:** 251S–259S.
3. SHEKELLE, R. B., M. LEPPER, S. LIU, C. MALIZA, W. J. RAYNOR, JR. & A. H. ROSSOF. 1981. Dietary vitamin A and risk of cancer in the Western Electric Study. Lancet **2:** 1185–1190.
4. NOMURA, A. M. Y., G. N. STEMMERMANN, L. K. HEILBRUN, R. M. SALKELD & J. P. VUILLEUMIER. 1985. Serum vitamin levels and the risk of cancer of specific sites in men of Japanese ancestry in Hawaii. Cancer Res. **45:** 2369–2372.
5. ZIEGLER, R. G., T. J. MASON, A. STEMHAGEN, R. HOOVER, J. B. SCHOENBERG, G. GRIDLEY, P. W. VIRGO & J. F. FRAUMENI, JR. 1986. Carotenoid intake, vegetables, and the risk of lung cancer among white men in New Jersey. Am. J. Epidemiol. **123:** 1080–1093.
6. ZIEGLER, R. G., L. E. MORRIS, W. J. BLOT, L. M. POTTERN, R. HOOVER & J. F. FRAUMENI, JR. 1981. Esophageal cancer among black men in Washington, D.C. II. Role of nutrition. J. Natl. Cancer Inst. **67:** 1199–1206.
7. BUIATTI, E., D. PALLI, A. DECARLI, D. AMADORI, C. AVELLINI, S. BIANCHI, R. BISERNI, F. CIPRIANI, P. COCCO, A. GIACOSA, E. MARUBINI, R. PUNTONI, C. VINDIGNI, J. FRAUMENI, JR. & W. BLOT. 1989. A case-control study of gastric cancer and diet in Italy. Int. J. Cancer **44:** 611–616.
8. BUIATTI, E., D. PALLI, A. DECARLI, D. AMADORI, C. AVELLINI, S. BIANCHI, C. BONAGURI, F. CIPRIANI, P. COCCO, A. GIACOSA, E. MARUBINI, C. MINACCI, R. PUNTONI, A. RUSSO, C. VINDIGNI, J. F. FRAUMENI, JR. & W. J. BLOT. 1990. A case-control study of gastric cancer and diet in Italy: II. Association with nutrients. Int. J. Cancer **45:** 896–901.
9. ZIEGLER, R. G., G. URSIN, N. E. CRAFT, A. F. SUBAR, B. I. GRAUBARD & B. H. PATTERSON. 1992. Does β-carotene explain why reduced cancer risk is associated with vegetable and fruit intake? New research directions. In Vitamins and Cancer Prevention. G. Bray & D. Ryan, Eds. 352–371. Louisiana State University Press. Baton Rouge, LA.
10. STEINMETZ, K. A. & J. D. POTTER. 1991. Vegetables, fruit, and cancer. I. Epidemiology. Cancer Causes Control **2:** 325–327.
11. STEINMETZ, K. A. & J. D. POTTER. 1991. Vegetables, fruit, and cancer. II. Mechanisms. Cancer Causes Control **2:** 427–442.
12. BLOCK, G., B. PATTERSON & A. SUBAR. 1992. Fruit, vegetables, and cancer prevention: a review of the epidemiologic evidence. Nutr. Cancer **18:** 1–29.
13. BRESLOW, N. E. & N. E. DAY. 1980. Statistical methods in cancer research. Vol. I. The analysis of Case-Control Studies. International Agency for Research on Cancer. Lyon, France.
14. ZIEGLER, R. G., A. F. SUBAR, N. E. CRAFT, G. URSIN, B. H. PATTERSON &

B. I. GRAUBARD. 1992. Does β-carotene explain why reduced cancer risk is associated with vegetable and fruit intake? Cancer Res. **52:** 2060S–2066S.

15. EPLER, K. S., L. C. SANDER, R. G. ZIEGLER, S. A. WISE & N. E. CRAFT. 1992. Evaluation of reversed-phase liquid chromatographic columns for recovery and selectivity of selected carotenoids. J. Chromatogr. **595:** 89–101.

16. EPLER, K. S., R. G. ZIEGLER & N. E. CRAFT. 1993. Liquid chromatographic determination of carotenoids, retinoids, and tocopherols in human serum and in food. J. Chromatogr. In press.

17. ZIEGLER, R. G., L. A. BRINTON, R. F. HAMMAN, H. F. LEHMAN, R. S. LEVINE, K. MALLIN, S. A. NORMAN, J. F. ROSENTHAL, A. C. TRUMBLE & R. N. HOOVER. 1990. Diet and the risk of invasive cervical cancer among white women in the United States. Am. J. Epidemiol. **132:** 432–445.

18. BLOCK, G. 1991. Vitamin C and cancer prevention: the epidemiologic evidence. Am. J. Clin. Nutr. **53:** 270S–282S.

19. LI, J. Y., P. R. TAYLOR, B. LI, S. DAWSEY, G. Q. WANG, A. G. ERSHOW, W. GUO, S. F. LIU, C. S. YANG, Q. SHEN, W. WANG, S. D. MARK, X. N. ZOU, P. GREENWALD, Y. P. WU & W. J. BLOT. 1993. Nutrition intervention trials in Linxian, China: multiple vitamin/mineral supplementation, cancer incidence, and disease-specific mortality among adults with esophageal dysplasia. J. Natl. Cancer Inst. **85:** 1492–1498.

20. BLOT, W. J., J. Y. LI, P. R. TAYLOR, W. GUO, S. DAWSEY, G. Q. WANG, C. S. YANG, S. F. ZHENG, M. GAIL, G. Y. LI, Y. YU, B. Q. LIU, J. TANGREA, Y. H. SUN, F. LIU, J. F. FRAUMENI, JR., Y. H. ZHANG & B. LI. 1993. Nutrition intervention trials in Linxian, China: supplementation with specific vitamin/mineral combinations, cancer incidence, and disease-specific mortality in the general population. J. Natl. Cancer Inst. **85:** 1483–1492.

21. ALBANES, D., J. VIRTAMO, M. RAUTALAHTI, J. PIKKARAINEN, P. R. TAYLOR, P. GREENWALD & O. P. HEINONEN. 1986. Pilot study: the US-Finland lung cancer prevention trial. J. Nutr. Growth Cancer **3:** 207–214.

Carotenoids, Cigarette Smoking, and Mortality Risk[a]

E. R. GREENBERG

Skin Cancer Prevention Study Group[b]
Dartmouth Medical School and Norris Cotton Cancer Center
Departments of Community and Family Medicine and Medicine
HB 7925
Hanover, New Hampshire 03756

INTRODUCTION

Epidemiological studies have repeatedly shown that cancer risk is lower among individuals with high intake of foods that contain carotenoids or with high blood levels of one particular carotenoid, beta-carotene.[1,2] There is also evidence, although considerably less extensive and conclusive, that beta-carotene may lower the risk of cardiovascular disease.[3,4] In industrialized countries cancer and cardiovascular disease together account for roughly two thirds of all deaths, and a strong protective effect of carotenoids should therefore translate into a lower risk of overall mortality. Nevertheless, virtually all of the studies published to date have focused on specific diseases rather than total mortality associated with beta-carotene or other carotenoids. Also, the health benefits observed in epidemiological studies among people who ingest more carotenoids and who have higher blood levels could be due to other components in their diets[5] or to nondietary factors. The most important concern in this regard is cigarette smoking, since smokers on average consume fewer fruits and vegetables than nonsmokers,[6,7] and their blood levels of carotenoids are also lower.[8,9] To examine further the possible relationship between mortality risk, beta-carotene intake, and smoking we have continued to follow patients enrolled in a clinical trial of beta-carotene to prevent nonmelanoma skin cancer. We present here the preliminary results of our posttreatment follow-up survey, for data through 1 March 1991.

METHODS

The design and principal results of the Skin Cancer Prevention Study were reported previously.[10,11] Briefly, this was a randomized, double-blind clinical trial

[a] Supported by US Public Health Service Grants #CA32934 and #CA23108. The capsules used in this study were provided without charge by BASF, Wyandotte, MI.
[b] The Skin Cancer Prevention Study Group consists of the following investigators: John A. Baron, MD; E. Robert Greenberg, MD; Margaret R. Karagas, PhD; Marguerite M. Stevens, PhD; Thérèse A. Stukel, PhD; Steven Spencer, MD; David Nierenberg, MD (Dartmouth-Hitchcock Medical Center); Nicholas Lowe, MD; Robert Haile, DrPH (The University of California, Los Angeles); Peter Elias, MD; Virginia Ernster, PhD; Nikolajs Lapins, MD (The University of California, San Francisco); Jack Mandel, PhD; J. Corwin Vance, MD; Garrett Bayrd, MD (The University of Minnesota).

involving four dermatology clinical centers: the Dartmouth-Hitchcock Medical Center in Hanover, NH; the University of California at Los Angeles School of Medicine; the University of California Medical School, San Francisco (including the Fort Miley Veterans Affairs Hospital and the Letterman Army Hospital); and the University of Minnesota Schools of Medicine and Public Health, Minneapolis (including Group Health, Inc., a health maintenance organization). We began to enroll patients in February 1983. Each had had at least one biopsy-proven basal cell or squamous cell carcinoma diagnosed and treated in the recent past. Reviews of dermatology office records and dermatopathology reports were the principal methods used to identify potential enrollees. Eligible patients were less than 85 years old, did not have an inherited predilection to skin cancer (*i.e.*, xeroderma pigmentosum), and were free of major medical conditions that might impair their ability to participate in the study. During the three-year recruitment period we enrolled 1,805 of the 5,232 potentially eligible persons identified through record review.[10]

At the time of their enrollment patients completed a questionnaire regarding personal characteristics, vitamin use, and habits including whether they had ever smoked cigarettes and the amount currently smoked. They also reported their height and weight. Upon enrollment, and annually thereafter, we obtianed a 20-ml specimen of venous blood using heparin-treated vacuum tubes. After centrifugation, plasma was stored and shipped to the central laboratory at Dartmouth where tubes were stored at $-75°C$ until analysis. Beta-carotene was measured using a high performance liquid chromatographic assay.[12]

We randomized patients to receive capsules containing either placebo or 50 mg beta-carotene to be taken daily. We continued to provide capsules to all cooperating patients until the end of the study treatment phase on September 30, 1989. Patients adhered well to the study protocol, and throughout the clinical trial the great majority of them took half or more of the recommended number of capsules.[11] Among the group of patients prescribed beta-carotene, the median plasma level of beta-carotene increased from the pretreatment value of 175 ng/ml to 1624 ng/ml after one year, and it remained elevated throughout the treatment phase of the study. The group of patients receiving placebo capsules showed almost no change in the median plasma level.[11]

Patients were followed through questionnaires every six months and with annual visits to the dermatologist. At each of these contacts we asked about the occurrence of hospitalizations and serious diseases. In winter of 1991 we sent an additional questionnaire to all patients, or their next-of-kin, asking about any diagnoses of cancer other than nonmelanoma skin cancer. All reports of cancer were validated through hospital discharge summaries and pathology reports. For patients who had died, we obtained a copy of the death certificate for coding as to cause of death by a trained nosologist.

The analyses presented here include 1,761 patients of the total of 1,805 randomized in the study. The 44 excluded patients did not have a plasma beta-carotene level determined before randomization. The included patients were predominantly male (69%), age 50–69 years (64%), and were not currently smoking cigarettes (81%) (TABLE 1).

At study entry plasma beta-carotene levels ranged from 9 to 2526 ng per ml. For analyses of risk associated with baseline beta-carotene, we divided patients into four quartiles according to their plasma levels, with means of 74, 143, 222, and 458 ng per ml respectively (TABLE 2).

For each patient, we calculated the length of time from randomization to the earliest of the following events: death (208 patients), loss to follow-up (33 patients),

TABLE 1. Characteristics of the 1761 Patients with Plasma Beta-Carotene Determined at Entry to the Skin Cancer Prevention Study

Characteristic	Number	%
Sex		
Male	1223	69
Female	538	31
Age		
<50	169	10
50–69	1131	64
70+	461	26
Smoking history[a]		
Never smoked	634	36
Former smoker	797	45
Current cigarettes		
1–39 per day	224	13
40+ per day	102	6

[a] Smoking history was incomplete for 4 patients.

or the closing date for this analysis (1 March 1991). Crude mortality rates for groups of patients were based on total person-years of follow-up and total numbers of deaths, and cumulative probability of death was estimated using actuarial methods.[13] We used the proportional hazards method[14] to compare risk of death among groups of patients classified according to quartile of plasma beta-carotene or to treatment assignment. For the analyses of risk associated with baseline beta-carotene levels we constructed three proportional hazards models: Model 1 adjusted for no covariables, Model 2 adjusted for age, sex, and study center only, and Model 3 adjusted for the covariables in Model 2 plus cigarette smoking history. Relative rates of death and 95% confidence limits were estimated from the coefficients and their standard errors in the proportional hazards model.

RESULTS

Patient characteristics differed according to baseline levels of beta-carotene (TABLE 3). Subjects in the lowest quartile of beta-carotene were more likely to be male, with body mass index greater than 27 kg/M², current smokers, and were less likely to use daily vitamins.

Patients in the three highest quartiles of plasma beta-carotene had mortality rates substantially lower than those in the lowest quartile (TABLE 4). The lower

TABLE 2. Skin Cancer Prevention Study; Number of Patients and Person-Years (PYR) of Follow-Up by Quartile of Plasma Beta-Carotene at Study Entry

	Quartile of Plasma Beta-Carotene			
	I	II	III	IV
Mean plasma level (ng/ml)	74	143	222	458
Number	437	436	443	445
PYR	2601	2629	2741	2706

TABLE 3. Characteristics of Patients according to Quartile of Plasma Beta-Carotene at Study Entry

	Quartile of Beta-Carotene (Plasma)			
	I (%)	II (%)	III (%)	IV (%)
Male	86	70	65	57
Age >70 yrs	23	23	29	29
Quetelet >27	37	28	22	15
Current smoker	29	20	16	8
Daily vitamins	21	20	27	31

risk of death in patients with higher levels of beta-carotene was apparent for up to seven years (data not shown). Overall, in an unadjusted analysis, the relative rate of death for patients in quartiles II, III, and IV was 38% to 52% lower than that for patients in quartile I. These results were altered little by adjustment in the proportional hazards model (Model 2) for age, sex, and study center. Further adjustment for the confounding effects of cigarette smoking (Model 3) diminished the apparent protective effect of beta-carotene somewhat but did not completely remove it. Patients in quartiles II, III, and IV still had estimated relative rates of death in this analysis which were 28%, 45%, and 29% lower respectively, compared to quartile I. In the analysis using Model 3, age, male gender, and smoking history were each strongly and statistically significantly related to overall mortality risk.

Despite the apparent protective effect of higher levels of plasma beta-carotene at study entry, there was no evidence of diminution in mortality risk over the seven-year follow-up period among subjects assigned to receive beta-carotene when compared to those assigned to receive placebo. The overall relative rate of death in the beta-carotene-treated group was 1.00 with a 95% confidence interval of 0.83–1.39. To determine whether a protective effect of supplemental beta-carotene might occur only in those with initially low plasma levels, we restricted our analysis to the 437 patients who, at study entry, were in the lowest quartile of plasma beta-carotene. Among these patients the relative rate of death associated with beta-carotene treatment was 1.21, 95% confidence interval 0.71–1.75.

DISCUSSION

The results of these preliminary analyses indicate a clearly elevated risk of death in persons whose plasma beta-carotene levels were in the lowest quartile

TABLE 4. Mortality from All Causes according to Quartile of Plasma Beta-Carotene at Study Entry

Quartile	Deaths	Rate (per thousand PYR)
I	75	28.8
II	47	17.9
III	38	13.9
IV	48	17.7

when they entered the study. This finding of a higher mortality is supported by the results of numerous earlier studies which showed a higher risk of cancer, especially lung cancer, in persons with lower carotenoid levels.[2] There are also indications that atherosclerosis may be impeded by carotenoids,[3] and thus carotenoids might lower cardiovascular disease risk. We found little difference in mortality risk among persons in the higher three quartiles of plasma beta-carotene. These results seem more indicative of an adverse effect of low plasma beta-carotene rather than a beneficial effect of having beta-carotene levels above the norm. However, more extensive data will be necessary to provide a clear picture of any dose-response relationship between plasma beta-carotene and risk of death.

Almost all prior reports of blood carotenoids and disease risk have focused on patients with a particular disease (or group of diseases such as cancer) rather than deaths from all causes. This may reflect the fact that these studies have usually involved a case-control (or "nested" case-control) approach in which blood carotenoids were measured only for individuals with the disease of interest and for a sample of undiseased individuals. In our study plasma levels were analyzed for all participants who provided blood specimens at the time of enrollment, and this feature of the study facilitated an analysis of all causes of death. The higher risk of death noted in persons with low plasma beta-carotene has potentially profound public health importance. The prospect of reducing death from all causes by 25%, or more, could strongly influence personal decisions and public policy regarding dietary change and nutritional supplementation, whereas a beneficial effect for single disease might carry less weight in these decisions.

Patients with initially low plasma levels of beta-carotene were more likely to be cigarette smokers, but smoking did not appear to account for much of their mortality risk elevation. Adjustment for cigarette smoking in the survival analysis produced only a modest diminution in the risk estimates differences compared to the unadjusted analyses. The effect of errors in measurement of variables in these analyses requires consideration, however. Firstly, imprecise measurement of cigarette smoking would result in incomplete control for this confounding variable. Nevertheless, we think it unlikely that patients' reports of smoking history were so unreliable as to account for the large remaining differences in risk among groups in the smoking-adjusted analyses. Secondly, measurement of a single blood specimen of beta-carotene provides an imprecise estimate of typical plasma levels over time.[15] However, this would lead our analyses to underestimate any true relationship between plasma levels and risk.

Despite the strong association between initial plasma beta-carotene and subsequent mortality, subsequent prescription of supplemental beta-carotene did not appear to diminish risk of death. Treated patients in our study received beta-carotene for over four years on average, and their follow-up observation extended as much as seven years after randomization. Those assigned to take beta-carotene received relatively large doses, 50 mg per day, and they increased their plasma levels about tenfold above pretreatment values. This pronounced elevation of plasma beta-carotene levels for a relatively prolonged period seemed to have no effect on risk of death, even among the group of patients whose pretreatment plasma beta-carotene levels were in the lowest quartile. However, the follow-up period did not extend past seven years, and further follow-up and disease-specific information from these patients will be helpful in assessing whether a benefit might occur after a more prolonged period. We are currently collecting such information. Also, results of other studies involving larger numbers of participants and longer periods of beta-carotene prescription should be available before long.

In summary, our findings indicate that lower blood levels of beta-carotene (and presumably other carotenoids) are associated with a higher risk of death and that this excess risk cannot be explained entirely by the lower beta-carotene levels found among cigarette smokers. The absence of a detectable effect of supplemental beta-carotene on mortality risk, however, does not support a strong direct benefit from having higher blood levels of this substance. Although we cannot exclude the possibility of benefits which were too small or too delayed to detect in this preliminary analysis, one must consider whether plasma beta-carotene may simply be a marker for other factors which lower the risk of death. Higher blood levels of beta-carotene principally identify persons who eat large amounts of fruits and vegetables, and many ingredients other than carotenoids in these foods conceivably could reduce risk of cancer and cardiovascular disease. For example, fruits and vegetables contain antioxidant vitamins, fiber, selenium, indoles, flavinoids, and numerous other substances, all of which have anticarcinogenic effects in laboratory experiments. While carotenoids themselves may eventually be shown to have disease preventive effects, they seem unlikely to account for all of the benefits associated with eating a diet high in fruits, vegetables, and grains. Indeed, there may be no single substance in foods which is both highly effective in reducing risk of heart disease and cancer and also entirely safe to consume as a supplement. A perhaps more plausible situation is that there are many aspects of diet which individually have only weak protective effects, but which act together to produce the impressive decrease in mortality risk we have seen in our analyses. If this is the case, programs to produce broad changes in dietary patterns would ultimately have more efficacy than attempts to alter intake of specific micronutrients.

ACKNOWLEDGMENTS

The author acknowledges with gratitude the indispensable help of the following colleagues: Margaret Karagas, PhD, Thérèse Stukel, PhD, and Leila Mott, MS, oversaw the statistical analyses; David Nierenberg, MD, developed and directed the laboratory analyses of blood plasma; John Baron, MD, Marguerite Stevens, PhD, and Loretta Pearson, MPhil, helped plan and organize the post-treatment follow-up effort; and lastly, the study dermatologists, co-investigators, and clinical coordinators at the four clinical sites provided help and advice over the many years of planning, data collection, and analysis in the original study.

REFERENCES

1. ZIEGLER, R. G. 1991. Vegetables, fruits, and carotenoids and the risk of cancer. Am. J. Clin. Nutr. **53:** 251S–259S.
2. BYERS, T. & G. PERRY. 1992. Dietary carotenes, vitamin C, and vitamin E as protective antioxidants in human cancers. Annu. Rev. Nutr. **12:** 139–159.
3. GERSTER, H. 1991. Potential role of beta-carotene in the prevention of cardiovascular disease. Int. J. Vitam. Nutr. Res. **61:** 277–291.
4. RIEMERSMA, R. A., D. A. WOOD, C. C. A. MACINTYRE, R. A. ELTON, K. F. GEY & M. F. OLIVER. 1991. Risk of angina pectoris and plasma concentrations of vitamins A, C, and E and carotene. Lancet **337:** 1–5.
5. STEINMETZ, K. A. & J. D. POTTER. 1991. Vegetables, fruits, and cancer. II. Mechanisms. Cancer Causes Cont. **2:** 427–442.
6. MORABIA, A. & E. L. WYNDER. 1990. Dietary habits of smokers, people who never smoked, and exsmokers. Am. J. Clin. Nutr. **52:** 933–937.

7. CADE, J. E. & B. M. MARGETTS. 1991. Relationship between diet and smoking—is the diet of smokers different? J. Epidemiol. Comm. Health **45:** 270–272.
8. STRYKER, W. S., L. A. KAPLAN, E. A. STEIN, M. J. STAMPFER, A. SOBER & W. C. WILLETT. 1988. The relation of diet, cigarette smoking, and alcohol consumption to plasma beta-carotene and alpha-tocopherol levels. Am. J. Epidemiol. **127:** 283–296.
9. NIERENBERG, D. W., T. A. STUKEL, J. A. BARON, B. J. DAIN, E. R. GREENBERG, AND THE SKIN CANCER PREVENTION STUDY GROUP. 1989. Determinants of plasma levels of beta-carotene and retinol. Am. J. Epidemiol. **130:** 511–521.
10. GREENBERG, E. R., J. A. BARON, M. M. STEVENS, T. A. STUKEL, J. S. MANDEL, S. K. SPENCER, P. M. ELIAS, N. LOWE, D. W. NIERENBERG, G. BAYRD, J. C. VANCE, AND THE SKIN CANCER PREVENTION STUDY GROUP. 1989. The Skin Cancer Prevention Study: design of a clinical trial of beta-carotene among persons at high risk for nonmelanoma skin cancer. Controlled Clin. Trials **10:** 153–166.
11. GREENBERG, E. R., J. A. BARON, M. M. STEVENS, T. A. STUKEL, J. S. MANDEL, S. K. SPENCER, P. M. ELIAS, N. LOWE, D. W. NIERENBERG, G. BAYRD, J. C. VANCE, D. H. FREEMAN, W. E. CLENDENNING, T. KWAN, AND THE SKIN CANCER PREVENTION STUDY GROUP. 1990. A clinical trial of beta-carotene to prevent basal-cell and squamous-cell cancers of the skin. N. Engl. J. Med. **323:** 789–795.
12. NIERENBERG, D. W. 1985. Serum and plasma beta-carotene levels measured with an improved method of high-performance liquid chromatography. J. Chromatogr. **339:** 273–284.
13. LEE, E. T. 1980. Statistical Methods for Survival Data Analysis. Lifetime Learning Publications. Belmont, CA.
14. COX, D. R. & D. OAKES. 1984. Analysis of Survival Data. 91–110. Chapman and Hall. New York.
15. CANTILENA, L. R., T. A. STUKEL, E. R. GREENBERG, S. NANN & D. W. NIERENBERG. 1992. Diurnal and seasonal variation of five carotenoids measured in human serum. Am. J. Clin. Nutr. **55:** 659–663.

Carotenoids in Erythropoietic Protoporphyria and Other Photosensitivity Diseases

MICHELINE M. MATHEWS-ROTH

Channing Laboratory
Harvard Medical School
and Brigham & Women's Hospital
180 Longwood Avenue
Boston, Massachusetts 02115

It is now well established that a crucial function of carotenoid pigments in green plants and photosynthetic bacteria is to protect these organisms against photosensitization by their own chlorophyll. In this paper I will describe how I employed this protective function of carotenoids to develop a treatment for the genetic disease, erythropoietic protoporphyria, and also how this treatment has been used in certain other photosensitivity diseases.

Carotenoid Function in Bacteria

Sistrom, Griffiths and Stanier[1] first suggested that carotenoids might be acting as protective agents against photosensitization as a result of observations they made on the wild-type and on a mutant of the photosynthetic bacterium *Rhodopseudomonas spheroides* which lacked colored carotenoids. They found that when these organisms were grown in the presence of light and air, the mutant was killed, but the wild-type, with its normal component of carotenoid pigments, survived. They showed that the cells' bacteriochlorophyll was responsible for the lethal photosensitization of the mutant, that both oxygen and light were necessary for the destructive reaction to occur, and that the carotenoid pigments were functioning as protective agents against this lethal photosensitization. These findings, that carotenoids can protect against chlorophyll photosensitization, have been confirmed in other photosynthetic bacteria, algae and green plants.[2]

Kunisawa and Stanier[3] showed that a colorless mutant of *Corynebacterium poinsettiae,* a nonphotosynthetic bacterium which contains carotenoids, is killed in the presence of an exogenous photosensitizer (toluidine blue), light and air, whereas the wild-type which contained colored carotenoids was not affected by this exposure. However, they could not demonstrate the presence of an endogenous photosensitizer in this organism, and so were not sure how useful carotenoid protection was to the cells. Sistrom and I[4–5] showed that nonphotosynthetic bacteria do indeed contain endogenous photosensitizers. When we exposed wild-type *Sarcina lutea,* another nonphotosynthetic carotenoid-containing organism, and its colorless mutant to natural sunlight in air for 4 hours, we found that, at these high light intensities, the mutant was killed and the wild-type was not, and that, here also, oxygen was needed for killing to occur. Other workers have since confirmed the protective function of carotenoid pigments in nonphotosynthetic bacteria.[6]

A Clinical Application?

Since carotenoid pigments could prevent photosensitization by porphyrins, it seemed sensible to me to see if the administration of carotenoid pigments could prevent photosensitization in patients with those diseases in which the photosensitizer had some resemblance to the endogenous photosensitizer in plants. Such a disease was light-sensitive porphyria, where the porphyrins produced are similar to the porphyrin group of chlorophyll. Preliminary studies in porphyria patients done in the summer of 1961 with Dr. L. C. Harber at New York University School of Medicine seemed to suggest that the onset of erythema to artificial light could be delayed by the oral administration of β-carotene. A search of the literature up to that time revealed that Kesten[7] had been able to delay the onset of erythema in a patient with urticaria solare by the use of β-carotene.

Studies in Animals

It seemed important to develop an animal model to test more thoroughly the hypothesis that carotenoids could protect against photosensitization. Eighteen to 24 hours before light exposure, a suspension of 3 mg of β-carotene in Tween-80[8] or the equivalent volume of Tween-80 alone was administered intraperitoneally to groups of mice, and just prior to light exposure, each mouse in both groups received 1 mg of hematoporphyrin derivative[9] intraperitoneally. I found that significantly more animals which received the β-carotene survived the treatment with hematoporphyrin and light than did those that had not received the β-carotene.[10] Thus, β-carotene was effective in mice in preventing the lethal photosensitivity induced by injection of hematoporphyrin and exposure to visible light.

Studies in a Human Photosensitivity Disease

The successful photoprotection studies in animals suggested to me that it would now be feasible to administer β-carotene to patients with photosensitivity. The disease chosen for study was erythropoietic protoporphyria (EPP). In EPP, ferrochelatase, the enzyme which inserts iron into protoporphyrin to make heme, is defective, resulting in the accumulation of protoporphyrin in blood and other tissues. Leakage of protoporphyrin from blood cells leads to a cascade of reactions resulting in itching, burning and ulceration of skin on exposure to visible light.[11]

The first patient with EPP who was treated, a 10-year-old girl, could tolerate only brief exposures to sunlight. Exposure to a carbon arc light (340–640 nm) produced erythema in 2 minutes. In June of 1968, she was given a preparation of concentrated carrot oil in doses approximately equivalent to 30 mg β-carotene per day. After a month of carrot oil ingestion, she could tolerate at least 30 min of carbon arc light, and more than one hour of sunlight. By the middle of the summer she could play outdoors in the afternoon without experiencing any symptoms of photosensitivity. In the summer of 1969, she and two other patients were given β-carotene in the form of 10% β-carotene "beadlets" (Hoffmann-La Roche). Here also, all three were found to have improved tolerance to sunlight exposure.[12,13] In 1970, I set up a collaborative study to include all the patients of Dr. Harber and those of other physicians who had contacted us concerning the use of β-carotene since the publication of our first three cases. By the summer of 1975, we had treated 133 patients suffering from EPP with β-carotene, using a standard protocol adhered to by all participating physicians.[14,15] In July, 1975, the U.S. Food and Drug Administration approved the use of β-carotene for the treatment of EPP and we terminated the collaborative study at that time.

In the collaborative study we used the starting dosage schedule for β-carotene given in TABLE 1. We found it to be effective,[14,15] and I still recommend it. The average dose for the patient's age should be administered for 4–6 weeks, and the patient should be instructed not to increase sun exposure either for 4 weeks or until some yellow discoloration of the skin, especially of the palms of the hand, is noted. Then, exposure can be increased cautiously and gradually until the patient determines the limits of exposure to light that can be tolerated without the development of symptoms. If the degree of protection is not sufficient, the daily dose of carotene should be increased by 30–60 mg for children under 16, and up to a total of 300 mg/day for those over 16 years of age. If after 3 months of therapy at these higher doses (blood carotene levels should reach at least 800 μg/dl) no significant increase in tolerance to sunlight exposure has occurred, it can be assumed that β-carotene therapy will not be effective for that patient, and the medication should be discontinued.

TABLE 1. Starting Dosages for β-Carotene in the Collaborative Study

Years of Age	β-Carotene (mg/Day)
1–4	60–90
5–8	90–120
9–12	120–140
13–15	150–180
16+	180

We found that eighty-four percent of the patients increased by a factor of 3 or more their ability to tolerate sunlight exposure without the development of symptoms.[14,15] On average, it took between 1 and 2 months for the patients who received benefit from carotene therapy to notice increased tolerance to sun exposure. The majority of patients reported that with β-carotene therapy, they could engage in outdoor activities which they were unable to do before therapy started. Children, who, previous to carotene therapy, could not play out of doors to any great extent, could now spend hours outside with their friends. Many patients stated that they were able to develop a suntan for the first time in their lives, some feeling that the acquisition of the tan, plus the β-carotene, added to their protection from the sun's effects. The majority of the patients noted that while they take β-carotene, those reactions from the sun that do occur are less severe in intensity and duration than before therapy, and that they also developed fewer cutaneous lesions during their increased exposure time.

We found that the patients' blood and stool porphyrin levels were not affected by the ingestion of large amounts of β-carotene. Thus, treatment with β-carotene ameliorates photosensitivity in EPP, but has no effect on the biochemical lesion in this disease.

Because of the difficulties in the subjective evaluation of therapeutic effect and of setting up a controlled double-blind study in the particular case of beta-carotene and EPP, we decided to use phototesting with polychromatic light from

380 to 560 nanometers (as opposed to monochromatic light) as an objective measure of clinical improvement. Using exposure to a xenon arc lamp under the conditions we have developed,[14,16] we found that tolerance to xenon arc light exposure increased in those patients who reported benefit from β-carotene therapy, but no increased tolerance to this radiation was found in patients reporting no improvement. Other workers also noted increased tolerance to polychromatic xenon arc light after treatment with β-carotene.[17-18] Thus, phototesting with polychromatic xenon arc light can serve as an objective method of determining improvement in tolerance to light.

Confirmation of Our Results

In previous reviews, I listed 27 other studies reporting increases in tolerance to sunlight in over three-quarters of patients with EPP treated with high doses of β-carotene, either alone or in combination with canthaxanthin:[19-22] in this paper I list an additional 18 reports.[23-40] All these reports describe either individual patients, or a group of patients, the majority of whom received benefit from carotenoid therapy. In some of these series, as well as in other reports,[41-45] there are patients who do not benefit from carotenoid therapy, in spite of adequate pigment dosage: this is most likely due to either poor absorption of pigment, or the patient having markedly elevated blood porphyrin levels. One controlled study of β-carotene therapy in EPP was performed, and reported little or no improvement in the subjects' photosensitivity:[46] unfortunately, these workers used a lower dosage of β-carotene than we had recommended as effective. Later, some of the patients from this unsuccessfully-treated study were given higher doses of β-carotene by another investigator, and the patients noted some increased tolerance to sun while taking the higher dose.[47] These results emphasize the importance, as mentioned above, of individualizing dosage to each patient, and increasing the dose until the patient reports some improvement. The problem of individualizing treatment is especially important to the conduct of a controlled trial and makes double-blinded designs almost impossible. At a minimum, such trials should use a dose of β-carotene large enough to produce amelioration of symptoms in the majority of patients (a minimum period of 3 months' treatment at doses giving blood levels of at least 800 μg/dl; for adults at least 180 mg/day should be given). To summarize, in spite of the occasional treatment failure, from our results, and those of the other workers listed above, it can be concluded that β-carotene, when administered in sufficiently high doses, can be an effective therapy for ameliorating photosensitivity in most patients with EPP.

Carotenoid Use in Other Photosensitivity Diseases

Since β-carotene seemed to be effective in preventing photosensitivity in EPP, it seemed logical to see if it could be an effective treatment for other photosensitivity diseases. Several workers, including ourselves, have investigated this possibility.

There have been 9 reports of some success in treating with carotenoids patients suffering from congenital porphyria (Gunther's disease).[48-56] New lesions were significantly decreased in number and severity, and the patients have been able somewhat to increase their sun exposure. In most cases, other treatment modalities, such as transfusions, and meticulous treatment of skin infections, must continue.

Several groups, including the author's, have used carotenoids to prevent photosensitivity in polymorphic light eruption (PMLE).[15,18,32,57–71] Reports of improvement range from one-third to two-thirds of the patients being able to tolerate light exposure without the development of new lesions. Usually, sunscreens must also be used to get a beneficial effect from carotenoid intake: sunscreens by themselves did not provide relief for these patients. One group used phototesting as an objective method of judging improvement: Wennersten and Swanbeck treated 8 patients with PMLE with β-carotene and found an increase in the minimal erythema dose (tested with an appropriately-filtered xenon arc lamp) of all the patients after treatment.[18,57]

Three controlled trials were done with β-carotene in PMLE. Suhonen and Plosila[65] found good to excellent results in 36 out of 50 patients. Corbett et al.[66] found only a small degree of improvement using either β-carotene or chloroquin as compared to placebo. Jansen[70] studied 40 patients in a trial comparing carotenoids, oxychloroquin and placebo, and concluded that chloroquine and carotenoids are both effective in alleviating the photosensitivity symptoms of PMLE, but since carotenoids have less toxicity than chloroquin, carotenoid treatment is to be preferred.

A few studies have reported the effects of carotenoid treatment in other photosensitivity diseases. Our group and Kobza et al.[15,72] found no benefit from carotenoid ingestion in Porphyria cutanea tarda, but Francescini et al.[73] reported excellent improvement in 3 cases, and Eales found some relief in 1 patient.[74] Aratari et al.[75] had some success in treating actinic reticuloid with carotenoids but Kobza et al.[72] and Wennesten[32] reported that β-carotene alone had no effect in the treatment of actinic reticuloid or solar urticaria. On the other hand, Saito et al.[76] reported improvement in 1 patient with solar urticaria Type IV. We treated 6 cases of solar urticaria, 3 cases of hydroa aestivale and 2 cases of actinic reticuloid with high doses of β-carotene.[15] Only 1 patient with solar urticaria and 1 patient with hydroa aestivale reported noticeable relief. Both stated that they obtained improvement without the use of a topical sunscreen. Bickers et al. noted that 2 patients with Hydroa vacciniforme developed no new lesions when taking β-carotene.[77] Carotenoid treatment seemed to offer some relief to a few patients with Porphyria variegata.[74,78–79] In two cases of sideroblastic anemia, where ferrochelatase was found to be defective and protoporphyrin accumulated, β-carotene administration prevented or lessened photosensitivity[80,81] (S. Bottomly, personal communication about case in [80]). In summary, β-carotene treatment may be of some use in congenital porphyria, if given in high doses starting when the patients are very young, and sideroblastic anemia, when photosensitivity is present. However, carotene treatment seems of limited use in PMLE, solar urticaria, Hydroa aestivale, Hydroa vaccineforme, Porphyria variegata, Porphyria cutanea tarda or actinic reticuloid; we would recommend it only after other treatment modalities have failed.

Two independent observations suggested that perhaps carotenemia might have an effect on a normal individual's response to sunlight. Bendes[82] had observed that the presence of carotenemia in children undergoing heliotherapy for tuberculosis prevented sunburn, and Sandler[83] found that carotenemia facilitated tanning of the skin. These observations, plus our success with β-carotene in the treatment of EPP led us to conduct a controlled trial to determine if the administration of high doses of β-carotene would alter the normal fair-skinned individual's response to sunlight. We found that high doses of β-carotene had a small but statistically significant effect in increasing the minimal erythema dose for eliciting erythema produced by natural sunlight.[84] However, the observed effects were too small to recommend the use of β-carotene as a protective agent for sunburn. It was also found that the men in the group taking carotene in this study developed more pigmentation (tanning) than did the men in the placebo group, thus confirming the findings of Bendes[82] and Sandler.[83]

Anyan[85] reported that a young girl who had been carotenemic while hypothyroid had not been able to tan while in this condition. Once she became euthyroid after appropriate treatment, her carotenemia disappeared, and the ability to tan returned. These findings are not necessarily at variance with ours: perhaps as Anyan suggests, marked, long-standing carotenodermia may protect the skin to such a degree that tanning may become hard to induce.

How Do Carotenoids Protect Against Photosensitization?

At this conference we have heard about the chemical and physical reactions carotenoids can undergo. Some of these are certainly involved in the mechanism of photoprotection. Krinsky[2] suggested four possible ways that carotenoid pigments could exert their protective functions: 1) a filter system in the cell envelope to filter out potentially harmful light, 2) systems that can interact with and quench photosensitizer triplet states, 3) systems that can serve as preferred substrates for photosensitized oxidations and 4) systems that can stabilize membranes or repair damaged membranes. Since that time, additional evidence has indicated that only the second suggested mechanism, now extended to include quenching of singlet oxygen by carotenoids, seems to be significantly associated with the pigments' protective function.[6] Mechanism 1) may have some function in certain plants, although it may not be the sole explanation for the pigments' protective effects in these organisms. This mechanism is also unlikely to be involved in carotenoid protection in humans, as the amounts deposited in skin are not sufficient to act as a physical sunscreen.[86-87] In addition, the photoprotective effect of the carotenoids seems to be independent of the absorption spectrum. The findings in photosynthetic organisms which led to the suggestion of mechanism 3) by several groups of workers are thought to be connected with reactions involved with photosynthesis rather than with the protective function of carotenoids.[6] The author and Krinsky showed that the presence of carotenoids does not seem to be involved with membrane stability in *Sarcina lutea*,[88] thus suggesting that mechanism 4) may not be of wide significance in the protective function of carotenoids.

Thus it would seem that the quenching of excited species is the most widely applicable mechanism for the carotenoids' protective effects. Since the first demonstration of the ability of carotenoids to quench the triplet state of chlorophyll[89] and to quench singlet oxygen,[90] many workers including ourselves have confirmed that porphyrins form these excited species when illuminated, and that carotenoids indeed can quench them.

Studies on the action at the cellular level of carotenoids have also been performed. Carotenoids can inhibit arachidonic acid and prostaglandin release,[91] although retinoic acid has a higher activity. The pigments can inhibit lipid peroxide formation caused by reactive oxygen species.[92,93] Using a method of detecting photochemical reactions in epidermis, the author has been able to show that the carotenoids present in the skin of mice made porphyric by the ingestion of collidine and also receiving supplementation of either β-carotene or canthaxanthin, could quench photochemical reactions occurring in isolated epidermis.[94] In nonporphyric mice supplemented with either of these carotenoids, or with the colorless carotenoid, phytoene, the pigments could also quench excited species formed in skin on irradiation with UV-B (290–320 nm) radiation.[95]

Recently, carotenoids have been found to affect T-cells,[96–97] natural killer cells[98] and cytokine production.[99] Bendich[100] postulates that carotenoids may enhance immune activity by 1) quenching excessive reactive species formed by various immunoactive cells, 2) quenching immunosuppressive peroxides and maintaining membrane fluidity, 3) helping to maintain membrane receptors essential for immune function, and 4) acting in the release of immunomodulatory lipid molecules such as prostaglandins and leukotrienes. These immune-protective functions may work in concert with excited species quenching to prevent photosensitization in EPP. Lim[101] postulates that protoporphyrin and light exposure can lead to the activation of complement, which will in turn cause the activation of mast cells, as well as cause the release of mast cell mediators. Peroxidation is involved in this process. He suggests that the release of mast cell mediators may account for the erythema, edema and urticaria which EPP patients develop when exposed to sunlight, and that the skin thickening sometimes seen may be formed as a result of the interactions of mast cells with fibroblasts in addition to the direct effects of protoporphyrin-induced excited species on fibroblast cell membrane components. Although more work needs to be done to determine the molecular mechanisms of photosensitization and photoprotection in humans, it is conceivable that carotenoids prevent the porphyrin-induced peroxidation and lipid oxidation of cellular components of endothelial and immune system cells, and thereby prevent the release of mediators which give rise to the symptoms associated with photosensitization in EPP and possibly other photosensitivity diseases.

Lack of Toxicity of Carotenoids

No serious side effects from β-carotene ingestion have been found either by us or by other workers. Some patients report gastrointestinal disturbances when they first start taking carotenoids. In most patients, these discomforts seem to clear up spontaneously, but some patients require that the dose be lowered. On rare occasions, a patient may have to stop β-carotene intake to obtain relief. Canthaxanthin, which has been used in conjunction with β-carotene in Europe, is also effective in preventing photosensitivity, but ingestion of large doses leads to the deposition of pigmented granules in the retinas of some patients, which occasionally may have some effect on night vision.[102] The granules have been found to disappear several months after cessation of canthaxanthin ingestion, with return of any visual changes to normal.[102] No such granules seem to form from β-carotene ingestion.[103] It should be noted that canthaxanthin, although approved by the U.S. Food & Drug Administration as a food coloring agent, has not yet been approved for use as a drug.

SUMMARY

Studies in bacteria, animals and humans have demonstrated that carotenoid pigments can prevent or lessen photosensitivity by endogenous photosensitizers such as chlorophyll or porphyrins, as well as by exogenous photosensitizers such as dyes (e.g., toluidine blue) or porphyrin derivatives. The carotenoids β-carotene and canthaxanthin have been found to be effective in the treatment of the photosensitivity associated with EPP and certain other photosensitivity diseases. No serious toxicity has been reported from their use, although the use of canthaxanthin is not recommended because of its propensity to form retinal granules. The pigments perform their protective function by quenching excited species formed by the interaction of porphyrins or dyes, light and air, thereby preventing the cellular damage which leads to the symptoms of photosensitivity.

REFERENCES

1. SISTROM, W. R., M. GRIFFITHS & R. STANIER. 1957. Biology of a photosynthetic bacterium which lacks colored carotenoids. J. Cell. Comp. Physiol. **48:** 473–515.
2. KRINSKY, N. I. 1968. The protective function of carotenoid pigments. *In* Photophysiology, Current Topics, A. C. Giese, Ed. Vol. **3:** 123–195. Academic Press. New York, NY.
3. KUNISAWA, R. & R. Y. STANIER. 1958. Studies on the role of carotenoid pigments in a chemoheterotropic bacterium, *Corynebacterium poinsettiae,* Arch. Mikrobiol. **31:** 146–159.
4. MATHEWS, M. M. & W. R. SISTROM. 1959. Function of carotenoid pigments in non-photosynthetic bacteria. Nature **184:** 1892.
5. MATHEWS, M. M. & W. R. SISTROM. 1960. The function of the carotenoid pigments of *Sarcina lutea.* Arch. Mikrobiol. **35:** 139–146.
6. KRINSKY, N. I. 1971. Function. *In* Carotenoids. O. Isler, Ed. 669–706. Birkhauser Verlag. Basel & Stuttgart.
7. KESTEN, B. M. 1951. Urticaria solare (4,200–4,900 A). Arch. Dermatol. Syphilol. **64:** 221–228.
8. FORSSBERG, A., C. LINGEN, L. ERNSTER & O. LINDBERG. 1959. Modification of X-irradiation syndrome by lycopene. Exp. Cell Res. **16:** 7–14.
9. LIPSON, R. L. & E. J. BALDES. 1960. Photodynamic properties of a particular hematoporphyrin derivative. Arch. Dermatol. **82:** 508–516.
10. MATHEWS, M. M. 1964. Protective effect of beta-carotene against lethal photosensitization by hematoporphyrin. Nature **203:** 1092.
11. A. KAPPAS, S. SASSA & K. E. ANDERSON. 1983. The porphyrias. *In* The Metabolic Basis of Inherited Disease. J. B. Stanbury, D. S. Fredrickson, J. L. Goldstein & M. S. Brown, Eds. 1301–1384. McGraw-Hill. New York, NY.
12. MATHEWS-ROTH, M. M., M. A. PATHAK, T. B. FITZPATRICK, L. C. HARBER & E. H. KASS. 1970. Beta-carotene as a photoprotective agent in erythropoietic protoporphyria. Trans. Assoc. Am. Phys. **83:** 176–184.
13. MATHEWS-ROTH, M. M., M. A. PATHAK, T. B. FITZPATRICK, L. C. HARBER & E. H. KASS. 1970. Beta-carotene as a photoprotective agent in erythropoietic protoporphyria. N. Engl. J. Med. **282:** 1231–1234.
14. MATHEWS-ROTH, M. M., M. A. PATHAK, T. B. FITZPATRICK, L. C. HARBER & E. H. KASS. 1974. Beta-carotene as an oral photoprotective agent in erythropoietic protoporphyria. J. Am. Med. Assoc. **228:** 1004–1008.
15. MATHEWS-ROTH, M. M., M. A. PATHAK, T. B. FITZPATRICK, L. C. HARBER & E. H. KASS. 1977. Beta-carotene therapy for erythropoietic protoporphyria and other photosensitivity diseases. Arch. Dermatol. **113:** 1229–1232.
16. MATHEWS-ROTH, M. M., E. H. KASS, T. B. FITZPATRICK, M. A. PATHAK & L. C. HARBER. 1979. Phototesting as an objective measure of improvement in erythropoietic protoporphyria. Arch. Dermatol. **115:** 1381–1382.
17. KROOK, G. & B. HAEGER-ARONSON. 1974. Erythrohepatic protoporphyria and its treatment with beta-carotene. Acta Dermatovener. **54:** 39–44.
18. WENNERSTEN, G. & G. SWANBECK. 1974. Treatment of light sensitivity with carotenoids: serum concentrations and light protection. Acta Dermatovener. **54:** 491–499.

19. MATHEWS-ROTH, M. M. 1982. Beta-carotene therapy for erythropoietic protopor-phyria and other photosensitivity diseases. *In* The Science of Photomedicine. J. D. Regan & J. Parrish, Eds. 409–440. Raven Press. New York, NY.
20. MATHEWS-ROTH, M. M. 1986. Beta-carotene therapy for erythropoietic protopor-phyria and other photosensitivity diseases. Biochimie **68:** 875–884.
21. MATHEWS-ROTH, M. M. 1990. Carotenoid functions in photoprotection and cancer prevention. J. Environ. Pathol. Toxicol. Oncol. **10:** 181–192.
22. MATHEWS-ROTH, M. M. 1991. Recent progress in the medical applications of carot-enoids. Pure Appl. Chem. **63:** 147–156.
23. BECKERT, E. & J. METZ. 1976. Erythropoetische protoporphyrie. Fortschr. Medizin **94:** 1981–1995.
24. NONAKA, S., T. HIROWATARI, T. HONDA, T. SHIMOYAMA, M. HORI, H. YAMAURA, N. FUJIWARA, I. TAKAHASHI, K. NISHIMOTO & M. NOGITA. 1977. Erythropoietic protoporphyria. Jap. J. Dermatol. **87:** 7–32.
25. MARSDEN, R. A. & R. P. R. DAWBER. 1977. Erythropoietic protoporphyria with onycholysis. Proc. R. Soc. Med. **70:** 572–574.
26. WESTON, W. L. 1978. Erythropoietic protoporphyria masquerading as angioedema. J. Allergy Clin. Immunol. **61:** 408.
27. ROSSI, E., D. H. CURNOW & H. SCHENBERG. 1978. The detection of porphyria in photosensitive patients. Pathology **10:** 17–26.
28. NIEBAUER, G., P. MISCHER & I. FORMANEK. 1978. Light-sensitive dermatoses in children. Mod. Probl. Paediat. **20:** 86–101.
29. HALPERN, G. M. 1978. Urticarie solaire: protoporphyrie erythropoietique. Allerg. Immunol. **10:** 19–25.
30. VASQUEZ BOTET, M. 1979. Erythropoietic protoporphyria. Bull. Assoc. Med. Puerto Rico **71:** 107–113.
31. HUSQUINET, H. & D. VAN NESTE. 1979. La protoporphyrie. Rev. Med. Liege **34:** 98–103.
32. WENNESTEN, G. 1980. Carotenoid treatment for light sensitivity. Acta Dermatovener. **60:** 251–255.
33. PEZZAROSSA, E., D. BENOLDI, A. ALINOVI & P. BASSISSI. 1985. La protoporfiria eritropoietica. G. Ital. Dermatol. Venereol. **120:** 351–353.
34. DE SELYS, R., J. DECROIX, M. FRANKART, A. HASSOUN, D. WILLOCX, C. PIRARD & A. BOURLOND. 1988. Protoporphyrie erythropoietique. Ann. Dermatol. Vener-eol. **115:** 555–560.
35. PRAVETTONI, C., S. PINELLI, S. VERALDI & E. BERTANI. 1988. Trattamento della protoporphyria eritropoietica con beta-carotene. Chron. Derm. **19:** 45–49.
36. POLSON, R. J., C. K. LIM, K. ROLLES, R. Y. CALNE & R. WILLIAMS. 1988. The effect of liver transplantation in a 13-year old boy with erythropoietic protoporphyria. Transplantation **46:** 386–389.
37. CROSBY, D. L., C. E. WHEELER & J. D. CHEESBOROUGH. 1989. An unusual case of erythropoietic protoporphyria. Arch. Dermatol. **125:** 846–847.
38. PIOTTE, M., A. HASSOUN, A. BOURLOND & C. CORNU. 1989. Erythropoietic proto-porphyria in a child. Eur. J. Pediatr. **148:** 507–509.
39. FALLON, J. D., J. C. KVEDAR, R. J. MARGOLIS & M. A. PATHAK. 1989. Erythropoietic protoporphyria presenting in adulthood. Arch. Dermatol. **125:** 1286–1287.
40. LEHMANN, P., K. SCHARFFETTER, P. KIND & G. GOERZ. 1991. Erythropoetische protoporphyrie: synopsis von 20 patienten. Hautarzt **42:** 570–574.
41. SMIT, A. F. D. 1980. Erythropoietic protoporphyria. Br. J. Dermatol. **102:** 743.
42. KUHLWEIN, A. & W. BEYKIRCH. 1980. Das β-carotin als therapeutikum der erythro-poetischen protoporphyrie (EPP), nicht der weisheit letzter schluss. Z. Hautkr. **55:** 817–820.
43. BECHTEL, M. A., S. J. BERTOLONE & S. J. HODGE. 1981. Transfusion therapy in a patient with erythropoietic protoporphyria. Arch. Dermatol. **117:** 99–101.
44. MURPHY, G. M., J. L. M. HAWK & I. A. MAGNUS. 1985. Late-onset erythropoietic protoporphyria with unusual clinical features. Arch. Dermatol. **121:** 1309–1310.
45. ROSS, J. B. & M. A. MOSS. 1990. Relief of the photosensitivity of erythropoietic protoporphyria by pyridoxine. J. Am. Acad. Dermatol. **22:** 340–342.

46. CORBETT, M. F., A. HERXHEIMER, I. A. MAGNUS, C. A. RAMSAY & A. KOBZA-BLACK. 1977. The long-term treatment with beta-carotene in erythropoietic proto-porphyria—a controlled trial. Br. J. Dermatol. **97:** 655–662.
47. SHAFRIR, A. 1977. Comment to Marsden Case Report. Proc. R. Soc. Med. **70:** 574.
48. SEIP, M., P. O. THUNE & L. ERIKSEN. 1974. Treatment of photosensitivity in congenital erythropoietic porphyria (CEP) with beta-carotene. Acta Dermatovener. **54:** 239–240.
49. SNEDDON, I. B. 1974. Congenital porphyria. Proc. R. Soc. Med. **67:** 593–594.
50. BAART DE LA FAILLE, H. & J. J. REMME. 1979. Congenital porphyria (Gunther). Br. J. Dermatol. **101:** 224–226.
51. STORCK, H. & J. KAUFMANN. 1978. Kongenitale erythropetische porphyrie morbus Gunther. Dermatologica **157:** 323–333.
52. MALEVILLE, J., P. BABIN, S. MOLLARD, C. MARTIN, Y. NORDMANN & G. GUILLET. 1982. Porphyrie erythropoietique congenitale de Gunther et carotenoides. Essai therapeutique de quatres ans. Ann. Dermatol. Venereol. (Paris) **109:** 883–887.
53. JUNG, E. C. 1977. Porphyria erythropoietica congenita Gunther. Dtsch. Med. Wochenschr. **102:** 279–280.
54. MATHEWS-ROTH, M. M., R. C. HAINING & T. R. KINNEY. 1977. Beta-carotene treatment of congenital porphyria. Am. J. Dis. Child. **131:** 366.
55. STRETCHER, G. S. 1978. Beta-carotene in congenital porphyria. Arch. Dermatol. **114:** 1242–1243.
56. HARRINGTON, C. I. 1986. Gunther's disease (congenital erythropoietic porphyria). Br. J. Dermatol. **115**(Suppl. 30): 87–88.
57. SWANBECK, G. & G. WENNERSTEN. 1972. Treatment of polymorphous light eruption with beta-carotene. Acta Dermatovener. **52:** 462–466.
58. JANSEN, C. T. 1974. Beta-carotene treatment of polymorphous light eruption. Dermatologica **149:** 363–373.
59. NORDLUND, J. J., S. N. KLAUS, M. M. MATHEWS-ROTH & M. A. PATHAK. 1973. New therapy for polymorphous light eruption. Arch. Dermatol. **108:** 710–712.
60. THUNE, P. 1976. Chronic polymorphic light eruption: particular wave bands and the effect of carotene therapy. Acta Dermatovener. **56:** 127–133.
61. BARTH, J. 1977. Chronisch-polymorphe lichtdermatose: endogenes ekzem. Dermatol. Monatsschr. **163:** 566–567.
62. PARRISH, J. A., M. J. LEVINE, W. L. MORRISON, E. GONZALEZ & T. B. FITZPATRICK. 1979. Comparison of PUVA and beta-carotene in the treatment of polymorphic light eruption. Br. J. Dermatol. **100:** 187–193.
63. HAEGER-ARONSEN, B., G. KROOK & M. ABDULLA. 1979. Oral carotenoids for photo-hypersensitivity in patients with erythropoietic protoporphyria, polymorphous light eruption and lupus erythematodes discoides. Int. J. Dermatol. **18:** 73–82.
64. FUSARO, R. M. & J. A. JOHNSON. 1980. Hereditary polymorphic light eruption in American Indians. J. Am. Med. Assoc. **244:** 1456–1457.
65. SUHONEN, R. & M. PLOSILA. 1981. The effect of beta-carotene in combination with canthaxanthin, Ro-8-8427 (Phenoro), in the treatment of polymorphic light eruption. Dermatologica **163:** 172–176.
66. CORBETT, M. F., J. L. M. HAWK, A. HERXHEIMER & I. A. MAGNUS. 1982. Controlled therapeutic trials in polymorphous light eruption. Br. J. Dermatol. **107:** 571–581.
67. TRONNIER, H. 1983. Zur schutzwirkung von β-carotin un xanthaxanthin gegen UV-reaktionen der haut. Z. Hautkr. **59:** 859–870.
68. BARTH, J., E. FICKWEILER, K. HARNACK, K. HERMANN, U. HUBNER, H. SCHAARSCHMIDT & F. SCHILLER. 1984. β-carotin in der behandlung von protoporphyrien und polymorphen lichdermatosen. Dermatol. Monatsschr. **170:** 244–248.
69. RABB, W. P., H. TRONNIER & A. WISKEMANN. 1985. Photoprotection and skin coloring by oral carotenoids. Dermatologica **171:** 371–373.
70. JANSEN, C. T. 1985. Oral carotenoid treatment in polymorphous light eruption: a cross-over comparison with oxychloroquine and placebo. Photodermatology **2:** 166–169.
71. DRAELOS, Z. K. & R. C. HANSEN. 1986. Polymorphic light eruption in pediatric patients with American Indian ancestry. Pediatr. Dermatol. **3:** 384–389.

72. Kobza, A., C. A. Ramsay & I. A. Magnus. 1973. Oral beta-carotene therapy in actinic reticuloid and solar urticaria. Br. J. Dermatol. **88:** 157–166.
73. Francescini, Ph., P. Godreau, B. Weschler, Ph. Giral & J. Weschler. 1981. Traitment de lupus erythemateux et des dermatoses photosensibles par les carotenoides. Nouv. Presse Med. **10:** 1938.
74. Eales, L. 1978. The effects of canthaxanthin on the photocutaneous manifestations of porphyria. S. Afr. Med. J. **54:** 1050–1052.
75. Aratari, E., G. Virno, G. Desirello & G. Nazzari. 1982. Associazione di beta-carotene e cantaxantina nel trattamento del reticuloideattinico. Acta Vitaminol. Enzymol. **4:** 319–324.
76. Saito, N., H. Kuboi, H. Moriwaki, E. Tomita, T. Takai & Y. Moriwaki. 1985. Therapeutic effect of β-carotene on solar urticara (Type IV): a case report. Nippon Naika Gakkai Zasshi. **74:** 66.
77. Bickers, D. R., L. K. Demar, V. DeLeo, M. B. Poh-Fitzpatrick, J. M. Aronberg & L. C. Harber. 1978. Hydroa vaccineforme. Arch. Dermatol. **114:** 1193–1196.
78. Husquinet, H., A. Noifalise & M-Th. Parent. 1978. Porphyria variegata. J. Genet. Hum. **26:** 367–383.
79. Muhlbauer, J. E., M. A. Pathak, P. V. Tischler & T. B. Fitzpatrick. 1982. Variegate porphyria in New England. J. Am. Med. Assoc. **247:** 3095–3102.
80. Bottomly, S. S. & M. Z. Moore. 1987. Acquired erythropoietic protoporphyria and sideroblastic anemia. Clin. Res. **35:** 38a.
81. Lim, H. W., D. Cooper, S. Sassa, H. Dosik, M. R. Buchness & N. A. Soter. 1992. Photosensitivity, abnormal porphyrin profile and sideroblastic anemia. J. Am. Acad. Dermatol. **27:** 287–292.
82. Bendes, J. H. 1926. Heliotherapy in tuberculosis. Minn. Med. **9:** 112–114.
83. Sandler, A. S. 1935. Carotene in prophylactic pediatrics. Arch. Pediatr. **52:** 391–406.
84. Mathews-Roth, M. M., M. A. Pathak, J. Parrish, T. B. Fitzpatrick, E. R. Kass, K. Toda & W. Clemans. 1972. A clinical trial of the effects of oral beta-carotene on the responses of human skin to solar radiation. J. Invest. Dermatol. **59:** 349–353.
85. Anyan, W. P. 1972. Carotenemia. Arch. Dermatol. **105:** 130.
86. Lamola, A. A. & W. Blumberg. 1976. The effectiveness of beta-carotene and phytoene as systemic sunscreens. Abstracts of the Annual Meeting of the American Society For Photobiology. Abstract No. FAM-C4.
87. Sayre, R. M. & H. S. Black. 1992. Beta-carotene does not act as an optical filter in skin. J. Photochem. Photobiol. B: Biol. **12:** 83–90.
88. Mathews-Roth, M. M. & N. I. Krinsky. 1970. Carotenoid pigments and the stability of the cell membrane of *Sarcina lutea*. Biochim. Biophys. Acta **203:** 357–359.
89. Fugimori, E. & M. Tavla. 1966. Light-induced electron transfer between chlorophyll and hydroquinone and the effect of oxygen and beta-carotene. Photochem. Photobiol. **5:** 877–887.
90. Foote, C. S. & R. W. Denny. 1968. Chemistry of singlet oxygen. VII. Quenching by beta-carotene. J. Am. Chem. Soc. **90:** 6233–6235.
91. Mufson, R. A., D. DeFeo & I. B. Weinstein. 1979. Effect of phorbol ester tumor promoters on arachidonic acid metabolism in chick embryo fibroblasts. Mol. Pharmacol. **16:** 569–578.
92. Dixit, R., M. Mukhtar & D. R. Bickers. 1983. Studies on the role of reactive oxygen species in mediating lipid peroxide formation in epidermal microsomes of rat skin. J. Invest. Dermatol. **81:** 369–375.
93. Kunert, K. J. & A. L. Tappel. 1983. The effect of vitamin C on *in vivo* lipid peroxidation in guinea pigs as measured by pentane and ethane production. Lipids **18:** 271–274.
94. Mathews-Roth, M. M. 1984. Porphyrin photosensitization and carotenoid protection in mice: *in vitro* and *in vivo* studies. Photochem. Photobiol. **40:** 63–67.
95. Mathews-Roth, M. M. 1986. Carotenoids quench evolution of excited species in epidermis exposed to UV-B (290-320 nm) light. Photochem. Photobiol. **43:** 91–93.
96. Prabhala, R. H., V. Maxey, M. J. Hicks & R. R. Watson. 1989. Enhancement

of the expression of activation markers on human peripheral blood mononuclear cells by *in vitro* culture with retinoids and carotenoids. J. Leukocyte Biol. **45:** 249–254.

97. BENDICH, A. & S. SHAPIRO. 1986. Effect of beta-carotene and canthaxanthin on the immune response of the rat. J. Nutr. **116:** 2254–2262.

98. LESLIE, C. A. & D. P. DUBY. 1982. Carotene and natural killer cell activity. Fed. Proc. **41:** 381.

99. ABRIL, E. R., J. A. RYBSKI, P. SCUDERI & R. R. WATSON. 1989. Beta-carotene stimulates the production of a tumor-necrosis factor (TNF)-like cytokine from human peripheral blood monocytes. J. Leukocyte Biol. **45:** 255–261.

100. BENDICH, A. 1989. Carotenoids and the immune response. J. Nutr. **119:** 112–115.

101. LIM, H. W. 1989. Mechanisms of phototoxicity in porphyria cutanea tarda and erythropoietic protoporphyria. *In* Immune Mechanisms in Cutaneous Disease. D. A. Norris, Ed. 671–685. Marcel Dekker, Inc. New York, NY.

102. ARDEN, G. B. & F. M. BARKER. 1991. Canthaxanthin and the eye: a critical ocular toxicologic assessment. J. Toxicol. Cutaneous Ocul. Toxicol. **10:** 115–155.

103. POH-FITZPATRICK, M. B. & L. BARBERA. 1984. Absence of crystalline retinopathy after long-term therapy with β-carotene. J. Am. Acad. Dermatol. **11:** 111–113.

Carotenoids in Oral Cancer Prevention[a]

HARINDER S. GAREWAL

University of Arizona Cancer Center
Tucson VA Medical Center
3601 S. 6th Avenue
Tucson, Arizona 85723

Oral cavity cancer is a common malignancy whose regional incidence varies from one part of the world to another. Overall oral cancers are the sixth most frequent cancers in the world with some of the highest rates being encountered in developing countries, where up to 25% of all malignancies are found in the oral cavity.[1-3] In the United States there are approximately 42,000 new cases of head and neck cancer annually leading to 12,000 deaths.[4] Most of these malignancies are caused by tobacco and alcohol use.[5,6] In developing countries, tobacco and betel quid chewing, usually mixed with other toxins such as slaked lime, is a common custom leading to many of these cancers. Tobacco, either smoked or chewed, results in more than 75% of oral cavity cancer.[5] Consequently, particularly in Western societies, the major risk factor for oral cancer is the same as that for some other common diseases, such as lung cancer and heart disease. Thus prevention strategies for oral cancer, such as discontinuing tobacco use, will have an impact on many life-threatening diseases. Furthermore, if most or all tobacco-related cancers, particularly those of the upper aerodigestive tract, result from similar tobacco-induced damage to the underlying mucosa, it may indeed be that other preventive strategies, such as the use of beta-carotene, will be beneficial for a number of cancer sites.

Even though the treatment of oral cancer has improved over the past few decades from the standpoint of reducing morbidity and disfigurement, there has been no demonstrable improvement in the survival of patients afflicted with this disease. In fact, the National Cancer Institute surveillance data, comparing outcomes in the 1980s to those that were achievable in the 1970s, are essentially identical.[7] Advanced disease patients, who account for over half the cases, have a dismal 5-year survival in the range of 25% or less. Early disease patients generally can achieve a high cure rate with local treatment modalities, such as surgery and radiotherapy, but they have a high risk of developing a second malignancy of the upper aerodigestive tract resulting in significant mortality despite cure of the primary lesion.[8-10] In the 1950s, the concept of "field cancerization" was proposed as an explanation for the coexistence of malignant and premalignant changes often seen in the same patient.[11] This refers to diffuse changes in the mucosa, presumably by exposure to carcinogens, leading to increased neoplastic growth.

The approach most likely to reduce morbidity and mortality from oral cancer is its prevention. Cessation of tobacco use is clearly a major objective in this endeavor. Additionally, there is now considerable evidence suggesting a potential role for nutritional agents, particularly the antioxidants beta-carotene and vitamin E, in preventing this disease. In this overview, I shall summarize this evidence,

---

[a] This work was partially supported by United States Public Health Service Grant CA-27501.

emphasizing data from the more recent clinical intervention trials in oral cavity premalignant lesions.

Carcinogenesis and Invasive Cancer

The disease process resulting in invasive cancer is called carcinogenesis. Carcinogenesis is now believed to occur through a series of several steps, named initiation, promotion, and progression. Our efforts in the area of cancer therapeutics have concentrated primarily on the final stage of this disease, *i.e.*, invasive cancer. Although this has resulted in an occasional success story, such an approach is inherently limited in its impact, because it focuses on the last stage of a continuous disease process, namely, carcinogenesis. As is the case with emphasis on the final stage of any chronic, ultimately fatal, disease, this approach leads to only modest, if any, effect on its control and eradication. Such is the case, for example, with cardiovascular heart disease in which emphasis on the management and treatment of myocardial infarction, the final step, will have considerably less impact on the morbidity from heart disease than effective prevention of the disease process of atherosclerosis. Such a re-focus on carcinogenesis as the disease, rather than invasive cancer as the endpoint, is particularly important when one thinks of strategies for prevention of cancer.

TABLE 1. Beta-Carotene and Oral Cancer Prevention

1. Laboratory studies, animal models (hamster cheek pouch).
2. Epidemiology: dietary correlations and use of supplements.
3. Pharmacology: high risk groups (tobacco) have low levels.
4. Ability to decrease micronucleated cells in very high risk groups (Stich *et al.*).
5. Beta-carotene reverses oral leukoplakia, a premalignant lesion.
6. Effect on incidence of second malignancies?

The most convincing and direct proof of cancer preventive activity for any intervention would be to demonstrate the actual reduction in cancer incidence via a clinical trial. Nevertheless, such an approach is impossible for most cancers for a number of logistical and practical reasons, including the fact that, although common, most individual cancers are infrequent events in an otherwise healthy population. Therefore, long trials, lasting decades and involving several thousands of subjects, would be necessary for each malignancy. A more practical approach to come to a conclusion regarding putative chemopreventive activity is to consider an accumulation of other, admittedly indirect, lines of evidence for or against each agent. TABLE 1 lists the various lines of evidence supporting such a role for beta-carotene in oral cancer prevention. Supportive evidence for each of these is discussed below with emphasis on the more recent clinical trial information.

Epidemiologic and Laboratory Evidence for an Inhibitory Role for Carotenoids and Antioxidants in Oral Carcinogenesis

A large number of epidemiologic studies have linked a low intake of carotenoids with increased risk of cancer, including that of the oral cavity.[12] This overall area is reviewed elsewhere in this symposium. Specifically for oral cancer, for example, a recent study undertaken by the Tata Memorial Institute in Bombay found a twofold increased risk in subjects consuming nondaily vegetables vs daily consumers.[13] Similar findings exist for vitamin C intake. Because of the difficulty in quantitating vitamin E in the diet, studies with this antioxidant are fewer in number, but also suggest protection.[14] A very important epidemiologic study was published recently by Gridley et al. reporting that subjects taking supplemental vitamin E had approximately half the risk of oral cavity cancer than those not taking the supplement.[15] This study is important, because it is the first epidemiologic study demonstrating a beneficial effect from *supplemental* vitamin E.

Another epidemiologic approach is to study the pharmacology of carotenoids and antioxidants in subjects at risk for oral malignancy. Although it has been known that heavy cigarette smokers have lower plasma levels of carotenoids and beta-carotene than nonsmokers, Stich et al., and more recently Peng et al., have further shown that buccal mucosal cell levels of beta-carotene are also lower in heavy smokers vs nonsmokers.[16,17] At our own institution Peng et al. have demonstrated that this difference exists despite similar dietary intakes and that the magnitude of the difference is likely to be too large for smokers to achieve nonsmoker levels simply by diet modification.[17] In another series of studies, Kaugars and colleagues, from the Medical College of Virginia, have studied plasma levels of carotenoids in tobacco chewers. In preliminary results they found lower dietary intakes and lower plasma levels in those subjects who developed premalignant lesions vs those who did not.[18,19] These latter findings need further study since, in subsequent reports, the same group failed to confirm a statistically significant difference, although a difference did exist.[20]

In laboratory studies retinoids and carotenoids have been shown to have antimutagenic activity in bacterial systems. Similarly, in many cell culture systems, they have a profound effect in preventing transformation induced by chemicals and radiation.[21,22] Of direct relevance to oral carcinogenesis are recent observations made on the capacity of these compounds to block genotoxic damage in Chinese hamster ovary cells caused by tumor promoters such as extracts of areca nut and other oral carcinogens.[23] The precise mechanism of action of retinoids and carotenoids in cancer inhibition has not yet been determined. They produce effects on cell differentiation, immunologic function, interaction of cells with growth factors such as epidermal growth factor, and changes in gene expression, all mechanisms which may be important in their anticarcinogenic activity.

An animal model of particular relevance to head and neck cancer is the hamster cheek pouch, in which precancerous and cancerous lesions are produced after application of the carcinogen, 7,12-dimethylbenz(a)anthracene. This model was first described in 1954 and has been extensively studied by Shklar, Schwartz and their colleagues.[24-30] The retinoids (13-cis-retinoic acid, retinyl acetate) and beta-carotene are all very active in inhibiting the formation of cancerous lesions in this system. Vitamin E also has inhibitory activity which is synergistic with beta-carotene.[31] This system has proved to be very useful for the study or oral carcinogenesis and its inhibition.

Beta-Carotene and Micronucleated Cell Frequency

Increased frequency of micronucleated cells is thought to reflect genotoxic damage produced by carcinogens. Stich and colleagues have reported a series of studies showing that beta-carotene, alone or in combination with vitamin A, can

TABLE 2. Beta-Carotene and Micronuclei Frequency

Population	Dose	Result	Reference
India	180 mg/week	Decrease	41
Philippines	180 mg/week	Decrease	42
Canada (Inuits)	180 mg/week	Decrease	43

decrease the incidence of micronucleated cells in exfoliated oral mucosal cells from populations considered to be at high risk for oral cancer (TABLE 2).[41–43] Preliminary results from studies in the West, where the lesion is primarily from smoking and not from chewing tobacco, have shown a much lower initial frequency of micronucleated cells than in the trials by Stich *et al.* No results on changes with treatment have yet been reported in "nonchewing" subjects, and such changes may be difficult to demonstrate because of the low initial, *i.e.*, pretreatment, frequency.

Beta-Carotene Reverses Oral Cavity Premalignancy

The reversal or suppression of premalignant lesions is an important strategy against carcinogenesis for the prevention of cancer. The basis for this approach is that premalignant lesions are often the first clinically identifiable clues that allow recognition of a mucosa that has been affected by carcinogenesis. *It should be emphasized that the ultimate goal of this strategy is to develop interventions applicable to the prevention of cancer and not merely to the eradication of premalignant lesions.* In general, the latter are not lethal or even morbid by themselves and are associated with rather low rates of transformation to cancer. Therefore, it is imperative that agents selected for trials in premalignant lesions, whose final goal is application for cancer prevention, should have minimal, or preferably no, toxicity, since a large number of subjects whose lesions are unlikely to progress to cancer in their lifetimes will necessarily be exposed to the intervention. Clearly, the type and number of side effects considered acceptable for any therapy depends on the severity of the condition being treated. High levels of toxicity are quite acceptable in treatments for overt malignancy. Similarly, a moderate degree of toxicity can be tolerated for some premalignant diseases, such as familial polyposis of the colon, which are associated with a very high cancer risk. However, for the majority of the commoner premalignant lesions, the cancer risk is often very low, and almost any side effects produced by a drug will generally be unacceptable.

Most oral cavity premalignant lesions come under the category of leukoplakia, *i.e.*, a white patch or plaque on the mucosa that cannot be rubbed off and is not attributable to a specific disease entity.[32] In general, they have a rather low malignant potential.[33] Oral erythroplakia and speckled leukoplakia have a higher transformation rate, but are relatively rare lesions.[33,34] Similarly, presence of severe dysplasia, demands a more aggressive treatment strategy.[33]

The objectives of intervention trials involving leukoplakia must therefore be kept in mind when designing chemoprevention studies. If the objective is to develop a treatment applicable to the small minority of patients with erythroplakia and/or high grade dysplasia that are not amenable to standard treatments, such as reduction in local irritants, surgical excision or cryosurgery, then some degree of toxicity in the therapy may be acceptable. In this category would be the use of toxic agents such as topical bleomycin, 5-fluorouracil, high-dose vitamin A and synthetic retinoids such as 13-cis-retinoic acid, which have been shown to be effective.[35-40] However, if the objective is to develop agents for generalized, population-based use for the primary prevention of oral cancer, then such agents are not practical, while the nontoxic antioxidants, such as beta-carotene and vitamin E, clearly are.

Interest in testing beta-carotene arose from the accumulated epidemiologic, laboratory and animal data. Furthermore, the activity of vitamin A and several synthetic retinoids was known, but their applicability was limited. Consequently, in the 1980s, a series of trials testing beta-carotene were accomplished, the results of which are summarized in TABLE 3.

As shown in TABLE 2, Stich et al. have reported clinical results on a series of trials in India using vitamin A and beta-carotene, alone or in combination.[41,44] It should be emphasized that this study population differs from the other trials in that the lesion in India is related primarily to chewing of betel nuts and other noxious substances. Furthermore, the study population may have had some degree of preexisting vitamin A deficiency. In one study, treatment consisted of beta-carotene (180 mg/week, Group I) or beta-carotene plus vitamin A (100,000 IU/week, Group II) or placebo (Group III) given twice weekly for six months. After six months, 15% of patients in Group I, 27.5% in Group II compared with only 3% in Group III had complete remissions of their lesions.[41] Furthermore, the appearance of new lesions was strongly inhibited in the treatment groups. (In a more recent trial using 200,000 IU of vitamin A alone per week for six months, Stich et al. have reported a 57% complete response rate with complete suppression of new lesions.[44] Although this moderately high dose of vitamin A did not produce clinically overt toxicity, potentially serious side effects such as liver function abnormalities were not specifically monitored.) Studies with beta-carotene in Western populations have been more recent. We have reported a pilot trial of beta-carotene alone, given at a dose of 30 mg/day daily for 3-6 months.[45] A response rate of 71% (95% confidence interval 53-89%) was observed in 24 evaluable patients. Of particular importance was the fact that no clinically significant toxicity was observed during this trial that could be attributed to beta-carotene.

In a carefully conducted crossover phase II trial by Malaker et al. in Canada, in which patients were initially treated with beta-carotene for 6-9 months, with nonresponders then receiving 13-cis-retinoic acid, a response rate of about 50% was noted with beta-carotene.[46]

Another study using a combination of antioxidant agents, including beta-caro-

TABLE 3. Oral Leukoplakia Trials Using Beta-Carotene[a]

Investigator	Agent	CR%	PR%	OR%	Country	Reference
Stich	BC	15	NS	NS	India	41
Stich	BC + vit A	27	NS	NS	India	41
Garewal	BC	8	63	71	USA	45
Toma	BC	33	11	44	Italy	49
Malaker	BC	28	22	50	Canada	46
Kaugars	BC + vit E + vit C	—	—	60	USA	48
Garewal	BC	—	—	56	USA	50

[a] BC = beta-carotene, CR = complete response, PR = partial response, OR = overall response, NS = not stated.

tene, is being conducted by Kaugars et al.[47] In this trial, patients are supplemented with a combination of beta-carotene, alpha-tocopherol and vitamin C. This combination is virtually nontoxic and a 60% response rate was recently reported from this trial.[48] Toma et al. from Italy have reported a response rate of 44% in 18 evaluable subjects treated with beta-carotene alone at a dose of 90 mg/day.[49]

We are presently conducting a multi-institutional trial that involves the University of California (Irvine), the University of Connecticut (Farmington) and the University of Arizona.[50] In this trial subjects are treated with beta-carotene at a dose of 60 mg/day for 6 months, at which point responding subjects are randomized in a blinded fashion to continue either beta-carotene or placebo for a subsequent 12 months. There are two main clinical objectives of this study: (1) Confirm the response rate to beta-carotene in a multi-institutional setting. (2) Establish whether continuation of beta-carotene will produce sustained remissions. It is well known from all previous studies that discontinuation of the intervention agent results in rapid recurrence of lesions, presumably because the initiating factors are still present. However, it needs to be established whether continued treatment will produce lasting remissions. The initial phase of this study was a feasibility trial to confirm whether a high response rate would be obtained when this treatment is used in a multi-institutional setting. This has been accomplished with a response rate of 56% (95% confidence interval 41–72%) being noted in the first 39 subjects completing six months of "induction."

Although the laboratory data is equally convincing for vitamin E as for beta-carotene, clinical intervention trials with vitamin E have been started more recently. In addition to the study by Kaugars et al. mentioned above, Benner et al. recently reported a multicenter study that showed a response rate of 46% (95% confidence interval 32–61%) in 43 subjects treated with 400 IU of vitamin E twice daily for 24 weeks.[51] The response rate for this study was 65% if calculated on the basis of evaluable subjects, of which there were 31. This result is extremely encouraging in that another nontoxic, nutritional agent, namely vitamin E, has been shown to be active in reversing oral leukoplakia.

CONCLUSIONS AND FUTURE TRIALS

In summary, numerous lines of evidence suggest a potential role for beta-carotene and other antioxidants in preventing oral cavity malignancy. Though it is recognized that the "ultimate" proof would be actual demonstration of oral cavity cancer reduction, trials with this as an endpoint will never be feasible. Therefore, all alternative, indirect lines of evidence need to be considered in arriving at a conclusion regarding a putative chemopreventive role. In this regard, the accumulated evidence in favor of these agents is quite strong and derives from a wide range of specialties, including epidemiology, laboratory studies, pharmacology and clinical intervention trials.

Another important group of subjects that has been targeted for testing for chemopreventive approaches are those that have had an early primary head and neck cancer that is considered cured. As mentioned earlier, these patients have a high risk for developing a second primary cancer of the aerodigestive tract.[8-10,52] It is reasonable to speculate that agents active in reversing preneoplastic lesions might be active in reversing the "field cancerization" defect thought to underlie this increased incidence of second cancers. Nontoxic agents are again preferred in this setting, inasmuch as prolonged treatment is anticipated and many of these patients will have received radiation treatment to the oral cavity resulting in chronic mucosal injury. Hence, they will be unable to tolerate any mucocutaneous toxicity associated with other active agents such as the retinoids. Trials using beta-carotene, alone or in combination with low doses of retinol, have recently been initiated in multicenter settings to test whether the incidence of second primaries can be reduced by these agents.

Finally, it is important to consider these results in the context of the ability of these agents to prevent other life-threatening, chronic diseases, particularly cardiovascular disease. The data from recent studies is indeed very exciting and is reviewed elsewhere in this symposium. The unifying mechanism underlying these diseases could very well be accumulating oxidative damage, thereby providing a theoretical basis for the potential of antioxidants to prevent a variety of seemingly unrelated diseases. The remarkable consistency of results from the various clinical trials reported thus far, such as those in oral leukoplakia or heart disease incidence reduction, has generated tremendous enthusiasm for conducting prospective trials to add to the array of evidence for a chemopreventive role for antioxidants. Indeed, the potential for making a significant impact on morbidity and mortality reduction is of such a magnitude that these innocuous, nontoxic, dietary components could very well emerge as one of the most important disease preventive modalities of the decade.

REFERENCES

1. PARKIN, S. M., E. LAARA & C. S. MUIR. 1988. Estimates of the worldwide frequency of sixteen major cancers. Int. J. Cancer (Philadelphia) **41:** 184–197.
2. DUNHAM, L. J. 1968. A geographic study of a relationship between oral cancer and plants. Cancer Res. **28:** 2369–2371.
3. BADEN, E. 1978. Tabac et cancers de la region oropharyngée et des bronches. Données actuelles. Rev. Med. Joulouse **14:** 549–560.
4. SILVERBERG, E., C. C. BORING & T. S. SQUIRES. 1990. Cancer statistics. CA Cancer J. Clin. **40:** 9–26.
5. US DEPARTMENT OF HEALTH AND HUMAN SERVICES. 1982. The Health Consequences of Smoking and Cancer. A Report of the Surgeon General. DHHS Publication (PSII) 5107. US Government Printing Office. Washington, DC.
6. MUIR, C. S. & R. KIRK. 1990. Betel, tobacco and cancer of the mouth. Br. J. Cancer **14:** 597–608.
7. US DEPARTMENT OF HEALTH AND HUMAN SERVICES. 1990. Cancer Statistics Review (1973–87). National Cancer Institute Division of Cancer Prevention and Control Surveillance Program. DHHS Publication 90-2789. National Cancer Institute, National Institutes of Health. Bethesda, MD.
8. KARP, D. D., E. GURALNICK, L. A. GUIDICE et al. 1985. Multiple primary cancers: a prevalent and increasing problem. Proc. Am. Soc. Clin. Oncol. **4:** 13.
9. KOTWALL, C., M. S. RAZACK, K. SAKO & U. RAO. 1990. Multiple primary cancers in squamous cell cancers of the head and neck. J. Surg. Oncol. **40:** 97–99.
10. McGUIRT, W. F., B. MATHEWS & J. A. KAUFMAN. 1982. Multiple simultaneous tumors in patients with head and neck cancer. Cancer (Philadelphia) **50:** 1195–1199.
11. SLAUGHTER, D. P., H. W. DOUTHWICH & W. SMEJKAL. 1953. Field cancerization in oral stratified squamous epithelium: clinical implications of multicentric origin. Cancer (Philadelphia) **5:** 963–968.
12. ZIEGLER, R. G. 1989. A review of epidemiologic evidence that carotenoids reduce the risk of cancer. J. Nutr. **119:** 116–122.
13. NOTANI, P. & K. JAYAAT. 1987. Role of diet in upper aerodigestive tract cancers. Nutr. Cancer **10:** 103–113.

14. BARONE, J., E. TAIOLI, J. R. HEBERT & E. L. WYNDER. 1992. Vitamin supplement use and risk for oral and esophageal cancer. Nutr. Cancer **18:** 31–41.

15. GRIDLEY, G., J. K. MCLAUGHLIN, G. BLOCK, W. J. BLOT, M. GLUCH & J. F. FRAUMENI. 1992. Vitamin supplement use and reduced risk of oral and pharyngeal cancer. Am. J. Epidemiol. **135:** 1083–1092.

16. STICH, H. F., A. P. HORNBY & B. P. DUNN. 1986. Beta-carotene levels in exfoliated mucosa cells of population groups at low and elevated risk for oral cancer. Int. J. Cancer **37:** 389–393.

17. PENG, Y. M., Y. PENG, T. MOON & D. ROE. 1993. Effect of multivitamin supplements and smoking on levels of carotenoids, retinoids and tocopherols in human plasma, skin and buccal mucosal cells. Proc. Am. Assoc. Cancer Res. In press.

18. KAUGARS, G. E., R. B. BRANDT, W. CHAN, S. J. KILPATRICK, P. CARCAISE-EDINBORO & S. MORAN. 1990. Risk factors in the development of oral lesions in smokeless tobacco users. J. Dent. Res. **69:** 345.

19. KAUGARS, G., R. BRANDT, W. CHAN, N. LANE & K. PECCATIELLO. 1989. Diet, serum carotenoids and oral lesions in smokeless tobacco users. J. Dent. Res. **68:** 254.

20. KAUGARS, G., R. B. BRANDT, W. CHAN & P. CARCAISE-EDINBORO. 1991. Evaluation of risk factors in smokeless tobacco-associated oral lesions. Oral Surg. Oral Med. Oral Pathol. **72:** 326–331.

21. SOM, S., M. CHATTERJEE & M. R. BANNERJEE. 1984. Beta-carotene inhibition of 7,12-dimethylbenz(a)anthracene-induced transformation of murine mammary cells *in vitro*. Carcinogenesis **5:** 937–940.

22. BERTRAM, J. S., A. PENG & J. E. RUNDHAUG. 1988. Carotenoids have intrinsic cancer preventive action. FASEB J. **2:** 1413A (abstract).

23. STICH, H. F. & B. P. DUNN. 1987. Relationship between cellular levels of beta-carotene and sensitivity to genotoxic agents. Int. J. Cancer **38:** 713–717.

24. BURGE-BOTTENBLEY, A. & G. SHKLAR. 1983. Retardation of experimental oral cancer development by retinyl acetate. Nutr. Cancer **5:** 121–129.

25. SCHWARTZ, J., D. SUDA & G. LIGHT. 1987. Beta-carotene is associated with the regression of hamster buccal pouch carcinoma and induction of tumor necrosis factor in macrophages. Biochem. Biophys. Res. Commun. **136:** 1130–1135.

26. SHKLAR, G., J. SCHWARTZ, D. GRAU *et al.* 1980. Inhibition of hamster buccal pouch carcinogenesis by 13-cis-retinoic acid. Oral Surg. Oral Med. Oral Pathol. **50:** 45–52.

27. SHKLAR, G., P. MAREFAT, A. KORNHAUSER *et al.* 1980. Retinoid inhibition of lingual carcinogenesis. Oral Surg. Oral Med. Oral Pathol. **49:** 325–332.

28. SHKLAR, G. 1982. Oral mucosal carcinogenesis in hamsters: inhibition by vitamin E. J. Natl. Cancer Inst. **68:** 791–797.

29. ODUKOYA, O., F. HAWACH & G. SHKLAR. 1984. Retardation of experimental oral cancer by topical vitamin E. Nutr. Cancer **6:** 98–104.

30. SUDA, D., J. SCHWARTZ & G. SHKLAR. 1986. Inhibition of experimental oral carcinogenesis by topical beta-carotene. Carcinogenesis **7:** 711–715.

31. SHKLAR, G., J. SCHWARTZ, D. TRICKLER & S. REID. 1989. Regression of experimental cancer by oral administration of combined alpha-tocopherol and beta-carotene. Nutr. Cancer **12:** 321–325.

32. KRAMER, I. R. H., R. B. LUERS, J. J. PINDBORG & L. H. SOBIN. 1978. Definition of leukoplakia and related lesions: an aid to studies on oral precancer. Oral Surg. Oral Med. Oral Pathol. **46:** 518–539.

33. SILVERMAN, S. & E. J. SHILLITOE. 1990. *In* Etiology and Predisposing Factors in Oral Cancer. 3rd Edit. S. Silverman, Ed. American Cancer Society. New York.

34. HANSEN, L. S., J. A. OLSON & S. SILVERMAN. 1985. Proliferative verrucous leukoplakia. A long-term study of thirty patients. Oral Surg. Oral Med. Oral Pathol. **60:** 285–298.

35. WONG, R., J. EPSTEIN & A. MILLNER. 1989. Treatment of oral leukoplakia with topical bleomycin. A pilot study. Cancer (Philadelphia) **64:** 361–365.

36. SILVERMAN, S., E. EISENBERG & G. RENSTRAP. 1965. A study of the effects of high doses of vitamin A on oral leukoplakia (hyperkeratosis), including toxicity, liver function and skeletal metabolism. J. Oral Ther. Pharmacol. **2:** 9.

37. Koch, H. F. 1978. Biochemical treatment of precancerous oral lesions: the effectiveness of various analogues of retinoic acid. J. Maxillofac. Surg. 6: 59–63

38. Koch, H. F. 1981. Effect of retinoids on precancerous lesions of oral mucosa. *In* Retinoids: Advances in Basic Research and Therapy. C. E. Orfanos, O. Braun-Falco, E. M. Farber *et al.*, Eds. 307–312. Springer, Berlin.

39. Shah, J. P., E. W. Strong, J. J. DeCosse *et al.* 1983. Effects of retinoids on oral leukoplakia. Am. J. Surg. 146: 466–470.

40. Hong, W. K., J. Endicott, L. M. Itri *et al.* 1986. 13-Cis-retinoic acid in the treatment of oral leukoplakia. N. Engl. J. Med. 315: 1501–1505.

41. Stich, H. F., M. P. Rosin, A. P. Hornby *et al.* 1988. Remission of oral leukoplakias and micronuclei in tobacco/betel quid chewers treated with beta-carotene and with beta-carotene plus vitamin A. Int. J. Cancer 42: 195–199.

42. Stich, H. F., W. Stich, M. P. Rosin & D. M. Vallejera. 1990. Use of the micronucleus test to monitor the effect of vitamin A, beta-carotene and canthaxanthin on the buccal mucosa of betel nut/tobacco chewers. Int. J. Cancer 34: 745–750.

43. Stich, H. F., A. P. Hornby & B. P. Dunn. 1985. A pilot beta-carotene intervention trial with Inuits using smokeless tobacco. Int. J. Cancer 36: 321–327.

44. Stich, H. F., A. P. Hornby, B. Mathew *et al.* 1988. Response of oral leukoplakias to the administration of vitamin A. Cancer Lett. 40: 93–101.

45. Garewal, H. S., F. L. Meyskens, D. Killen *et al.* 1990. Response of oral leukoplakia to beta-carotene. J. Clin. Oncol. 8: 1715–1720.

46. Malaker, K., B. J. Anderson, W. A. Beecroft & D. I. Hodson. 1991. Management of oral mucosal dysplasia with beta-carotene retinoic acid: a pilot crossover study. Cancer Detect. Prev. 15: 335–340.

47. Kaugars, G., R. Brandt, P. Carcaise-Edinboro, R. Strauss & J. Kilpatrick. 1990. Beta-carotene supplementation in the treatment of oral lesions. Oral Surg. Oral Med. Oral Pathol. 70: 607–608.

48. Brandt, R., G. Kaugars, S. Silverman, J. Lovas, W. Chan, V. Singh, B. Dezzutti & Q. Dao. 1991. Regression of oral lesions with the use of antioxidant vitamins and beta-carotene supplements. *In* Pennington Symposium "Vitamins and Cancer Prevention." Louisiana State University Press. Baton Rouge, LA.

49. Toma, S., S. Benso, E. Albanese, R. Palumbo, G. Nicolo & P. Mangiante. 1991. Response of oral leukoplakia to β-carotene treatment. *In* Pennington Symposium "Vitamins and Cancer Prevention." Louisiana State University Press. Baton Rouge, LA.

50. Garewal, H. S., J. Pitcock, S. Friedman, D. Alberts, F. Meyskens, L. Ramsey, Y. M. Peng & K. Girodias. 1992. Beta-carotene in oral leukoplakia. Proc. Am. Soc. Clin. Oncol. (28th meeting) 11: 141.

51. Benner, S. E., R. W. Winn, S. M. Lippman, J. Poland, K. S. Hansen, M. A. Luna & W. K. Hong. 1993. Regression of oral leukoplakia with alpha-tocopherol: a community clinical oncology program chemoprevention study. J. Natl. Cancer Inst. 85: 44–47.

52. Shapshay, W., W. K. Hong, M. Fried *et al.* 1980. Simultaneous carcinomas of the esophagus and upper aerodigestive tract. Otolaryngol. Head Neck Surg. 88: 373–377.

The Role of Beta-Carotene in the Prevention of Cardiovascular Disease

J. MICHAEL GAZIANO[a,b,d] AND
CHARLES H. HENNEKENS[a,c]

[a]Division of Preventive Medicine
[b]Cardiovascular Division
Department of Medicine
Brigham and Women's Hospital and Harvard Medical School
900 Commonwealth Avenue East
Boston, Massachusetts 02215-1204

[c]Department of Ambulatory Care and Prevention
Harvard Medical School
Boston, Massachusetts

[d]Department of Medicine
Veterans Administration Medical Center
West Roxbury, Massachusetts

INTRODUCTION

Recent evidence suggests that oxidative damage may be involved in the promotion of atherosclerotic disease. This raises the possibility that antioxidants, such as beta-carotene, may prevent or delay the progression of atherosclerosis. In this review, we will first discuss the functions of beta-carotene as an antioxidant, and then cite the evidence of the possible role of beta-carotene in the prevention of atherosclerotic disease. Finally, we will explore the possible mechanisms by which beta-carotene may impede the progression of atherosclerosis.

Beta-Carotene as an Antioxidant

Carotenoids, of which beta-carotene is the most abundant, are found in high concentrations in many fresh fruits and vegetables such as carrots, squash, melons, spinach, and broccoli. Beta-carotene is a vitamin precursor, which is converted to vitamin A as is needed by the body. Because of its lipid solubility, it is transported to the peripheral tissues via circulating lipoproteins.

In addition to its provitamin function, beta-carotene also functions as an antioxidant. The ability of beta-carotene to quench singlet oxygen and terminate lipid peroxidation relies on the series of conjugated double bonds.[1,2] The additional energy derived from the singlet oxygen molecule can be transferred to beta-carotene and eventually dissipated as heat, restoring oxygen to its stable form. In this process the beta-carotene molecule is not damaged and can therefore neutralize many singlet oxygen molecules. Beta-carotene is also a chain-breaking antioxidant under certain conditions.[2] The many adjacent double bonds provide a stable environment for the lone electron to reside. Beta-carotene stops the chain reaction by a mechanism similar to that of the tocopherols. It is effective at physiologic oxygen tension. Because beta-carotene is found in lipoproteins and

148

can accumulate in atherosclerotic plaque[3] it may prevent various oxidative processes that appear to be important steps in atherogenesis.

Epidemiologic Evidence

Descriptive and Cross-Sectional Studies

Several descriptive, or ecologic, studies have shown a correlation of per capita consumption of dietary antioxidants with cardiovascular disease. The consumption of fresh fruits and vegetables, which contain carotenoids, was inversely associated with the risk of heart disease in two British studies.[4,5] Verlangieri hypothesized that cardiovascular mortality is declining in the United States, in part, due to greater year-round availability of fruits and vegetables.[6]

Several blood-based descriptive and cross-sectional studies have also reported association between various antioxidants and atherosclerotic disease. Two population studies compared mortality rates of a given European population with mean plasma antioxidant levels, determined by obtaining plasma from a random sample of men in that population. In one study, carotenoids exhibited weak inverse trends with population cardiovascular mortality rates.[7-10] Remiersma compared plasma beta-carotene as well as other antioxidant levels in angina patients with those of healthy controls.[11,12] There was a significant trend for beta-carotene which was attenuated after controlling for smoking. These descriptive and cross-sectional studies are useful for formulating research questions, but analytic studies are necessary to test hypotheses.

Observational Cohort Studies

Prospective observational cohort studies are less subject to the biases of retrospective studies because investigators ascertain exposures before the onset of disease. Several prospective cohort studies have examined the role of intake of beta-carotene and cardiovascular disease, and all have shown a risk reduction associated with beta-carotene intake. The largest of these is the Nurses' Health Study, in which a cohort of 121,000 U.S. female nurses aged 30–55 is followed.[13,14] A semiquantitative food frequency questionnaire was administered in 1980 to 87,245 subjects who were free of cancer, stroke, and heart disease.

After eight years of follow-up, there were 552 cases of coronary disease, including 115 coronary deaths and 437 nonfatal myocardial infarctions, as well as 168 (15 fatal) strokes. Women who consumed the most antioxidant vitamins were compared with those who consumed the least. For coronary events, those in the highest quintile of beta-carotene consumption had a 22% risk reduction (p, trend = 0.02) when compared to women in the lowest quintile.[13] For stroke, there was a statistically significant 39% reduction in risk in the highest intake category (p, trend = 0.01).[14]

Another large-scale prospective cohort study, the Health Professionals Follow-Up Study, examined dietary antioxidants based on four-year follow-up data.[15] Of 39,000 men who had no history of vascular disease or other condition which would have necessitated dietary changes, there were 667 major coronary events (360 revascularizations, 209 nonfatal myocardial infarctions, and 106 fatal myocardial infarctions). When men in the highest quintile of intake of beta-carotene were compared with men in the lowest quintile, the relative risk was 0.75 (p, trend = 0.04).

The Massachusetts Elderly Cohort Study also examined dietary information, obtained through in-person interviews.[16] The 1,299 participants were followed for an average of 4.75 years through annual mailings, and were interviewed in 1976 and again in 1980. Of the participants, 151 died from cardiovascular deaths, and 47 of these were fatal myocardial infarctions. Comparing the lowest to the highest quartile of beta-carotene intake, the relative risk of cardiovascular deaths was 0.57 (p, trend = 0.02), after controlling for confounders such as age, sex, smoking, alcohol consumption, cholesterol intake, and functional status. The corresponding relative risk for fatal MI was 0.32 (p, trend = 0.02).

Blood-Based Observational Studies

In three nested case-control studies, blood samples were collected and frozen at baseline. Subjects who later developed cardiovascular disease were matched with healthy controls, and their baseline blood samples were compared. Street found a significant inverse association between baseline beta-carotene levels and subsequent myocardial infarction.[17] Two other nested case-control studies found no association between vitamin A level and subsequent vascular mortality;[18,19] however, vitamin A level may not accurately reflect beta-carotene status. In addition, the blood samples in these two studies were stored at $-20°C$, and the stability of antioxidants at this temperature is questionable.

Three studies measured plasma carotenoid levels at baseline for the entire cohort. Careful collection and immediate analysis can prevent decay of plasma antioxidants. After 14 years of follow-up in the Lipid Research Clinic Coronary Primary Prevention Trial, baseline carotenoid level was inversely correlated with risk of myocardial infarction after adjustment for age, smoking, HDL, and LDL.[20] The Basel Prospective Study measured baseline beta-carotene and followed a population of 2974 middle-aged men revealing an increased risk of death from coronary heart disease among those in the lowest quartile of carotene level compared with those with higher carotenoid levels (relative risk = 1.53; 95% confidence interval 1.07–2.20).[21] Plasma beta-carotene levels were inversely related to progression of carotid artery wall thickness in the Kupio Ischemic Heart Disease Study.[22]

Randomized Trials

While the data from both prospective blood-based and dietary intake studies are compatible with a possible benefit of beta-carotene, the available observational data are sparse. Observational investigations are limited in their ability to provide reliable estimates of the potential small-to-moderate benefits of antioxidants. It may be, for example, that greater dietary intake of beta-carotene, measured by blood levels or a diet assessment questionnaire, is only a marker for some other dietary practice or even nondietary life-style variable that is truly protective. It is, in fact, possible that intake of carotene-rich foods is indeed protective, but the benefit results not from their carotene content, but from some other component these foods have in common. In addition, the intake of individual dietary antioxidants is often highly correlated, making it difficult to determine the specific benefit of any one. Observational studies can control for the effects of known potential confounding variables, but they cannot take into account unknown or unmeasured confounding factors. In searching for small-to-moderate effects, the amount of uncontrolled confounding in observational studies may be as large as the likely risk reduction. For these reasons, reliable data can only emerge from large-scale randomized trials, in which investigators allocate subjects at random to either active treatment or placebo.

At present, randomized trial data on beta-carotene are limited. The Physicians' Health Study enrolled 333 doctors who had no prior history of myocardial infarction, transient ischemic attack, stroke or cancer but did have a history of chronic stable angina or who had a prior coronary revascularization procedure.[23] The Physicians' Health Study is a randomized, double-blind, placebo-controlled two-by-two factorial trial of 22,071 U.S. male physicians aged 40–84 testing aspirin in the primary prevention of cardiovascular disease and beta-carotene in the primary prevention of cardiovascular disease and cancer.

In analyses of the 333 men, two endpoints were defined: major coronary events and major vascular events. Major coronary events include coronary revascularization, fatal coronary disease, and nonfatal MI. Major vascular events included nonfatal and fatal stroke. Among subjects who received beta-carotene, there was a 51% reduction in risk of major coronary events, and a 54% reduction in risk of major vascular events ($p = 0.014$). Furthermore, the effect of beta-carotene was time-dependent, which is consistent with the theory that antioxidant intake slows the progression of atherosclerosis. Relative risk was analyzed by year of follow-up, and no effect appeared during the first year, but did appear in the second year and persisted thereafter.

There are currently several large-scale randomized trials of beta-carotene, as well as other antioxidants, testing their role in the prevention of cardiovascular disease and cancer. The Physicians' Health Study is testing beta-carotene in about 22,000 apparently healthy U.S. male physicians. The Women's Health Study (WHS) is testing beta-carotene as well as vitamin E and low-dose aspirin in the primary prevention of cardiovascular disease and cancer in 44,000 healthy U.S. female nurses.[24] The interactions between vitamin E and beta-carotene will be examined in this study. A secondary prevention trial of vitamin C, vitamin E, and beta-carotene in a factorial design is currently underway among 8,000 female nurses excluded from the WHS due to preexisting atherosclerotic disease.

The CARET study is testing a combination of beta-carotene and retinoic acid in 18,000 asbestos workers. The SU.VI.M.AX trial is a French initiative that will test the impact of supplementation of a cocktail of antioxidant vitamins at relatively lower dose. Later this year the Finnish Alpha-Tocopherol/Beta-Carotene Study and a Chinese antioxidant vitamin cocktail study will present results for both cardiovascular disease and cancer; both of these studies may be lacking in power to adequately detect small-to-moderate benefits due to sample size in the case of the Chinese study and short duration in the case of the Finnish study.

Biologic Mechanisms

Elevated LDL is clearly associated with increased risk of cardiovascular disease but, until recently, the mechanisms by which LDL acts were unclear. Data from *in vitro* and *in vivo* studies suggest that oxidative damage to LDL significantly increases atherogenicity.[25] Oxidized LDL (Ox-LDL) may have several different mechanisms of promoting atherogenicity including endothelial damage,[26,27] foam cell accumulation,[28–30] and growth.[31,32] In addition, Ox-LDL may stimulate the synthesis of autoantibodies which may play a role in atherogenesis.[33] By several mechanisms, then, Ox-LDL may initiate and propagate a cascade of reactions which result in atherosclerosis.

When incubated, LDL will become oxidized,[34-36] but this oxidative damage is inhibited by some dietary antioxidants. While vitamin E can inhibit the oxidation of LDL,[37] the ability of beta-carotene to protect LDL against oxidation remains unclear. Four studies have examined the ability of beta-carotene to inhibit the oxidation of LDL, and data are conflicting.

Two *in vitro* studies have reported protection of LDL from both cell oxidative modification after *in vitro* supplementation with beta-carotene.[37,38] Jialal *et al.*,[38] as well as Lavy *et al.*,[39] reported that *in vitro* supplementation of LDL with beta-carotene inhibited oxidation induced both by copper and human monocyte macrophages. In contrast, two researchers, Princen *et al.*[40] and Reaven *et al.*,[41] found that beta-carotene supplementation did not confer increased protection to LDL to *ex vivo* copper-mediated oxidation of LDL despite 17- to 20-fold increases in LDL beta-carotene levels.

It remains possible that beta-carotene contained within the LDL particle may inhibit LDL oxidation *in vivo,* but the *ex vivo* assay of LDL oxidation does not readily mimic the *in vivo* process. On the other hand, beta-carotene may inhibit oxidation of LDL not from within the particle but by reducing oxidative stress in the atherosclerotic plaque where carotenoids clearly accumulate.[42] Pretreatment of an endothelial cell preparation with beta-carotene has been shown to inhibit LDL oxidation.[43]

Alternatively, beta-carotene may not inhibit oxidation of LDL but may instead function in completely different ways. There is some evidence that beta-carotene may preserve endothelial function, reduce platelet aggregability, or even alter the lipoprotein profile. These potential mechanisms require further study.

CONCLUSIONS

In summary, available basic research as well as epidemiologic evidence are consistent with the possibility that beta-carotene may have a protective effect in cardiovascular disease. Only large-scale randomized trials of sufficient size and duration, such as the Physicians' Health Study and the Women's Health Study will provide reliable information on the role of beta-carotene, as well as other antioxidants, in reducing risks of cardiovascular disease and cancer. The precise mechanisms by which beta-carotene may protect against atherosclerotic disease remain unclear and warrant further basic research. Several small-scale blood-based studies nested within these larger trials may also provide valuable mechanistic information.

REFERENCES

1. FOOTE, C. S., R. W. DENNY, L. WEAVER, Y. CHANG & J. PETERS. 1970. Quenching of singlet oxygen. Ann. N.Y. Acad. Sci. **171:** 139–148.
2. BURTON, G. W. & K. U. INGOLD. 1984. Beta-carotene: an unusual type of lipid antioxidant. Science **224:** 569–573.
3. PRINCE, M. R., G. M. LaMURAGLIA & E. F. MacNICHOL. 1988. Increased preferential absorption in human atherosclerotic plaque with oral beta carotene: implications for laster endarterectomy. Circulation **78:** 338–444.

4. ACHESON, R. M. & D. R. R. WILLIAMS. 1983. Does consumption of fruit and vegetables protect against stroke? Lancet **1:** 1191–1193.

5. ARMSTRONG, B. K., J. L. MANN, A. M. ADELSTEIN & F. ESKIN. 1975. Commodity consumption and ischemic heart disease mortality, with special reference to dietary practices J. Chronic. Dis. **36:** 673–676.

6. VERLANGIERI, A. J., J. C. KAPEGHIAN, S. EL-DEAN & M. BUSH. 1985. Fruit and vegetable consumption and cardiovascular disease mortality. Med. Hypoth. **16:** 7–15.

7. GEY, K. F., G. B. BRUBACHER & H. B. STAHELIN. 1987. Plasma levels of antioxidant vitamins in relation to ischemic heart disease and cancer. Am. J. Clin. Nutr. **45:** 1368–1377.

8. GEY, K. F. & P. PUSKA. 1989. Plasma vitamins E and A inversely correlated to mortality from ischemic heart disease in cross-cultural epidemiology. Ann. N.Y. Acad. Sci. **570:** 254–282.

9. GEY, K. F., H. B. STAHELIN, P. PUSKA & A. EVANS. 1987. Relationship of plasma vitamin C to mortality from ischemic heart disease. Ann. N.Y. Acad. Sci. **498:** 110–123.

10. RIEMERSMA, R. A., M. OLIVER, R. A. ELTON, G. ALFTHAN, E. VARTIAINEN, M. SALO, P. RUBBA, M. MANCICI, H. GEORGI, J. VUILLEUMIER & K. F. GEY. 1990. Plasma antioxidants and coronary heart disease: vitamins C and E and selenium. Eur. J. Clin. Nutr. **44:** 143–150.

11. RIEMERSMA, R. A., D. A. WOOD, C. C. H. MACINTYRE, R. A. ELTON, K. F. GEY & M. F. OLIVER. 1991. Risk of angina pectoris and plasma concentrations of vitamins A, C, E, and carotene. Lancet **337:** 1–5.

12. RIEMERSMA, R. A., D. A. WOOD, C. C. H. MACINTYRE, R. A. ELTON, K. F. GEY & M. F. OLIVER. 1989. Low plasma vitamin E and C increased risk of angina in Scottish men. Ann. N.Y. Acad. Sci. **570:** 291–295.

13. MANSON, J. E., M. J. STAMPFER, W. C. WILLET, G. A. COLDITZ, B. ROSNER, F. E. SPEIZER & C. H. HENNEKENS. 1991. A prospective study of antioxidant vitamins and incidence of coronary heart disease in women. Circulation **84**(4, Suppl. II): 2168(abstr.).

14. MANSON, J. E., M. J. STAMPFER, W. C. WILLET, G. A. COLDITZ, F. E. SPEIZER & C. H. HENNEKENS. 1993. Antioxidant vitamins and incidence of stroke in women. Circulation **87**(2): 2(abstr.).

15. RIMM, E. B., M. J. STAMPFER, A. ASCHERIO, E. GIOVANNUCCI, G. A. COLDITZ & W. C. WILLETT. 1993. Dietary intake and risk of coronary heart disease among men. N. Engl. J. Med. **328:** 1450–1456.

16. GAZIANO, J. M., J. E. MANSON, L. G. BRANCH, F. LaMOTT, G. A. COLDITZ, J. E. BURING & C. H. HENNEKENS. 1992. Dietary beta carotene and decreased cardiovascular mortality in an elderly cohort. J. Am. Coll. Cardiol. **19**(3, Suppl. A): 377A(abstr.).

17. STREET, D. A., G. W. COMSTOCK, R. M. SALKELD, W. SCHUEP & M. KLAG. 1991. A population based case-control study of serum antioxidants and myocardial infarction. Am. J. Epidemiol. **134:** 719–720.

18. KOK, F. J., A. M. DE BRUIJN, R. VERMEEREN, A. HOFMAN, A. VANLAAR, M. DE-BRUIN, R. J. T. HERMUS & H. A. VALKENBERG. 1987. Serum selenium, vitamin antioxidants and cardiovascular mortality: a 9 year follow-up study in the Netherlands. Am. J. Clin. Nutr. **45:** 462–468.

19. SALONEN, J. T., R. SALONEN, I. PENTTILA, J. HERRANEN, M. JAUHIAINEN, M. KANTOLA, R. LAPPETELAINEN, P. MAENPAA, G. ALFTHAN & P. PUSKA. 1985. Serum fatty acids, apolipoproteins, selenium and vitamin antioxidants and risk of death from coronary artery disease. Am. J. Cardiol. **56:** 226–231.

20. MORRIS, D. L., S. B. KRITCHEVSKY & C. E. DAVIS. 1993. Serum carotenoids and coronary heart disease in the Lipid Research Clinics Coronary Primary Prevention Trial. Circulation **87**(2): 2(abstr.).

21. GEY, K. F., H. B. STAHELIN & M. EICHOLZER. 1993. Poor plasma status of carotene and vitamin C is associated with higher mortality from ischemic heart disease and stroke: Prospective Basel Study. Clin. Invest. **71:** 3–6.

22. SALONEN, J. T., K. NYYSSONEN, M. PARVIAINEN, M. KANTOLA, H. KORPELA & R. SALONEN. 1993. Low plasma beta-carotene, vitamin E and selenium levels associated with accelerated carotid atherogenesis in hypercholesterolemic eastern Finnish men. Circulation **87**(2): 1(abstr.).
23. GAZIANO, J. M., J. E. MANSON, P. M. RIDKER, J. E. BURING & C. H. HENNEKENS. 1990. Beta carotene therapy for chronic stable angina. Circulation **82**(4, Suppl. III): 202(abstr.).
24. WOMEN'S HEALTH STUDY RESEARCH GROUP. 1992. The Women's Health Study: summary of the study design. J. Myocardil. Ischemia **4:** 27–29.
25. STEINBERG, D., S. PARTHASARATHY, T. CAREW, J. KHOO & J. WITZTUM. 1989. Beyond cholesterol—modifications of low-density lipoprotein that increase its atherogenicity. N. Engl. J. Med. **320**(14): 915–924.
26. HESSLER, J. R., D. W. MOREL, L. J. JAMES & G. M. CHISOLM. 1983. Lipoprotein oxidation and lipoprotein-induced cytotoxicity. Arteriosclerosis **3**(3): 215–222.
27. YAGI, K. 1984. Increased serum lipid peroxides initiate atherogenesis. Bioessays **1:** 58–60.
28. QUINN, M. T., S. PARTHASARATHY & D. STEINBERG. 1985. Endothelial cell-derived chemotactic activity for mouse peritoneal macrophages and the effects of modified forms of low density lipoprotein. Proc. Natl. Acad. Sci. USA **82:** 5949–5953.
29. SCHAFFNER, T., K. TAYLOR, E. J. BARTUCCI, K. FISHER-DZOGA, J. H. BEESON, S. GLAGOV & R. W. WISSLER. 1980. Arterial foam cells with distinctive immunomorphologic and histochemical features of macrophages. Am. J. Pathol. **100:** 57–73.
30. GERRITY, R. G. 1981. The role of the monocyte in atherogenesis: I. Transition of blood-borne monocytes into foam cells in fatty lesions. Am. J. Pathol. **103:** 181–190.
31. FOGELMAN, A. M., I. SCHECHTER, M. HOKOM, J. S. CHILD & P. A. EDWARDS. 1980. Malondialdehyde alteration of low density lipoproteins leads to cholesterol ester accumulation in human monocyte macrophages. Proc. Natl. Acad. Sci. USA **77:** 2214–2218.
32. GOLDSTEIN, J. L., Y. K. HO, S. K. BASU & M. S. BROWN. 1979. Binding site on macrophages that mediates uptake and degradation of acetylated low density lipoprotein, producing massive cholesterol deposition. Proc. Natl. Acad. Sci. USA **76:** 333–337.
33. SALONEN, T., S. YLA-HERTTUALA, R. YAMAMOTO, S. BUTLER, H. KORPELA, R. SALONEN, K. NYYSSONEN, W. PALINSKI & J. L. WITZTUM. 1992. Autoantibody against oxidized LDL and progression of carotid atherosclerosis. Lancet **339:** 883–887.
34. FONG, L. G., S. PARTHASARATHY, J. L. WITZTUM & D. STEINBERG. 1987. Nonenzymatic oxidative cleavage of peptide bonds in apoprotein B-100. J. Lipid Res. **28:** 1466–1477.
35. MOREL, D. W., P. E. DiCORLETO & G. M. CHISOLM. 1984. Endothelial and smooth muscle cells alter low density lipoprotein in vitro by free radical oxidation. Arteriosclerosis **4:** 357–364.
36. CATHCORT, M. K., D. W. MOREL & G. M. CHISOLM. 1985. Monocytes and neutrophils oxidize low density lipoproteins making it cytotoxic. J. Leukocyte Biol. **38:** 341–350.
37. ESTERBAUER, H., M. DIEBER-ROTHENEDER, G. STRIEGL & G. WAEY. 1993. Role of vitamin E in preventing the oxidation of low density lipoprotein. Am. J. Clin. Nutr. **53:** 314s–321s.
38. JIALAL, I., E. NORKUS, L. CRISTOL & S. M. GRUNDY. 1991. Beta-carotene inhibits the oxidative modification of low-density lipoprotein. Biochim. Biophys. Acta **1086:** 134–138.
39. LAVY, A., A. B. AMOTZ & M. AVIRAM. 1993. Preferential inhibition of LDL oxidation by the all-trans isomer of beta-carotene in comparison with 9-cis beta-carotene. Eur. J. Clin. Chem. Clin. Biochem. **31:** 83–90.
40. PRINCEN, H. M. G., G. VAN POPPEL, C. VOGELEZANG, R. BUYTENHEK & F. J. KOK. 1992. Supplementation with vitamin E but not beta-carotene in vivo protects low density lipoprotein from lipid peroxidation in vitro: effect of cigarette smoking. Artheriosclerosis and Thrombosis. **12:** 554–562.

41. REAVEN, P. D., A. KHOUW, W. F. BELTZ, S. PARTHASARATHY & J. J. WITZTUM. 1993. Effect of dietary antioxidant combinations in humans: protection of LDL by vitamin E but not by beta-carotene. Arterioscler. Thromb. **13:** 590–600.

42. PRINCE, M. R., G. M. LaMURAGLIA & E. F. MacNICHOL. 1988. Increased preferential absorption in human atherosclerotic plaque with oral beta carotene: implications for laser endarterectomy. Circulation **78:** 338–344.

43. NAVAB, M., S. S. IMES, S. Y. HAMA, G. P. HOUGH, L. A. ROSS, R. W. BORK, A. J. VALENTE, J. A. BERLINER, D. C. DRINKWATER, H. LAKS & A. M. FOGELMAN. 1991. Monocyte transmigration induced by modification of low density lipoprotein in cocultures of human aortic wall cells is due to induction of monocyte chemotactic protein 1 synthesis and is abolished by high density lipoprotein. J. Clin Invest. **88:** 2039–2046.

Molecular Actions of Carotenoids[a]

JAMES ALLEN OLSON

Department of Biochemistry and Biophysics
3252 Molecular Biology Building
Iowa State University
Ames, Iowa 50011

INTRODUCTION

More than 600 carotenoids of established structure have been identified in nature, exclusive of isomeric forms. Isomers, however, play important specific biological roles among carotenoids and their cleavage products. In the case of α-carotene, for example, a total of 512 possible isomers exist. Although the number of possible isomers of symmetric carotenoids like β-carotene is much less, the total family of possible specific compounds in the carotenoid class numbers in the hundreds of thousands. Both carotenoids and their metabolites play crucial roles in biological systems, including essentially all forms of life. In this paper, some metabolic transformations of carotenoids will first be considered, followed by the biological functions of carotenoids and of selected metabolic products, and, then, by a discussion of various types of activities that carotenoids show in nature. The biosynthesis, metabolism, and actions of carotenoids have been judiciously considered in recent reviews.[1-8]

Metabolic Transformations of Carotenoids

The structure of β-carotene is given in FIGURE 1, together with the appropriate numbering of the carbon atoms. In nature, almost all of the positions in the β-carotene molecule, or its analogs, are the site of enzymatic reactions, namely, at C2, 3, 4, 5:6, 7:8, 9:10, 11:12, 13:14, 15:15', and 16. The other methyl groups, *i.e.*, C18, C19, and C20, are much less frequently attacked. Needless to say, the other half of the symmetrical molecule, *i.e.*, C1'–C20', are equally susceptible to enzymatic attack.

Hydrocarbon carotenoids are predominantly attacked initially by oxidative enzymes (TABLE 1). After oxygen has been introduced into the molecule, however, a variety of both oxidative and nonoxidative processes can occur (TABLE 1). The chemical transformation of carotenoids is extraordinarily dependent on the ambient conditions. Thus, in the presence of a catalyst, like activated SiO_2, oxygen and light, carotenoids are degraded very rapidly. On the other hand, carotenoids have been found in ancient fossil deposits in the bottom of China Lake in California, and their metabolic transformations *in vivo* tend to be slower than those of many

[a] Some of the research findings reported in this paper were supported by the National Institutes of Health (CA 46406) and by the US Department of Agriculture, CDFIN (91-34115-5903).

156

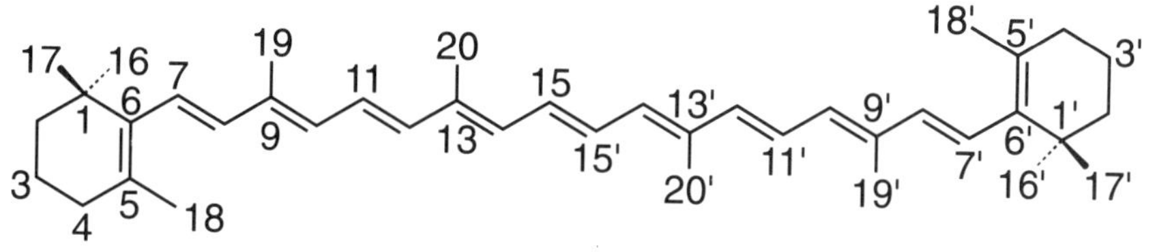

FIGURE 1. Structure of all-*trans* β-carotene.

other biological reactions. Thus, the precise conditions that are used in studying the transformation of carotenoids are of crucial importance.

In addition to the chemical transformation of carotenoids, the dioxocarotenoids readily form carotenoproteins in certain species, *e.g.*, crustacyanin in the lobster and in other crustacea. On the other hand, hydrocarbon carotenoids, which obviously do not have the ability to form Schiff bases, seem to bind to hydrophobic regions of proteins nonspecifically. In vertebrates, carotenoids are primarily carried in lipoproteins or are associated with membranes. Thus far, no specific well-characterized binding protein for hydrocarbon carotenoids has been convincingly shown to exist.

The Vitamin A Family

Various members of the vitamin A family are presented in FIGURE 2. The generally recognized parent of the family is 2A, or all-*trans* retinol. The interesting hydroxylated *retro* derivative (2B) plays a role in the growth of lymphoblastoid cells. The product of β-carotene oxidation is all-*trans* retinal (2C), which might be formed either directly by central cleavage of the β-carotene molecule or by step-wise cleavage via a group of β-apo-carotenals. Much attention has been devoted to all-*trans* retinoic acid (2D) and, in some instances, such as in the skin and in embryologic development, to its 3,4-didehydro derivative (2E). 9-*Cis* retinoic acid (2F) is an important ligand for the RXR group of nuclear transcription factors, 11-*cis* retinal (2G) plays an essential role in vertebrate vision, 13-*cis* retinal (2H) is involved in the bacteriorhodopsin cycle, and 13-*cis* retinoic acid (2I) both is a naturally occurring form of retinoic acid and has useful therapeutic effects on the skin.

The manner in which many of these compounds are formed in nature is given

TABLE 1. Enzymes Acting on Carotenoids

Oxidative	Nonoxidative
Dioxygenases	Aldehyde reductases
Epoxidases	Ketone reductases
Hydroxylases	Epoxide reductases
Dehydrogenases	Dehydrases
Aldehyde oxidases	Racemases
	Ene saturases
	Methoxy synthetases
	Fatty acyl transferases
	UDP-glucose transferases

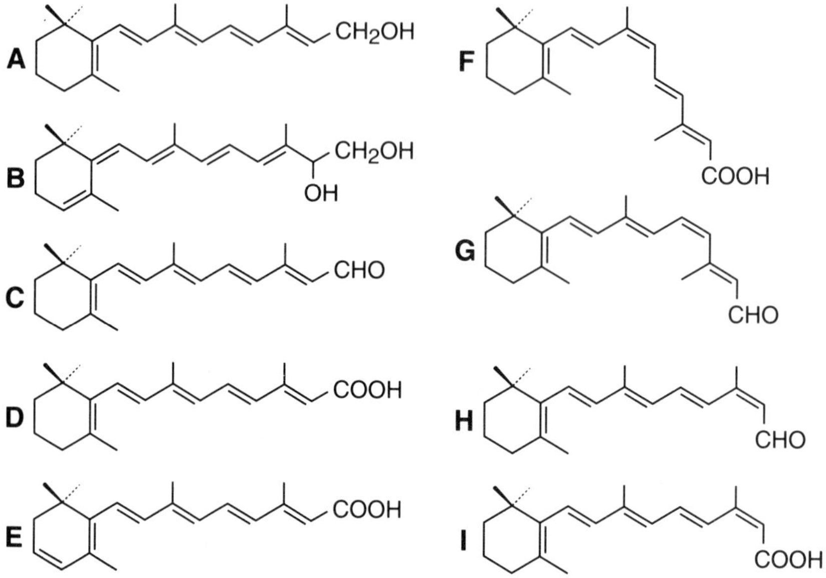

FIGURE 2. The vitamin A family. **(A)** all-*trans* retinol, **(B)** all-*trans* 14-hydroxyretroretinol, **(C)** all-*trans* retinaldehyde, **(D)** all-*trans* retinoic acid, **(E)** all-*trans*, 3,4-didehydroretinoic acid, **(F)** 9-*cis* retinoic acid, **(G)** 11-*cis* retinoic acid, **(H)** 13-*cis* retinal, **(I)** 13-*cis* retinoic acid.

in FIGURE 3. Ultimately, all forms of vitamin A are derived from carotenoids. In mammals, dioxygenases that attack one or more of the central double bonds ultimately give rise to all-*trans* retinal. Interestingly, fish are more versatile, in that both ketocarotenoids and xanthophylls can be reduced to provitamin A carotenoids before cleavage. Except for the formation of 11-*cis* retinol from all-*trans* retinol via retinyl ester in the eye,[9] the biological pathway for the synthesis of other isomers of retinol is not known. In the presence of light, of course, a mixture of most of the mono-*cis* isomers and, indeed, some of the di-*cis* and even tri-*cis* isomers are formed from the all-*trans* isomer in chemical studies. Although all-*trans* retinol is readily converted to 13-*cis* retinol *in vivo*, little is known about the mechanism of synthesis of the 9-*cis* isomer. The enzymes responsible for esterification and for oxidation-reduction reactions in this family, however, have been extensively studied.

The Trisporic Acid Family

Major members of the trisporic acid family are depicted in FIGURE 4. These compounds are produced when plus and minus strains of the fungal order *Mucorales* are incubated together. The trisporic acids, in turn, enhance the synthesis of β-carotene and related carotenoids by 15- to 24-fold.[10–12] The synthesis of sterols

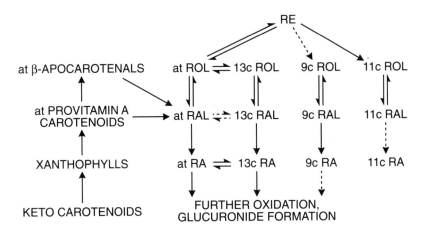

FIGURE 3. Biological formation of vitamin A from carotenoids. RE, retinyl ester; ROL, retinol; RAL, retinal; RA, retinoic acid; at, all-*trans*; 9c, 9-*cis*; 11c, 11-*cis*; 13c, 13-*cis*. *Full arrows* are demonstrated reactions; *dotted arrows* are proposed reactions.

is also enhanced by trisporic acids, even in noncarotenoid producing fungi.[12] As a result of the sexual fusion of these strains, zygospores are also produced.[10,11]

The putative pathway for the formation of trisporic acids from all-*trans* β-carotene[10,11] is given in FIGURE 5. β-Carotene is oxidatively cleaved, either directly to a C18 ketone analog or via retinal. The β-ionone ring is then oxidized through the hydroxy-derivative to the 4-oxo group. Thereafter, the 16 methyl group is oxidized through several stages to a carboxyl group. The 11:12 double bond is then saturated to yield all-*trans* trisporic acid B, which might then be isomerized

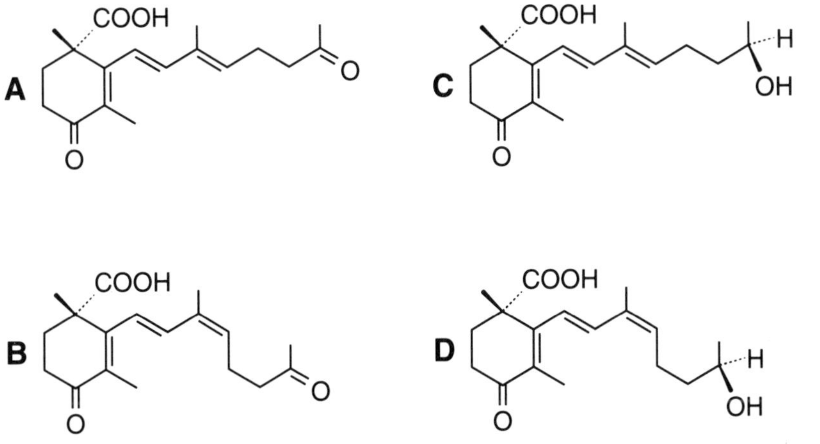

FIGURE 4. The trisporic acid family. **(A)** all-*trans* trisporic acid B, **(B)** 9-*cis* trisporic acid B, **(C)** all-*trans* trisporic acid C, **(D)** 9-*cis* trisporic acid C.

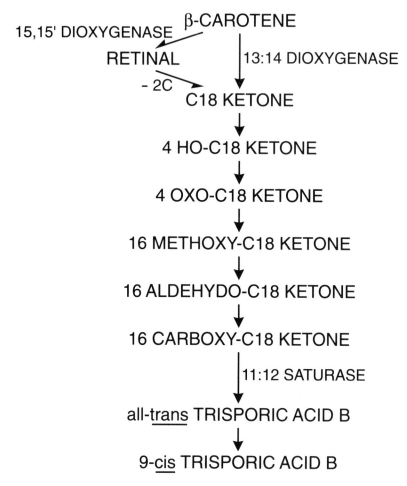

FIGURE 5. Putative pathway for the formation of trisporic acid from all-*trans* β-carotene.

to the 9-*cis* isomer. The sequence of some of these steps may be different, or, indeed, multiple pathways to the product may exist. Interestingly, the 9-*cis* trisporic acid B is approximately twice as active as the other three forms given in FIGURE 4 in stimulating zygospore formation.[10]

The Abscisic Acid Family

The structures of abscisic acid and of two of its derivatives, the 16-hydroxy compound and phaseic acid, are depicted in FIGURE 6. Abscisic acid, which is produced in plants in response to low temperature or water stress, is involved both in leaf abscission and in physiological responses to preserve water. A large number of genes, termed the RAB (responsive to abscisic acid) genes, are expressed in the presence of abscisic acid. The expression of various proteins in response to abscisic acid and the interaction of abscisic acid with gibberellin and other plant hormones is being actively explored at this time.[14,15]

Although abscisic acid might be derived directly from farnesyl pyrophosphate, a more probable source is violaxanthin. A possible pathway for its biosynthesis from violaxanthin is given in FIGURE 7. A 13:14 dioxygenase would yield a C18 ketone derivative (7B), which, by a sequence of several oxidative steps, would lose CO_2 and be converted to the all-*trans* 17-carbon precursor of abscisic acid (7C). After formation of the 9-*cis* product (7D), a rearrangement in the 5:6 epoxide and dehydrogenation of the C4 hydroxy to a keto group would yield abscisic acid. The sequence of biosynthetic steps, of course, could be different.

Although abscisic acid is known to have marked effects on gene expression, the transcription factors for it have not as yet been identified. Similarly, none of the enzymes involved has been isolated and studied.

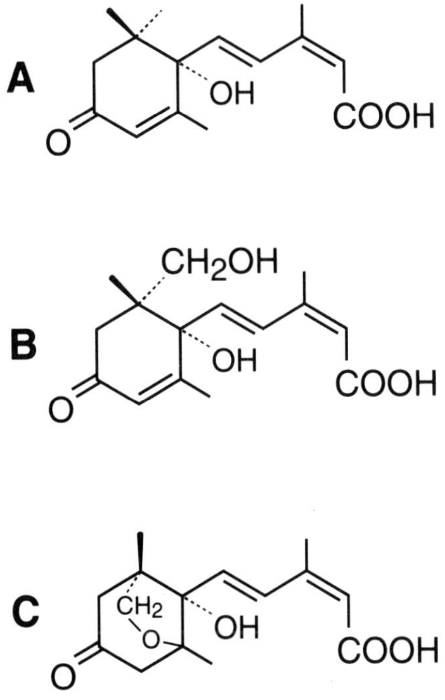

FIGURE 6. The abscisic acid family. (**A**) abscisic acid, (**B**) 16-hydroxyabscisic acid, (**C**) phaseic acid.

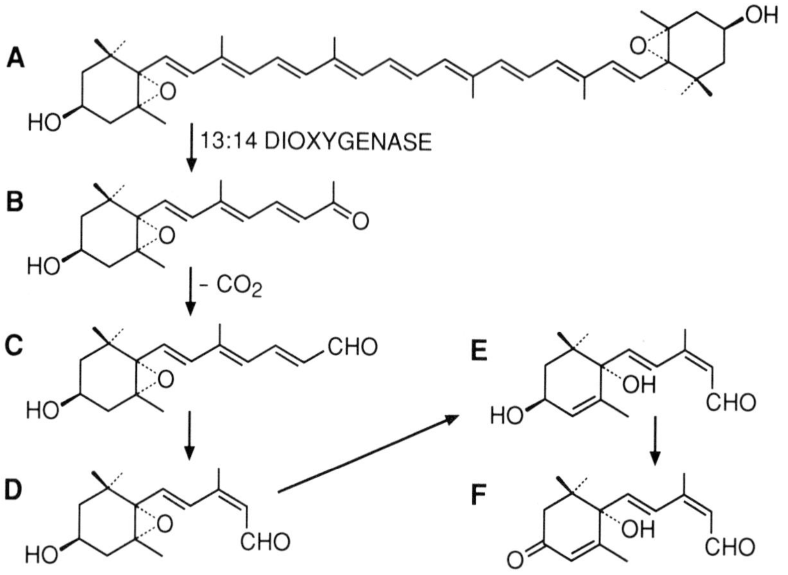

FIGURE 7. A possible pathway for the formation of abscisic acid from carotenoids. **(A)** violaxanthin, **(B)** C18 ketone of violaxanthin, **(C)** C17 aldehyde intermediate, **(D)** 9-*cis* xanthoxin, **(E)** 3-hydroxyabscisic acid, **(F)** abscisic acid.

Metabolism of Carotenoid Analogs

As indicated above, both in plants and in animals, a given carotenoid may be metabolized in quite different ways. In studies with human volunteers, the appearance in the plasma of several quite different carotenoids was examined.[16] When ethyl β-apo-8′carotenoate, β-apo-8′carotenal and 4,4′dimethoxy-β-carotene were administered to humans, all three appeared in the blood in reproducible but different kinetic patterns.[16] Of interest in a metabolic context, ethyl-β-apo-8′carotenoate was not detectably converted to any product. In contrast, β-apo-8′carotenal was rapidly reduced and esterified with long-chain fatty acids, as

TABLE 2. Major Metabolites of Carotenoid Analogs Detected in Human Serum

Compound	Metabolites
Ethyl-β-apo-8′carotenoate	none
β-Apo-8′carotenal	β-apo-8′carotenol β-apo-8′carotenyl esters β-apo-8′carotenoic acid retinyl ester
4,4′Dimethoxy-β-carotene	4′monomethoxyisozeaxanthin isozeaxanthin canthaxanthin

TABLE 3. Probable Biological Functions of Carotenoids and Their Metabolites

Compound	Organism	Function
Many carotenoids	plants, funghi, bacteria	light absorption and antioxidant protection in photosynthesis
cis-Canthaxanthin	artemia	cyst development and sexual maturation
Canthaxanthin	crustacea	carapace coloration and protein stability
Many carotenoids	birds, fish	sex-related protective coloration
Trisporic acid	mucorales, other funghi	carotenoid and sterol synthesis, sexual maturation
Abscisic acid	plants	abscission, responses to water-stress and wounding
Retinal	halobacteria	light-induced ion pumping, phototaxis
Vitamin A family	vertebrates	vision, cell differentiation
Canthaxanthin, β-carotene, lycopene	human and mouse cells	gap junction communication

well as being oxidized to carotenoic acid. Furthermore, β-apo-8′carotenal was converted by oxidative cleavage reactions to retinal, which was then reduced to retinol and esterified. In the case of 4,4′dimethoxy-β-carotene, no cleavage reactions were observed, but the methoxy groups were removed, and the resultant free hydroxyl groups could also be converted to oxo groups (TABLE 2). In essence, each of these carotenoids was metabolized by the human intestine in very different ways. Thus, generalizations about preferred pathways of carotenoid metabolism are fraught with peril.

Biological Functions

The probable biological functions of carotenoids and their metabolites are summarized in TABLE 3. Many carotenoids in plants, funghi and bacteria are involved both in trapping light, which is then transferred quite efficiently to the photosynthetic reaction center, and also in protecting chlorophyll and other photosensitive molecules from free radical degradation.[17] In the brine shrimp *Artemia,* the ratio of *cis* to *trans* canthaxanthins increases with the development of cysts and seems to be enriched in sexual-related tissues.[18] In crustacea, canthaxanthin, as already mentioned, makes precise covalent linkages with specific lysine residues in protein, and many carotenoids provide both dramatic and protective coloration in birds and fish. The biological functions of trisporic acid[10-12] and of abscisic acid[13-15] have already been discussed. In halobacteria, all-*trans* and 13-*cis* retinal are ligands for bacteriorhodopsin, halorhodopsin, and other pigments that are involved in ion pumping, in phototaxis and possibly in other light-sensitive functions.[20,21]

The effects of various members of the vitamin A family, and particularly the roles of 11-*cis* retinal in vision and of all-*trans* and 9-*cis* retinoic acid in cell differentiation, have been reviewed.[3,22,23] Finally, the interesting recent finding that carotenoids as well as retinoids can stimulate gap junction communication, particularly by the induction of the connexin-43 gene,[24,25] is of great current interest. In the latter case, whether these carotenoids must be converted to a retinoid-like molecule or are acting per se in binding to some transcription factor in the nucleus is still unclear.

Functions, Actions and Associations

Carotenoids and their metabolites act in various ways on biological systems. In this context, it is useful to distinguish those activities that are established *functions*, those that are *actions*, often induced by the administration of large doses of carotenoids, and those that are *associations*, mainly of an epidemiological nature. Different activities of carotenoids and a tentative classification of each activity are provided in TABLE 4.

TABLE 4. Some Biological Activities of Carotenoids

Nature	Example
Functions	Light gathering in plants and photosynthetic bacteria Protection against light-induced peroxidation Vitamin A formation Coloration related to protection and sexual processes
Actions	Reduced skin reactions in photosensitivity diseases Reduced leukoplakia Reduced buccal micronuclei in betel-nut chewers Reduced free-radical formation in some ambients Reduced photo-induced neoplasm Reduced mutagenesis Reduced sister chromatid exchange Reduced cell transformation *in vitro* Increased immune responsiveness *in vivo* Increased quenching of singlet oxygen
Associations	Reduced lung cancer incidence Possible reduction in other precancerous and cancerous conditions, *e.g.*, cervical dysplasia Possible reduction in atherosclerosis

Various functions of carotenoids and their metabolites have already been summarized. A large variety of effects, including those seen in purely chemical systems, in various types of biological systems, and in experimental animals and humans *in vivo* are listed under actions. Some of these observations may be very relevant to physiological events and to the prevention of chronic diseases, and others may not be.

Finally, associations, largely in epidemiological studies, have been made between carotenoid intake and a lowered risk of various diseases. While worthwhile as a starting point for the development of public health measures, causal relationships cannot be inferred on the basis of such studies. After such associations have been shown, the next logical step is an intervention trial, in which the effects of a given carotenoid on the incidence of a given disease in a population is tested.[26] If a protective effect is shown in such intervention studies, the relative risk of different groups in the population must then be assessed. The effect must also be in keeping with the known biochemical and physiological roles of the compound. Clearly, the establishment of a public health policy first requires the most judicious consideration of all available information.

SUMMARY

Carotenoids can be attacked enzymatically at almost every position in the molecule. On the other hand, under dark nonoxidative conditions, they can be very stable. Thus, the precise chemical and biological environment is of crucial importance in determining whether, and how, they are transformed.

Three important biologically active derivatives of carotenoids, vitamin A, trisporic acid and abscisic acid, all of which serve as hormones in appropriate cells, are, or can be, formed from precursor carotenoids. Highly active forms of all three hormones are 9-*cis* isomers. In all cases, the products are involved both in light-induced reactions as well as in cellular differentiation, often related to sexual maturation.

Each of these hormones is formed by an initial dioxygenase attack on the central conjugated chain of carotenoids followed by a series of specific reactions. Indeed, when various carotenoids of different structure are studied in humans, each shows a characteristic, if not unique, set of metabolites. Thus, generalizations about carotenoid metabolism must be constrained by precise metabolic information about given compounds.

In dealing with the manifold biological activities of carotenoids, it is useful to categorize them as functions, actions or associations. In the hope of gaining greater insight into the relationship between carotenoids, health and longevity, these distinctions should be helpful.

REFERENCES

1. ISLER, O., Ed. 1971. Carotenoids. Birkhäuser Verlag, Basel, Switzerland.
2. PORTER, J. W. & S. L. SPURGEON, Eds. 1983. Biosynthesis of Isoprenoid Compounds. Vol. 2. John Wiley & Sons, New York, NY.
3. OLSON, J. A. 1993. Vitamin A, retinoids and carotenoids. *In* Modern Nutrition in Health and Disease. M. E. Shils, J. A. Olson & M. Shike, Eds. 8th edit. 287–307. Lea & Febiger. Philadelphia, PA.
4. SANDMANN, G. 1991. Biosynthesis of cyclic carotenoids: biochemistry and molecular genetics of the reaction sequence. Physiol. Plant. **83:** 186–193.
5. OLSON, J. A. 1992. Carotenoids and vitamin A: an overview. *In* Lipid Soluble Antioxidants: Biochemistry and Clinical Applications. A. S. H. Ong & L. Packer, Eds. 178–191. Birkhäuser Verlag. Basel, Switzerland.
6. OLSON, J. A. 1989. Provitamin A function of carotenoids: the conversion of β-carotene into vitamin A. J. Nutr. **119:** 105–108.
7. BENDICH, A. & J. A. OLSON. 1989. Biological actions of carotenoids. FASEB J. **3:** 1927–1932.
8. BRITTON, G., Ed. 1991. 9th International Symposium on Carotenoids. Pure Appl. Chem. **63:** 1–176.
9. RANDO, R. R. 1990. The chemistry of vitamin A in vision. Angew. Chem. Int. Ed. Engl. **29:** 461–480.
10. BU'LOCK, J. D. 1983. Trisporic acids. *In* Biosynthesis of Isoprenoid Compounds. J. W. Porter & S. L. Spurgeon, Eds. Vol. **2:** 437–462. John Wiley & Sons. New York, NY.

11. LAMPILA, L. E., S. E. WALLEN & L. B. BULLERMAN. 1985. A review of factors affecting biosynthesis of carotenoids by the order *Mucorales*. Mycopathologia **90:** 65–80.
12. YANG, S. S., C. K. LIN & C. Y. LIU. 1986. Sexuality and steroid distribution in *Mucorales*. Proc. Natl. Sci. Counc. Repub. China, Part B: Life Sci. **10:** 13–19.
13. MILBORROW, B. V. 1983. Biosynthesis of abscisic acid and related compounds. *In* Biosynthesis of Isoprenoid Compounds. J. W. Porter & S. L. Spurgeon, Eds. Vol. **2:** 413–436. John Wiley & Sons. New York, NY.
14. SKRIVER, K. & J. MUNDY. 1990. Gene expression in response to abscisic acid and osmotic stress. Plant Cell **2:** 503–512.
15. MARCOTTE, W. R., JR., N. J. GUILTINAN & R. S. QUATRANO. 1992. ABA-regulated gene expression, *cis*-acting sequences and *trans*-acting factors. Biochem. Soc. Trans. **20:** 93–96.
16. ZENG, S., H. C. FURR & J. A. OLSON. 1992. Metabolism of carotenoid analogs in humans. Am. J. Clin. Nutr. **56:** 433–439.
17. KRINSKY, N. I. 1989. Antioxidant functions of carotenoids. Free Radical Biol. Med. **7:** 617–635.
18. NELIS, H. J. C. F., P. LAVENS, M. M. Z. VAN STEENBERG, P. SORGELOOS, G. R. CRIEL & A. P. DE LEENHEER. 1988. Qualitative and quantitative changes in the carotenoid during development of the brine shrimp *Artemia*. J. Lipid Res. **29:** 491–499.
19. BRUSH, A. H. 1990. Metabolism of carotenoid pigments in birds. FASEB J. **4:** 2969–2977.
20. MATHIES, R. A., S. W. LIN, J. B. AMES & W. T. POLLARD. 1991. From femtoseconds to biology: mechanism of bacteriorhodopsin's light-driven proton pump. Annu. Rev. Biophys. Biophys. Chem. **20:** 491–518.
21. OESTERHELT, D., J. TITTOR & E. BAMBERG. 1992. A unifying concept for ion translocation by retinal proteins. J. Bioenerg. Biomembr. **24:** 181–191.
22. HASHIMOTO, Y. & K. SHUDO. 1991. Retinoids and their nuclear receptors. Cell Rev. **25:** 209–235.
23. DE LUCA, L. M. 1991. Retinoids and their receptors in differentiation, embryogenesis and neoplasia. FASEB J. **5:** 2924–2933.
24. ZHANG, L.-X., R. V. COONEY & J. S. BERTRAM. 1991. Carotenoids enhance gap junctional communication and inhibit lipid peroxidation in C3H/10T1/2 cells: relationship to their cancer chemopreventive action. Carcinogenesis **12:** 2309–2314.
25. HOSSAIN, M. Z., L.-X. ZHANG & J. S. BERTRAM. 1992. Mechanistic studies of cancer chemoprevention by retinoids and carotenoids. *In* Retinoids: Progress in Research and Clinical Applications. M. A. Livrea & L. Packer, Eds. 361–381. Marcel Dekker Inc. New York, NY.

Mechanism of Carotenoid Cleavage to Retinoids[a]

NORMAN I. KRINSKY,[b,d] XIANG-DONG WANG,[b,c]
GUANGWEN TANG,[c] AND ROBERT M. RUSSELL[c]

[b]Department of Biochemistry
Tufts University School of Medicine
and
[c]Human Nutrition Research Center on Aging at Tufts University
Boston, Massachusetts 02111

INTRODUCTION

Within one year of the discovery by Moore in 1930 that β-carotene could be converted *in vivo* to vitamin A (retinol),[1] Karrer proposed that retinol is formed by a hydrolytic cleavage of the central 15, 15'-double bond of β-carotene.[2] Then, in the late 1940s, investigators discovered that the intestine was the major site for β-carotene metabolism, forming retinal, which was subsequently reduced to retinol. As no other products were observed, a consensus developed that the original Karrer hypothesis required a modification, which involved an oxidative cleavage of the central double bond of β-carotene. However, Glover and his associates, starting in 1954,[3–5] presented a series of observations that culminated in the hypothesis that β-carotene could undergo cleavage at the 15, 15'-double bond (central cleavage), as well as at the other double bonds in the polyene chain (excentric cleavage).[6] This hypothesis was partially supported by observations that the apo-carotenals (8'-, 10'-, and 12'-) were effectively converted into retinol in rats, as well as being oxidized to their corresponding carotenoic acids.[3,4,7–10] In addition, these apo-carotenals were identified in the intestine of chickens after the administration of β-carotene,[11] and could serve as substrates for a partially purified enzyme preparation from both rabbit and guinea pig intestine.[12–14] Ganguly and Sastry claimed that the "weight of the evidence so far is overwhelmingly in favor of random cleavage and is against any specific attack at the central double bond of the carotene molecule."[15] However, even recent reviews of both pathways are ambiguous in their conclusions.[16,17] Olson stated that "to remain viable as an alternative pathway in mammals, the excentric cleavage hypothesis clearly requires unambiguous direct supporting evidence."[18] Several recent publications have taken advantage of the ability of citral to differentiate between these two pathways, and offer this direct supporting evidence.[19–21] The topic has been the

[a] This study was funded by Grant R01CA49195-01A3 from the National Institutes of Health, Bethesda, MD, and in part by Federal funds from the U.S. Department of Agriculture, Agricultural Research Service under contract number 53-3K06-01. The contents of this publication do not necessarily reflect the views or policies of the U.S. Department of Agriculture, nor does mention of trade names, commercial products, or organizations imply endorsement by the U.S. Government.

[b] Address correspondence to: Dr. Norman I. Krinsky, Department of Biochemistry, Tufts University School of Medicine, 136 Harrison Avenue, Boston, MA 02111.

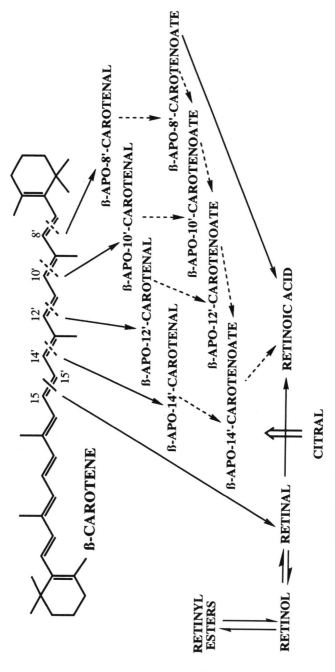

FIGURE 1. The central and excentric cleavage mechanism for converting β-carotene to retinoids.

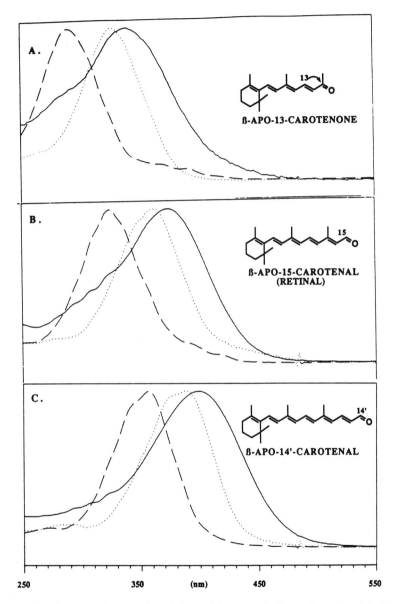

FIGURE 2. The spectral properties of β-apo-14′-carotenal, β-apo-15-carotenal (retinal), and β-apo-13-carotenone (————), their reduction products (·······), and their O-ethyl-oximes (— — —). (From Handelman *et al.*[27] Reprinted by permission from Pergamon Press.)

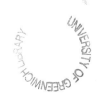

subject of a recent review,[22] and is summarized in FIGURE 1. The β-apo-carotenoic acids corresponding to the β-apo-14'-, 12'-, 10'-, and 8'-carotenal have been isolated and characterized in rat and chicken tissues,[11,15] and it is anticipated that these compounds will be found in human tissues in the near future. It has also been suggested that the excentric cleavage activity can metabolize xanthophylls such as canthaxanthin, isozeaxanthin and astaxanthin.[23]

Other tissues may not be as active with respect to excentric cleavage. For example, the hybrid rat intestinal epithelial cell line, hBRIE 380, converts β-carotene to retinol and retinoic acid, without the appearance of either retinal or retinyl esters.[24] However, it is not clear if these investigators monitored their experiments for β-apo-carotenal production. Other experiments with rat intestinal homogenates have detected the conversion of β-carotene to retinoic acid, without the formation of retinal.[25]

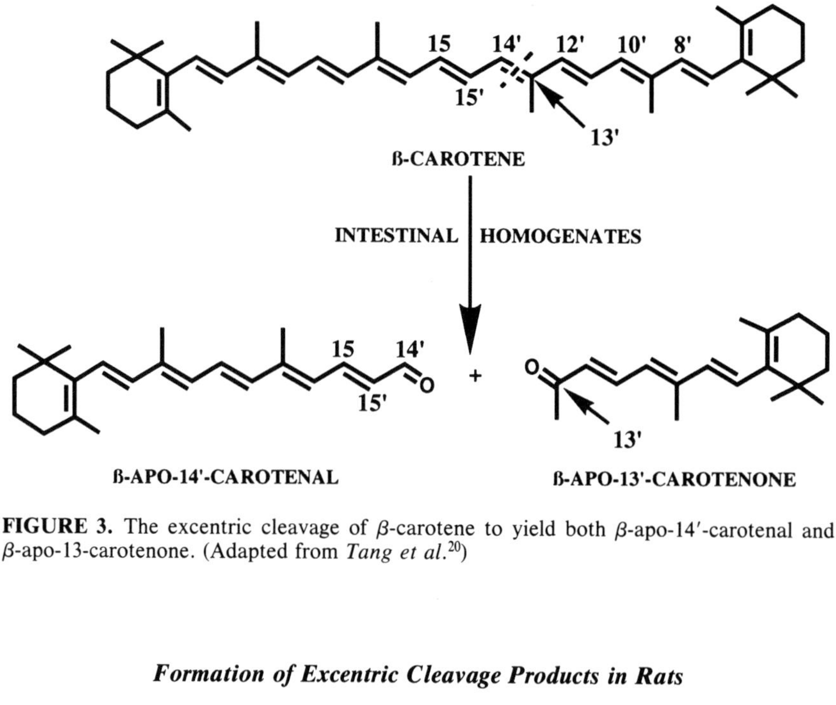

FIGURE 3. The excentric cleavage of β-carotene to yield both β-apo-14'-carotenal and β-apo-13-carotenone. (Adapted from *Tang et al.*[20])

Formation of Excentric Cleavage Products in Rats

We demonstrated earlier that the incubation of homogenates of rat intestinal mucosa with β-carotene resulted in the formation of retinal, retinoic acid, and the β-apo-12'-, 10'-, and 8'-carotenals.[19] Our controls, lacking either 2 μM β-carotene or the intestinal homogenate, did not produce any apo-carotenals, unlike other reports.[26] However, the sample incubated with β-carotene in the absence of the intestinal homogenate did show minor peaks that were less polar than the apo-carotenals, and might represent spontaneous oxidation products such as epoxides.[27–29] We have not attempted to further characterize these peaks.

The conversion of β-carotene to apo-carotenals in this system is completely

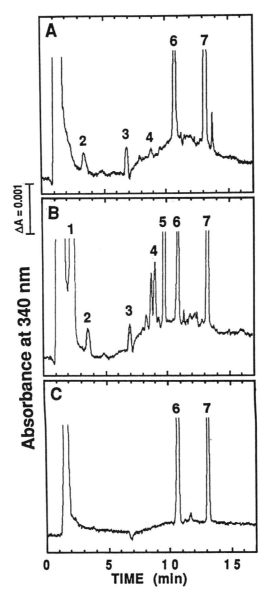

FIGURE 4. HPLC chromatography of extracts of human intestinal homogenates incubated with 2 μM β-apo-8′-carotenal in the absence **(A)** or presence **(B)** of 2 mM citral, and in a control vial lacking the homogenate **(C)**. Peak identification: (1) citral, (2) retinoic acid, (3) β-apo-13-carotenone, (4) retinal, (5) metabolite of citral, (6) retinyl acetate as the internal standard, and (7) β-apo-8′-carotenal. (From Wang *et al.*[21] Reprinted by permission from Academic Press.)

TABLE 1. β-Carotene, β-Apo-Carotenals, Retinol and Retinyl Esters in Ferret Intestinal Mucosa before and after Perfusion of β-Carotene[35,a]

	Perfusion Time (Hr)			
	0 ($n = 5$)	1 ($n = 3$)	4 ($n = 4$)	6 ($n = 3$)
β-Carotene	ND*	1590 ± 278†	800 ± 218†	Trace*
β-Apo-12'-carotenal	ND*	105 ± 11†	117 ± 21†	ND*
β-Apo-10'-carotenal	ND*	42 ± 4†	51 ± 17†	ND*
Retinol	0.8 ± 0.8*	19 ± 10†‡	30 ± 4†	6 ± 4*‡
Retinyl esters	50 ± 22*	1014 ± 101†	781 ± 63†	265 ± 85*

[a] Data shown (in pmol/g mucosa) are means ± SE; n, no. of animals. For each compound, data not sharing a common superscript are significantly different at $p < 0.05$. Time 0, including biopsy from 3 ferrets before the perfusion and 2 ferrets without successful lymph cannulation; time 6, additional 2 hr perfusion of 5% dextrose after 4 hr perfusion of β-carotene. ND: not detected. Retinyl esters include retinyl oleate, linoleate, palmitate and stearate.

dependent on the presence of dithiothreitol, and is somewhat enhanced by the addition of NAD^+. Disulfiram completely blocks these reactions.[19]

In addition to the apo-carotenals listed above, two prominent peaks appeared in our HPLC separations.[19] Based on their spectral properties, retention times, reduction with sodium borohydride to a more polar product, and ease of formation of an oxime derivative after treatment with O-ethyl-hydroxylamine, we suspected that these compounds were the larger (β-apo-14'-carotenal) and smaller (β-apo-13-carotenone) homologues of retinal, as seen in FIGURE 2.[27] A GC-MS analysis of these isolated peaks confirmed that they were these homologues, and could be formed by oxidative cleavage of the 13, 14-double bond of β-carotene, as seen in FIGURE 3.[20]

Formation of Excentric Cleavage Products in Human Tissue

In addition to the rat, intestinal mucosal homogenates from humans, monkeys and ferrets were also able to convert β-carotene to the β-apo-14'-, 12'-, 10'-, and 8'-carotenals, β-apo-13-carotenone, retinal and retinoic acid.[19,20] However, these observations did not prove unambiguously that the retinoic acid arose *via* excentric cleavage, for it could have come from a central cleavage process. In order to resolve this issue, we used citral, a monoterpene (3,7-dimethyl-2,6-octadienal) that inhibits the oxidation of retinal to retinoic acid, both *in vivo* and *in vitro*.[30,31] We were able to confirm that 1 mM citral completely inhibited the conversion of added retinal to retinoic acid in human intestinal mucosa homogenates, without affecting the conversion of β-carotene to retinoic acid.[21] As seen in FIGURE 4, β-apo-8'-carotenal could also be converted to retinoic acid, again without any interference by added 2 mM citral.[21]

Ferret Intestinal Perfusion

One of the basic problems in studying carotenoid metabolism is the absence of an adequate experimental model that mimics human β-carotene metabolism.

Most common laboratory animals do not absorb carotenoids such as β-carotene, unless they are administered in very large doses.[32] Recently, it was demonstrated that the domesticated ferret (*Mustela putorius furo*) can absorb β-carotene from the diet,[33,34] and we set out to measure the rate of uptake and absorption of β-carotene after perfusion through the small intestine.[35] As with the *in vitro* experiments described above, we were able to observe the appearance of β-apocarotenals, in addition to retinol and retinyl esters, in the intestinal mucosa during perfusion with β-carotene (TABLE 1). When 15, 15'-[^{14}C]-β-carotene was perfused through the intestine, considerable amounts of products more polar than retinol were found in the intestinal mucosa, and these polar products were preferentially absorbed through the portal venous system, whereas retinol and retinyl esters were absorbed mainly in the mesenteric lymph. The rate of absorption of β-carotene was determined to be 54 ng/hr/100 cm intestine,[35] which compares very favorably with the values of 38–120 ng/hr/100 cm intestine reported in humans.[36,37]

To demonstrate that retinoic acid was among the polar products absorbed through the portal venous system, we isolated the single retinoic acid fraction by HPLC, derivatized it to its methyl ester, and used GC/MS for further characterization. As can be seen in FIGURE 5, the GC/MS retention time and molecular ion of m/z 314 matched that of authentic methylretinoate. Although the HPLC separation did not resolve cis-trans isomers of retinoic acid, it is apparent from FIGURE 5, that four bands, all with the same molecular ion, m/z 314, are present in the retinoic acid fraction obtained by HPLC, and presumably represent four different cis-trans isomers.[38]

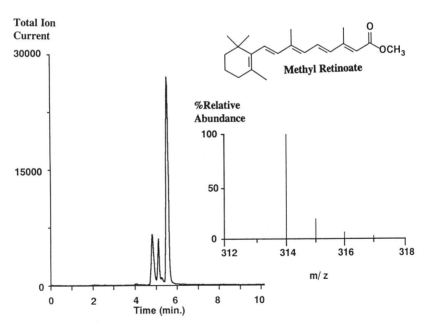

FIGURE 5. GC/MS total ion chromatography and negative ion chemical ionization mass spectrum (*inset*) of the methylated retinoic acid peak from ferret portal blood. The GC/MS retention time matched that of authentic methylretinoate, as did the molecular ion at m/z 314. (From Wang *et al.*[38] Reprinted by permission from Elsevier Press.)

During the period of β-carotene perfusion, the portal blood retinoic acid concentration increased 3-fold, while there was no change in the concentration of retinyl esters. However, during this perfusion period, there was a significant drop in the concentration of retinol, which may indicate some regulatory function of serum retinoic acid on serum retinol levels.[38]

CONCLUSION

An excentric cleavage pathway exists for the conversion of β-carotene to β-apo-carotenoids and retinoic acid in intestinal homogenates of humans, ferrets, monkeys and rats. The formation of retinoic acid occurs even in the presence of citral, an inhibitor of retinal oxidation. Furthermore, when β-carotene is perfused through the small intestine of ferrets, it is absorbed at a rate comparable to that of humans, and β-apo-carotenoids are found in the intestinal mucosa, along with polar retinoid products. Among the polar products in the perfused ferret small intestine is retinoic acid, which on GC/MS analysis, consists of a mixture of four cis-trans isomers. Thus, β-carotene can be converted to retinoic acid by an excentric cleavage process, and this process may be involved in the formation of cis-trans isomers of retinoic acid.

REFERENCES

1. MOORE, T. 1930. Vitamin A and carotene. VI. The conversion of carotene to vitamin A *in vivo*. Biochem. J. **24:** 696–702.
2. KARRER, P., R. MORF & K. SCHÖPP. 1931. Zur kenntnis des vitamins-A aus fischtranen II. Helv. Chim. Acta **14:** 1431–1436.
3. GLOVER, J. & E. R. REDFEARN. 1954. The mechanism of the transformation of β-carotene into vitamin A *in vivo*. Biochem. J. **58:** xv–xvi.
4. FAZAKERLEY, S. & J. GLOVER. 1957. The provitamin A activity of some possible intermediates in β-carotene metabolism. Biochem. J. **65:** 38P–39P.
5. FISHWICK, M. J. & J. GLOVER. 1957. The metabolism of uniformly ^{14}C-labelled· β-carotene in the rat. Biochem. J. **66:** 36P–37P.
6. GLOVER, J. 1960. The conversion of β-carotene into vitamin A. *In* Vitamins and Hormones. R. S. Harris & D. J. Ingle, Eds. Vol. 18: 371–386. Academic Press. New York and London.
7. KARRER, P. & U. SOLMSSEN. 1937. β-Carotinal, ein abbauprodukt des β-carotins. Helv. Chim. Acta **20:** 682–691.
8. BRUBACHER, G., U. GLOOR & O. WISS. 1960. Zum stoffwechsel von β-apo-8'-carotenal (C_{30}). Chimia **14:** 19–20.
9. AL-HASANI, S. M. & D. B. PARRISH. 1968. Vitamin A activity of β-apo-carotenals in Coturnix Coturnix Japonica. J. Nutr. **94:** 402–406.
10. SHARMA, R. V., S. N. MATHUR & J. GANGULY. 1976. Studies on the relative biopotencies and intestinal absorption of different apo-β-carotenoids in rats and chickens. Biochem. J. **158:** 377–383.
11. SHARMA, R. V., S. N. MATHUR, A. A. DIMITROVSKII, R. DAS & J. GANGULY. 1977. Studies on the metabolism of β-carotene and apo-β-carotenoids in rats and chickens. Biochim. Biophys. Acta **486:** 183–194.
12. LAKSHMANAN, M. R., J. L. POPE & J. A. OLSON. 1968. The specificity of a partially purified carotenoid cleavage enzyme of rabbit intestine. Biochem. Biophys. Res. Commun. **33:** 347–352.
13. LAKSHMANAN, M. R., H. CHANSANG & J. A. OLSON. 1972. Purification and properties of carotene 15,15'-dioxygenase of rabbit intestine. J. Lipid Res. **13:** 477–482.

14. SINGH, H. & H. R. CAMA. 1974. Enzymatic cleavage of carotenoids. Biochim. Biophys. Acta **370:** 49–61.

15. GANGULY, J. & P. S. SASTRY. 1985. Mechanism of conversion of β-carotene into vitamin A-central cleavage versus random cleavage. World Rev. Nutr. Diet. **45:** 198–220.

16. GERBER, L. E. & K. L. SIMPSON. 1990. Carotenoid cleavage: alternate pathways. Methods Enzymol. **189:** 433–436.

17. OLSON, J. A. & M. R. LAKSHMAN. 1990. Carotenoid conversions. Methods Enzymol. **189:** 425–432.

18. OLSON, J. A. 1989. Provitamin A function of carotenoids: the conversion of β-carotene into vitamin A. J. Nutr. **119:** 105–108.

19. WANG, X.-D., G.-W. TANG, J. G. FOX, N. I. KRINSKY & R. M. RUSSELL. 1991. Enzymatic conversion of β-carotene into β-apo-carotenals and retinoids by human, monkey, ferret, and rat tissues. Arch. Biochem. Biophys. **285:** 8–16.

20. TANG, G., X.-D. WANG, N. I. KRINSKY & R. M. RUSSELL. 1991. Characterization of β-apo-13-carotenone and β-apo-14'-carotenal as enzymatic products of the excentric cleavage of β-carotene. Biochemistry **30:** 9829–9834.

21. WANG, X.-D., N. I. KRINSKY, G. TANG & R. M. RUSSELL. 1992. Retinoic acid can be produced from excentric cleavage of β-carotene in human intestinal mucosa. Arch. Biochem. Biophys. **293:** 293–304.

22. KRINSKY, N. I., X.-D. WANG, G. TANG & R. M. RUSSELL. 1993. Conversion of carotenoids to retinoids. *In* Retinoids: Progress in Research and Clinical Applications. M. A. Livrea & L. Packer, Eds. 1–16. Marcel Dekker. New York.

23. DIMITROVSKII, A. A. 1991. Metabolism of natural retinoids and their functions. *In* New Trends in Biological Chemistry. T. Ozawa, Ed. 297–308. Japan Sci. Soc. Press. Tokyo.

24. SCITA, G., G. W. APONTE & G. WOLF. 1992. Uptake and cleavage of β-carotene by cultures of rat small intestinal cells and human lung fibroblasts. J. Nutr. Biochem. **3:** 118–123.

25. NAPOLI, J. L. & K. R. RACE. 1988. Biogenesis of retinoic acid from β-carotene. Differences between the metabolism of β-carotene and retinal. J. Biol. Chem. **263:** 17372–17377.

26. HANSEN, S. & W. MARET. 1988. Retinal is not formed *in vitro* by enzymatic central cleavage of β-carotene. Biochemistry **27:** 200–206.

27. HANDELMAN, G. J., F. J. G. M. VAN KUIJK, A. CHATTERJEE & N. I. KRINSKY. 1991. Characterization of products formed during the autoxidation of β-carotene. Free Radical Biol. Med. **10:** 427–437.

28. KENNEDY, T. A. & D. C. LIEBLER. 1991. Peroxyl radical oxidation of β-carotene: formation of β-carotene epoxides. Chem. Res. Toxicol. **4:** 290–295.

29. MORDI, R. C., J. C. WALTON, G. W. BURTON, L. HUGHES, K. U. INGOLD, D. A. LINDSAY & D. J. MOFFATT. 1993. Oxidative degradation of β-carotene and β-apo-8'-carotenal. Tetrahedron **49:** 911–928.

30. CONNOR, M. J. & M. H. SMIT. 1987. Terminal-group oxidation of retinol by mouse epidermis. Inhibition *in vitro* and *in vivo*. Biochem. J. **244:** 489–492.

31. CONNOR, M. J. 1988. Oxidation of retinol to retinoic acid as a requirement for biological activity in mouse epidermis. Cancer Res. **48:** 7038–7040.

32. GOODWIN, T. W. 1984. The Biochemistry of the Carotenoids. II. Animals, 2nd edit. Chapman and Hall. London.

33. RIBAYA-MERCADO, J. D., S. C. HOLMGREN, J. G. FOX & R. M. RUSSELL. 1989. Dietary β-carotene absorption and metabolism in ferrets and rats. J. Nutr. **119:** 665–668.

34. GUGGER, E. T., T. L. BIERER, T. M. HENZE, W. S. WHITE & J. W. ERDMAN, JR. 1992. β-Carotene uptake and tissue distribution in ferrets (*Mustela putorius furo*). J. Nutr. **122:** 115–119.

35. WANG, X.-D., N. I. KRINSKY, R. MARINI, G. TANG, J. YU, J. G. FOX & R. M. RUSSELL. 1992. Intestinal uptake and lymphatic absorption of β-carotene in ferrets: a model for human β-carotene metabolism. Am. J. Physiol. **263:** G480–G486.

36. BLOMSTRAND, R. & B. WERNER. 1967. Studies on the intestinal absorption of radioactive β-carotene and vitamin A in man. Scand. J. Clin. Lab. Invest. **19:** 339–345.

37. GOODMAN, D. S., R. BLOMSTRAND, B. WERNER, H. S. HUANG & T. SHIRATORI. 1966. The intestinal absorption and metabolism of vitamin A and β-carotene in man. J. Clin. Invest. **45:** 1615–1623.
38. WANG, X.-D., R. M. RUSSELL, R. MARINI, G. TANG, G. DOLNIKOWSKI, J. G. FOX & N. I. KRINSKY. 1993. Intestinal perfusion of β-carotene in the ferret raises retinoic acid levels in portal blood. Biochim. Biophys. Acta **1167:** 159–164.

Cancer Prevention by Carotenoids

Mechanistic Studies in Cultured Cells[a]

JOHN S. BERTRAM

Cancer Research Center of Hawaii
University of Hawaii
1236 Lauhala Street
Honolulu, Hawaii 96813

INTRODUCTION

Biological Effects of Carotenoids

In multiple epidemiologic studies (reviewed in Ref. 1) the consumption of dietary carotenoids has been statistically linked to decreased risk of cancer. In experimental animals certain carotenoids such as β-carotene and canthaxanthin have shown activity against chemical carcinogen- or UV-induced carcinogenesis.[2,3] However, studies in most experimental animals are hindered by the limited absorption of these compounds as intact molecules and by their rapid metabolism. Studies in cell culture have until recently also been hindered by difficulties in supplying carotenoids in a bioavailable form because of their highly lipophilic nature. We have overcome this problem by the development of tetrahydrofuran (THF) as solvent, allowing the delivery of diverse carotenoids to cells in culture at high concentration in a bioavailable, micelle-like form.[4] Using this delivery system, and the 10T1/2 line of transformable mouse fibroblasts, we have demonstrated that many dietary carotenoids can inhibit neoplastic transformation in the post-initiation phase of carcinogenesis.[4,5] The 10T1/2 cell culture system has been widely employed in studies of chemical and physical carcinogenesis, and mirrors whole animal studies in many important respects.[6,7]

Because of the persuasive epidemiologic evidence that dietary carotenoids are associated with decreased risk of cancer at several important anatomic sites, β-carotene is currently being tested in a number of clinical studies of cancer chemoprevention. Previously, it showed activity against precancerous lesions of the buccal mucosa.[8,9]

The mode of action of carotenoids as cancer chemopreventives is not understood at the cellular or molecular level. Carotenoids have been considered to have two possible functions in mammals: to be metabolized to retinoids for that limited group of compounds capable of such conversion (the provitamin A carotenoids); and to act as lipid-phase antioxidants.[10] This latter activity is shared by all carotenoids but to differing degrees. Because retinoids are potent chemopreventive agents, and because β-carotene (the carotenoid with the highest provitamin A activity) has been the carotenoid most extensively investigated, the question of whether the intact carotenoid molecule possesses intrinsic activity is unclear. Our demonstration that a series of carotenoids, both with and without provitamin A activity, have the ability

[a] This work was supported by grants from the American Cancer Society (BC 686) and the National Cancer Institute (CA 39947).

to suppress chemically-induced neoplastic transformation and to upregulate gap junctional intercellular communication suggests that certain carotenoids possess novel biological properties unrelated to their provitamin A status.

Gap Junctions: Structure and Function

Gap junctions have been shown to link virtually all cells within an organ to form a communicating syncytium. Genes coding for gap junctions have been highly conserved in evolution and are found in organisms as simple as hydra. They are known to: i/ transmit the ionic signals for contraction in heart and myometrium, and ii/ act as substitutes for chemical synapses in neurons when speed is essential. Furthermore, there is growing evidence that gap junctions have a role in regulating: iii/ morphogenesis, iv/ differentiation, v/ secretion of hormones, especially in the pancreatic islets, vi/ transfer of nutrients and waste products in the avascular cornea and lens, and vii/ growth control. It is this aspect of the proposed functions of gap junctions that will concern us here. The full spectrum of their activities are not yet fully understood (for reviews see Refs. 11–17).

A family of closely related genes, with organ and developmental specific expression have been described.[14,18] Connexin 43, first cloned from rat heart cDNA, and now known to be expressed in many tissues,[14] codes for a transmembrane protein, six copies of which form a hexameric array surrounding a central water-filled pore. Two such arrays in adjacent cells create a gap junction capable of transferring molecules of up to about 1,000 daltons between communicating cells.[12,18] The chemical nature of the signals and their physiological functions are beginning to be explored. It is known that intracellular messengers such as Ca^{++}, cAMP and inositol phosphates can travel through the junction.[19,20] We have proposed that one such function is the transfer of growth regulatory signals from nontransformed cells to adjacent carcinogen-initiated cells, thereby preventing their transformation.[21–24] The demonstrated ability of retinoids and carotenoids to upregulate gap junctional intercellular communication could in this model explain their activity as cancer chemopreventive agents.

MATERIALS AND METHODS

Chemicals

Tetrahydrofuran (THF) was analytical grade obtained from Fischer (Fair Lane, NJ). Butylated hydroxytoluene (BHT), 3-methylcholanthrene (MCA), Lucifer Yellow CH and other chemicals were obtained from Sigma Chemical Co. (St. Louis, MO). Canthaxanthin was a gift from Hoffmann-La Roche, Basel.

Cells and Cell Culture

C3H 10T1/2 cells were cultured as previously described[5] in basal Eagle's medium (GIBCO) with calf serum and 25 μg/ml gentamycin. They were exposed to 3 μg/ml methylcholanthrene (MCA) in acetone for 24 hr one day after seeding, then 7 days after removal of the carcinogen[5] to the stated concentration of carotenoid dissolved in tetrahydrofuran (THF). Cultures were refed and retreated with carotenoid every 7 days. Control cultures received acetone plus MCA or acetone plus THF. Numbers of morphologically transformed foci were evaluated 42 days after seeding the cultures as described.[25]

Communication Assays

Cell cultures were seeded as above and treated with carotenoids as in the transformation experiments. After 14, 24 and 34 days of treatment intercellular communication was assessed by microinjection of the junctionally permeable fluorescent dye Lucifer Yellow into approximately 20 randomly chosen cells. Communication, measured as the number of fluorescent cells surrounding each injected donor cell, was assessed 10 minutes after injection as described.[26]

Measurements of Lipid Peroxidation

Thiobarbituric acid reactive material was measured in 10T1/2 cells as previously described.[26]

Molecular Studies

Western blotting and immunofluorescence studies on intact cells were performed using a rabbit polyconal antibody raised against a synthetic peptide corresponding to the C-terminal 15 residues of the predicted sequence of connexin 43.[27] Northern blotting of total cellular RNA was performed at high stringency with P^{32}-labelled full-length cDNA to connexin 43, a gift of E. Beyer.[27] Methodology was as described in Ref. 28.

RESULTS

Carotenoids Inhibit Chemically- and Physically-Induced Neoplastically Transformed Foci in C3H10T1/2 Cells

Neoplastic transformation was induced in 10T1/2 cells by exposure to either a chemical carcinogen, 3-methylcholanthrene, or to 600 rad X-irradiation. The addition of nontoxic concentrations of carotenoids to 10T1/2 cells 7 days after removal of 3-methylcholanthrene or 8 days after X-irradiation, and maintained in the cultures for the remaining 4-week duration of the experiment, resulted in a dose-dependent reduction in the formation of carcinogen-induced neoplastically transformed foci (FIG. 1). A concentration of 10^{-5} M beta-carotene or canthaxanthin virtually completely eliminated transformed foci; however, continuous treatment was required. Removal of carotenoids after four weeks' treatment resulted in the appearance of foci in carcinogen-treated cultures after a 3–5-week latent period (FIG. 2). Addition of carotenoids prior to and during X-irradiation, or after neoplastic transformation had occurred, did not influence the formation of carcinogen-induced neoplastically transformed foci.[5] It may therefore be concluded that carotenoids act in the post-initiation phase of carcinogenesis by reversibly suppressing the ability of carcinogen-initiated cells to undergo neoplastic transformation.

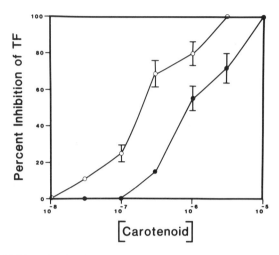

FIGURE 1. Inhibition of MCA-induced neoplastic transformation in 10T1/2 cells by carotenoids. Beta-carotene (●) or canthaxanthin (○) were added to cultures treated 7 days previously with MCA (1 μg/ml). Control cultures received MCA then vehicle. Data are expressed as transformation frequency (TF) as a % of these controls. (From Pung et al.[5] Reprinted by permission from *Carcinogenesis*.)

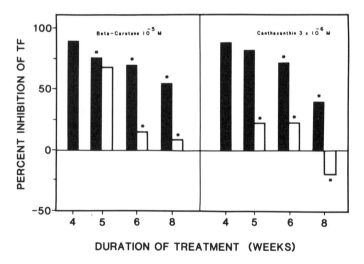

FIGURE 2. Reversibility of carotenoid effect on MCA-induced neoplastic transformation. Beta-carotene (*left panel*) or canthaxanthin (*right panel*) were added to MCA-treated cultures as in FIGURE 1 for 4 weeks; carotenoids were then withdrawn from half the cultures (*open bars*) or were maintained during an additional 4 weeks. The transformation frequency (TF) as a % of control was then calculated. * *over open bars*, significantly different from 4-week-treated cultures and cultures maintained with carotenoids; *over solid bars*, significantly different from 4-week-treated cultures. (From Pung et al.[5] Reprinted by permission from *Carcinogenesis*.)

The activity of carotenoids in this respect mirrors the actions of retinoids in C3H10T1/2 cells. Here too transformation is reversibly inhibited when retinoids are added after exposure to carcinogen, yet can be expressed after a 4–5-week latent period after drug withdrawal.[29] Is the action of carotenoids thus due to their conversion to retinoids in cell cultures? This explanation appears improbable; canthaxanthin, which is marginally more active than beta-carotene in 10T1/2 cells, is not a provitamin source in mammals, and we have furthermore demonstrated that lycopene[30] and a synthetic C-22 carotenoid (8,13-dimethyl-2,2,19,19-tetramethoxy-eicosa-4,6,8,10,12,14,16-heptaene-3,18-dione, a C-22-polyene-tetrone-diacetal[31]) are active in 10T1/2 cells as inhibitors of transformation. Conversion of these compounds to retinoids seems unlikely. Even for beta-carotene, the carotenoid with the highest provitamin A activity in mammals, we were not able to detect the expected products of conversion to retinoids after exposure of 10T1/2 cells to ^{14}C-labelled material.[32] Since the provitamin A properties of the carotenoids tested did not correlate with their activities as inhibitors of neoplastic transformation, we next examined their potential to act as lipid-phase antioxidants.

Carotenoid Inhibition of Oxidative Damage

To determine if the antioxidant properties of carotenoids correlate with their abilities to inhibit carcinogen-induced neoplastic transformation, we measured thiobarbituric acid-reactive material (TBA) in carotenoid-treated 10T1/2 cells. This assay, though nonspecific for the type of oxidative damage, has been widely used to measure lipid peroxidation in biological samples. As shown in FIGURE 3, while all carotenoids tested inhibited the formation of TBA-reactive material in 10T1/2 cells, there was no correlation between the potency of individual carotenoids in this assay and their potencies as inhibitors of carcinogen-induced neoplastic transformation.[26] For example, methyl-bixin was among the most potent of the carotenoids tested in the TBA assay, yet was inactive in the transformation assay.[30] Similar conclusions resulted from studies of the relative potencies of synthetic carotenoids to quench singlet oxygen in a chemical system and to protect against carcinogen-induced neoplastic transformation.[31] Thus, while prevention of oxidative damage by carotenoids may play a role in protection from neoplastic transformation, other factors must predominate.

Carotenoids Upregulate Gap Junctional Intercellular Communication

We previously demonstrated that gap junctional communication plays a crucial role in 10T1/2 cell transformation. The evidence is as follows: i/ when fully transformed cells are forced into gap junctional communication with nontransformed cells, the transformed cell becomes growth-arrested and the transformed phenotype latent;[21] ii/ chemopreventive retinoids induce a dramatic increase in gap junctional communication, and this increase is statistically highly correlated with their activities as inhibitors of carcinogen-induced neoplastic transformation[23] and their ability to enhance growth control in 10T1/2 cells;[22] iii/ carcinogen-initiated cells when placed in small colonies in intimate junctional contact with nontransformed cells fail to transform, whereas transformation approaches 100% when present in large colonies under the usual conditions of the transformation assay.[33] These data demonstrating the role of intercellular signalling in growth control

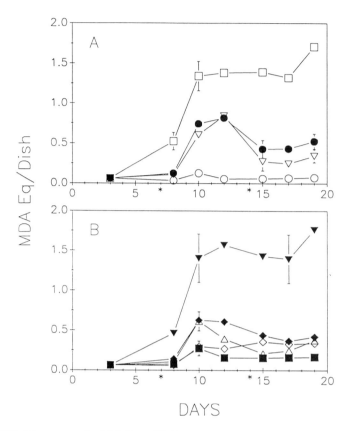

FIGURE 3. Time course for inhibition of lipid peroxidation by carotenoids in 10T1/2 cells. Values expressed as malondialdehyde-equivalents/dish. **(A)** Provitamin A carotenoids; alpha-carotene, ●; beta-carotene, ▽; and alpha-tocopherol, ○; and acetone control, □. **(B)** Non-provitamin A carotenoids; canthaxanthin, ◆; lutein, ■; methyl-bixin, ◇; THF solvent control, ▼. All compounds tested at 3×10^{-6} M. (From Zhang et al.[26] Reprinted by permission from *Carcinogenesis*.)

suggest that the action of retinoids may be to maintain initiated cells in junctional communication with surrounding nontransformed cells.[24] To determine if carotenoids share with retinoids this ability to upregulate junctional communication, 10T1/2 cells were exposed to carotenoids under the conditions of the transformation assay, and at various periods thereafter junctional communication was measured by dye injection.

As shown in FIGURE 4, carotenoid treatment caused a progressive increase in junctional communication after a delay of about 4 days. This increase was maintained over the 4-week experimental period; the same treatment period used in the transformation assays. Dose-response studies demonstrated that a good correlation existed between the ability to inhibit transformation and to induce gap junctional communication.[26] Thus beta-carotene and canthaxanthin were approximately equipotent in both assays, while methyl-bixin, for example, was without activity in either of the assays (FIG. 5).

In FIGURE 6 are shown the correlations between the three biological end points measured. Only induction of gap junctional communication correlated with inhibition of neoplastic transformation (r value -0.75), indicating a strong statistical association between the two events.

Mechanism of Enhanced Gap Junctional Communication: Measurements of Connexin 43 Gene Expression

Previous studies had shown that the increased gap junctional communication observed after retinoid treatment was a consequence of the upregulated expression of connexin 43 at the protein and message level. This is the only connexin known to be expressed in 10T1/2 cells.[34] When Northern and Western blots were performed on total mRNA and protein isolated from beta-carotene- or canthaxanthin-treated 10T1/2 cells, a major increase in connexin 43 gene products was observed in response to both carotenoids tested (FIGS. 7 and 8).[28] On Western blots an increased immunolabelling of two bands in the 43–45-kD region by anticonnexin 43 antibody was seen. The higher Mr band, also seen after retinoid treatment of 10T1/2 cells, was shown to represent a phosphorylated form of connexin 43.[34] Northern blotting of total RNA extracted from 10T1/2 cells probed with full-length connexin 43 cDNA demonstrated a major increase in hybridization to a *3.1*-kb band in carotenoid-treated cells (FIG. 8). This corresponds to the reported transcript size of connexin 43.[27] Control cultures treated with THF as solvent expressed only low amounts of connexin 43 mRNA or protein. This is in accord with their low level of communication seen in the dye transfer experiments.[26] It will be noted that the antioxidants alpha-tocopherol and methyl-bixin did not upregulate connexin 43 expression.

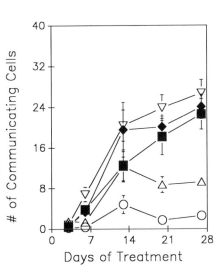

FIGURE 4. Time course for induction of gap junctional intercellular communication in 10T1/2 cells by carotenoids. Beta-carotene, ▽; canthaxanthin, ◆; lutein, ■; lycopene, △; THF solvent control, ○. All compounds were tested at 10^{-5} M. (From Zhang et al.[26] Reprinted by permission from *Carcinogenesis*.)

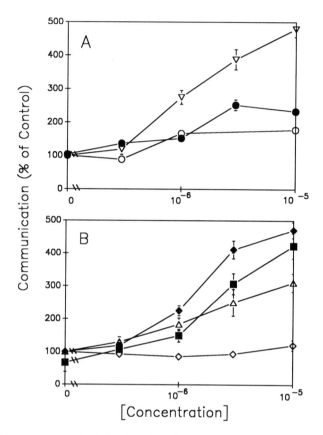

FIGURE 5. Dose response for induction of gap junctional intercellular communication by carotenoids and alpha-tocopherol in 10T1/2 cells. **(A)** Provitamin A carotenoids; alpha-carotene, ●; beta-carotene, ▽; alpha-tocopherol, ○. **(B)** Non-provitamin A carotenoids; canthaxanthin, ◆; lutein, ■; methyl-bixin, ◇; lycopene, △. (From Rundhaug *et al.*[32] Reprinted by permission from *Carcinogenesis*.)

Immunofluorescence Studies

When carotenoid-treated cells were processed for indirect immunofluorescence using the same connexin 43 antibody as used in the Western blots, a major increase in immunofluorescent plaques was observed in regions of cell-cell contact (FIG. 9C,D).[28] These plaques are the presumed sites of aggregation of individual connexins to form the junctional complexes which have been visualized by electron

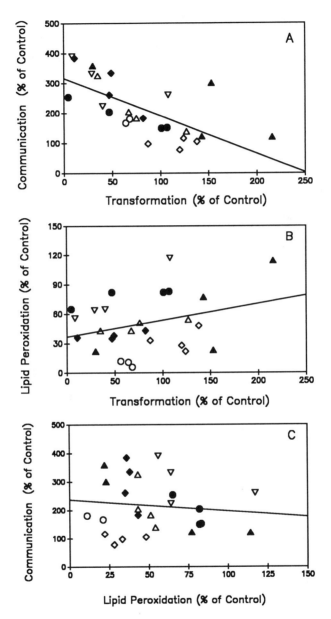

FIGURE 6. Correlations between effects of carotenoids on **(A)** gap junctional communication, **(B)** lipid peroxidation and **(C)** neoplastic transformation. (From Zhang *et al.*[26] Reprinted by permission from *Carcinogenesis*.)

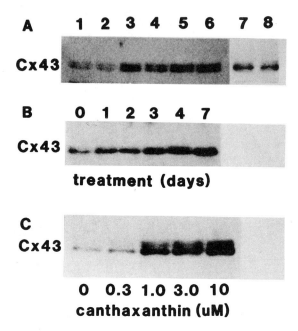

FIGURE 7. Carotenoids increase expression of connexin 43 gene products. 10T1/2 cells were treated with carotenoids 10^{-5} M, tetrahydrotetramethylnaphthalenylpropylbenzylbenzoic acid (TTNPB) 10^{-8} M or THF 0.5% as solvent control as in FIGURE 4. After 7 days cultures were harvested and prepared for Western blotting as described.[34] **(A)** *Lanes*: 1, solvent control; 2, alpha-tocopherol; 3, canthaxanthin; 4, lycopene; 5, beta-carotene; 6, synthetic retinoid TTNPB; 7,8, separate experiment: 7, methyl-bixin; 8, THF solvent control. **(B)** Time course; canthaxanthin 10^{-5} M. **(C)** Dose response; canthaxanthin treatment for 7 days. (From Zhang *et al.*[28] Reprinted by permission from *Cancer Research*.)

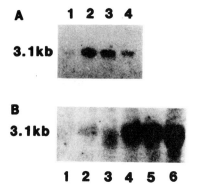

FIGURE 8. Induction of Cx43 mRNA by carotenoids. **(A)** Northern blot: *Lanes*: 1, THF solvent control; 2, beta-carotene; 3, canthaxanthin; 4, lycopene. All treatments 10^{-5} M for 7 days. **(B)** Time course for canthaxanthin 10^{-5} M. *Lanes* 1–6; 0, 1, 2, 3, 4, 7 days respectively. (From Zhang *et al.*[28] Reprinted by permission from *Cancer Research*.)

microscopy of other junctionally communicating cells.[35] Thus the increased amounts of connexin 43 detected by Western blotting became localized in regions of the cell where they could contribute to the carotenoid-enhanced junctional communication detected by the dye transfer experiments (FIG. 9A,B).

Effects in Human Cells

Addition of beta-carotene, canthaxanthin or lycopene to early passage human dermal fibroblast cells was recently shown to upregulate gap junctional communication and the expression of connexin 43. These effects were produced at concentrations between 10^{-6} and 10^{-5} M as in 10T1/2 cells. Effects on carcinogenesis could not be determined because human cells have so far resisted attempts to transform them with carcinogens. Addition of these compounds to human keratinocytes, derived from the same source, did not alter gap junctional communication or connexin 43 expression (Zhang et al., in preparation).

DISCUSSION

Retinoids and Carotenoids as Chemopreventive Agents: Comparisons of Cellular and Molecular Effects

As discussed above both types of molecules inhibit transformation in the postinitiation phase of carcinogenesis; an action which is reversible upon drug withdrawal. Furthermore, both agents upregulate gap junctional communication by increasing the steady-state levels of connexin 43. Differences, however, exist of a qualitative and quantitative nature. Carotenoids are less potent on a molar basis than are the retinoids. For example canthaxanthin, the most potent carotenoid yet tested, will completely inhibit carcinogen-induced neoplastic transformation at 10^{-5} M, whereas the most potent of the retinoids, the benzoidal compound TTNPB, is active at 10^{-10} M. Retinoic acid, which is active at 10^{-8} M,[23] it would probably exhibit greater potency if it were not rapidly metabolized.[32] Similar concentrations are required for upregulation of gap junctional communication. Secondly, the effects of carotenoids are only measurable after delay of about 24 hours posttreatment in the case of connexin 43 synthesis,[28] and of 48–72 hours for increases in gap junctional communication;[26] retinoids, however, increase connexin 43 mRNA levels within 6 hours and gap junctional communication within 24 hours of treatment.[34] It is tempting to speculate that this delay reflects the need for metabolic activation of carotenoids; however, other possibilities exist.

In addition to these quantitative differences, qualitative differences exist in the spectrum of genes activated by these agents: in 10T1/2 and F9 cells, retinoids upregulate expression of both connexin 43 and RAR-beta, whereas canthaxanthin does not activate this latter gene.[28] RAR-beta is retinoid-inducible in a wide variety of cell types and has been shown to possess a retinoic acid responsive element (RARE) in its promoter region.[36] These results imply that carotenoids and retinoids function through separate but overlapping pathways. We are currently investigating whether retinoid and/or carotenoid responsive elements exist in the promoter region of the connexin 43 gene.

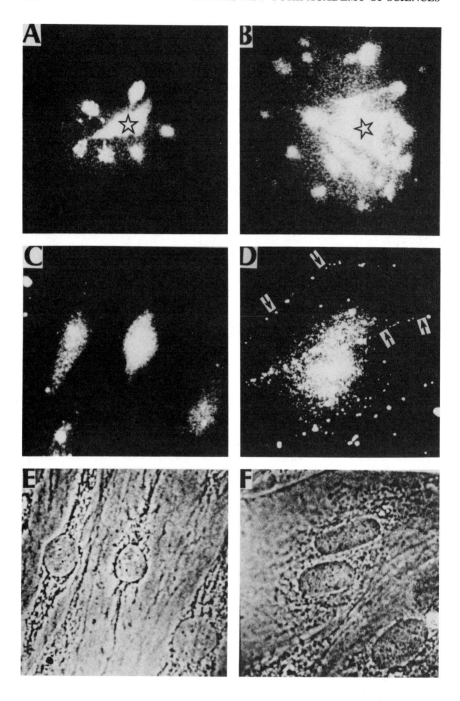

Proposed Significance of Upregulated Gap Junctional Communication

The consistent association between enhanced gap junctional communication, suppression of neoplastic transformation and augmented growth control of both normal and neoplastic cells[21-23] strongly supports the argument for a functional role for junctionally transmitted signals in these events. In a negative sense, too, junctional communication can be correlated with transformation; tumor promoters such as TPA and phenobarbital cause profound decreases in junctional communication in target cells such as fibroblasts and hepatocytes respectively (reviewed in Ref. 11). Certain oncogenes also inhibit junctional communication, for example a major early event upon activation of v-src is the downregulation of junctional communication[37]–an action which appears dependent on the tyrosine phosphorylation of connexin 43.[38,39]

In our proposed model of carotenoid and retinoid action, the increased gap junctional communication caused by these compounds places carcinogen-initiated cells within an expanded communicating network. This will usually be dominated by normal cells since, both *in vitro* and *in vivo*, initiation appears to be a rare event. This increased communication, which as discussed above is associated with enhanced growth control, acts to stabilize the initiated cell and prevent its neoplastic transformation.

Once neoplastic transformation has occurred, retinoids (carotenoids have not yet been tested) are unable to enhance the low level of heterologous communication that exists between normal and transformed 10T1/2 cells.[21,40] Accordingly retinoids in most circumstances do not act as chemotherapeutic agents, but act as chemopreventive agents against preneoplastic cells. These conclusions, derived from studies in cell cultures, have received support from a recent clinical trial of 13-cis-retinoic acid in which the drug failed to influence the growth of existing head and neck tumors but strongly suppressed the development of new primary tumors.[41]

A major question not addressed in these studies is the chemical nature of the putative growth regulatory signal(s) that is transferred through gap junctions. Because of the constraints of the junctional pore such signals must be below about 1500 daltons in size; because the pore is water-filled the signals should be water-soluble, and, to exclude passive transfer through adjacent plasma membranes, the signals should be electrically charged. Clearly, properties of physiologically active ions such as Ca^{++}, or second messengers such as cAMP, satisfy these criteria and both are known to traverse the junction.[19,20] One of the next phases of research in this area will be to devise appropriate techniques to test the effects of such ions and molecules on growth control and neoplastic transformation.

FIGURE 9 (*opposite*). Carotenoids upregulate gap junctional communication and increase the number of junctional plaques recognized by anti-connexin 43 antibody in monolayer cultures of 10T1/2 cells. *Left-hand panels*; solvent controls; *right-hand panels*, after treatment for 7 days with canthaxanthin 10^{-5} M. (**A, B**) Gap junctional communication assay; photomicrographs under fluorescence optics were taken 10 minutes after microinjection of the central cell (*marked* ☆) with the fluorescent, junctionally permeable dye Lucifer Yellow. The increased dye spread to neighboring cells is clearly visible in the treated cultures. (**C, D**) Immunofluorescence micrographs. Cell monolayers were stained with anti-connexin 43 antibody, then with goat, FITC-conjugated, anti-rabbit IgG, as secondary antibody. Immunofluorescent plaques are indicated by *arrows*. (**E, F**) Phase contrast micrographs of the cells shown in C, D above. (From Zhang *et al.*[28] Reprinted by permission from *Cancer Research*.)

SUMMARY

In 10T1/2 cells several dietary carotenoids have been shown to be capable of inhibiting carcinogen-induced neoplastic transformation. Their action appears qualitatively similar to the previously documented action of retinoids in this cell system; however, higher concentrations (10–1000-fold) are required. Both types of compound were found to strongly upregulate gap junctional intercellular communication, and these activities were statistically correlated. Upregulation of gap junctional intercellular communication was caused by the increased expression of connexin 43, a structural protein of the gap junction. Increased junctional communication has been proposed to be mechanistically linked to inhibition of transformation in 10T1/2 cells. In this model the gap junction serves as a conduit for growth regulatory signals from normal to initiated cells. These putative signals act to suppress transformation of the carcinogen-initiated cell.

REFERENCES

1. BERTRAM, J. S., L. N. KOLONEL & F. L. MEYSKENS. 1987. Cancer Res. **47:** 3012–3031.
2. MATHEWS ROTH, M. M. 1990. J. Environ. Pathol. Toxicol. Oncol. **10:** 181–192.
3. MOON, R. C. 1989. J. Nutr. **119:** 127–134.
4. BERTRAM, J. S., A. PUNG, M. CHURLEY, T. J. I. KAPPOCK, L. R. WILKINS & R. V. COONEY. 1991. Carcinogenesis **12:** 671–678.
5. PUNG, A., J. E. RUNDHAUG, C. N. YOSHIZAWA & J. S. BERTRAM. 1988. Carcinogenesis **9:** 1533–1539.
6. BERTRAM, J. S., M. Z. HOSSAIN, A. PUNG & J. E. RUNDHAUG. 1989. Prev. Med. **18:** 562–575.
7. BERTRAM, J. S. 1985. IARC Sci. Pub. **67:** 77–91.
8. STICH, H. F., M. P. ROSIN, A. P. HORNBY, B. MATHEW, R. SANKARANARAYANAN & M. K. NAIR. 1988. Int. J. Cancer **42:** 195–199.
9. GAREWAL, H. S., F. L. MEYSKENS, JR., D. KILLEN, D. REEVES, T. A. KIERSCH, H. ELLETSON, A. STROSBERG, D. KING & K. STEINBRONN. 1990. J. Clin. Oncol. **8:** 1715–1720.
10. KRINSKY, N. I. 1989. Free Radical Biol. Med. **7:** 617–635.
11. YAMASAKI, H. 1990. Carcinogenesis **11:** 1051–1058.
12. LOEWENSTEIN, W. R. 1987. Cell **48:** 725–726.
13. BENNETT, M. V. L., L. C. BARRIO, T. A. BARGIELLO, D. C. SPRAY, E. HERTZBERG & J. C. SÁEZ. 1991. Neuron **6:** 305–320.
14. BEYER, E. C., D. L. PAUL & D. A. GOODENOUGH. 1990. J. Membr. Biol. **116:** 187–194.
15. RASMUSSEN, H. 1991. Issues Biomed. **15:** 33–68.
16. GARFIELD, R. E., M. G. BLENNERHASSETT & S. M. MILLER. 1988. Oxf. Rev. Reprod. Biol. **10:** 436–490.
17. BRUZZONE, R. & P. MEDA. 1988. Eur. J. Clin. Invest. **18:** 444–453.
18. WILLECKE, K., H. HENNEMANN, E. DAHL, S. JUNGBLUTH & R. HEYNKES. 1991. Eur. J. Cell Biol. **56:** 1–7.
19. SÁEZ, J. C., J. A. CONNOR, D. C. SPRAY & M. V. L. BENNETT. 1989. Proc. Natl. Acad. Sci. USA **86:** 2708–2712.
20. FLETCHER, W. H., C. V. BYUS & D. A. WALSH. 1987. Adv. Exp. Med. Biol. **219:** 299–323.
21. MEHTA, P. P., J. S. BERTRAM & W. R. LOEWENSTEIN. 1986. Cell **44:** 187–196.
22. MEHTA, P. P., J. S. BERTRAM & W. R. LOEWENSTEIN. 1989. J. Cell Biol. **108:** 1053–1065.
23. HOSSAIN, M. Z., L. R. WILKENS, P. P. MEHTA, W. R. LOEWENSTEIN & J. S. BERTRAM. 1989. Carcinogenesis **10:** 1743–1748.
24. BERTRAM, J. S. 1990. Radiat. Res. **123:** 252–256.

25. REZNIKOFF, C. A., J. S. BERTRAM, D. W. BRANKOW & C. HEIDELBERGER. 1973. Cancer Res. **33:** 2339–2349.
26. ZHANG, L.-X., R. V. COONEY & J. S. BERTRAM. 1991. Carcinogenesis **12:** 2109–2114.
27. BEYER, E. C., D. L. PAUL & D. A. GOODENOUGH. 1987. J. Cell Biol. **105:** 2621–2629.
28. ZHANG, L.-X., R. V. COONEY & J. S. BERTRAM. 1992. Cancer Res. **52:** 5707–5712.
29. MERRIMAN, R. & J. S. BERTRAM. 1979. Cancer Res. **39:** 1661–1666.
30. BERTRAM, J. S., A. PUNG, M. CHURLEY, T. J. KAPPOCK, L. R. WILKINS & R. V. COONEY. 1991. Carcinogenesis **12:** 671–678.
31. PUNG, A., A. FRANKE, L-X. ZHANG, H. IPPENDORF, H-D. MARTIN, H. SIES & J. S. BERTRAM. 1993. Carcinogenesis. In press.
32. RUNDHAUG, J. E., A. PUNG, C. M. READ & J. S. BERTRAM. 1988. Carcinogenesis **9:** 1541–1545.
33. MORDAN, J. L., J. E. MARTNER & J. S. BERTRAM. 1983. Cancer Res. **43:** 4062–4067.
34. ROGERS, M., J. M. BERESTECKY, M. Z. HOSSAIN, H. GUO, R. KADLE, B. J. NICHOLSON & J. S. BERTRAM. 1990. Mol. Carcinog. **3:** 335–343.
35. YAMAMOTO, T., A. OCHALSKI, E. L. HERTZBERG & J. I. NAGY. 1990. Brain Res. **508:** 313–319.
36. HOFFMANN, B., J. M. LEHMANN, X. ZHANG, T. HERMANN, M. HUSMANN, G. GRAUPNER & M. PFAHL. 1990. Mol. Endocrinol. **4:** 1727–1736.
37. AZARNIA, R. & W. R. LOEWENSTEIN. 1984. J. Membr. Biol. **82:** 191–205.
38. CROW, D. S., W. E. KURATA & A. F. LAU. 1992. Oncogene **7:** 999–1003.
39. CROW, D. S., E. C. BEYER, D. L. PAUL, S. S. KOBE & A. F. LAU. 1990. Mol. Cell. Biol. **10:** 1754–1763.
40. MEHTA, P. P. & W. R. LOEWENSTEIN. 1991. J. Cell Biol. **133:** 371–379.
41. HONG, W. K., S. M. LIPPMAN, L. M. ITRI, D. D. KARP, J. S. LEE, R. M. BYERS, S. P. SCHANTZ, A. KRAMER, R. LOTAN, L. J. PETERS, I. W. DIMERY, B. W. BROWN & H. GOEPFERT. 1990. N. Engl. J. Med. **323:** 795–800.

Cooxidations: Significance to Carotenoid Action in Vivo[a]

LOUISE M. CANFIELD AND JESUS G. VALENZUELA

University Department of Biochemistry
University of Arizona
Biological Sciences West Building, Room 436
Tucson, Arizona 85721

INTRODUCTION

Cooxidation of fatty acids and carotenoids by soybean flour was first observed in 1928[1,2] as bleaching of carotene. This activity was subsequently determined to be due to the simultaneous oxidation (cooxidation) of lipids and carotenoids by lipoxygenases in soybeans.[3] In the last 35 years, this problem has received considerable attention and recent reviews are available.[1,3-5] Two possible mechanisms have been proposed for the cooxidation of carotenoids and fatty acids: (a) stepwise oxidation, first of the fatty acid to the lipid peroxyl radical which then oxidizes the carotenoid, and (b) simultaneous oxidation of the lipid substrate and the carotenoid. The latter hypothesis apparently involves binding of the carotenoid either to the enzyme or the substrate, although this has not been clearly substantiated in any system so far tested. Neither has it yet been possible to clearly distinguish between the two mechanisms. The possible biological significance of these reactions is of great interest, although this has not yet been investigated. However, a decrease in the production of lipoxygenase products (H(P)ETE) in bovine seminal vesicles by β-carotene as well as vitamin A and vitamin E has been noted.[6] Carotenoid products of these reactions have not previously been described.

Lipoxygenases are dioxygenases which use polyunsaturated fatty acids as substrates.[4] They are ubiquitous in plants and are found in a wide variety of mammalian cells, particularly cells of the immune system; *e.g.*, lymphocytes, platelets, reticulocytes, eosinophils, and macrophages.[1,3-5] A basic *cis, cis,* non-conjugated diene system is a required structure of all fatty acid substrates and the usual product is a *cis, trans,* conjugated hydroperoxy acid. Oxygenation sites of lipoxygenase substrates are enzyme-specific; *e.g.*, soybean lipoxygenase oxygenates linoleic acid at the 13-position and arachidonic acid at the 15-position. Mammalian tissues contain 5, 12, and 15 lipoxygenases, the numbers denoting the position of arachidonic acid at which the oxygenation occurs.

Although soybean lipoxygenase has been extensively studied,[3-5] the mechanism is exceedingly complex and important details are not yet clear. The enzyme contains non-heme iron which participates in catalysis. In the first minute of the reaction there is a lag phase and nonlinear kinetics, which is thought to be related to the generation of catalytic lipid hydroperoxide. Soybean lipoxygenase is also

[a] This work was supported by grants from the Wyeth Foundation and from the University of Arizona Undergraduate Research Program, a program funded by the Howard Hughes Medical Institute and the National Science Foundation.

thought to experience self-catalyzed inhibition by peroxyl radical. Production of singlet oxygen in the mechanism has been proposed but this is still controversial. However, in spite of the lack of precise details of the mechanism, soybean lipoxygenase has received far more study than mammalian enzymes, and has thus been used as a model for human lipoxygenases,[5] particularly for the 15-lipoxygenase.

Lipoxygenases are on the pathway of metabolism of arachidonic acid to leukotrienes via hydroperoxide intermediates H(P)ETEs. Leukotrienes act as growth or differentiation factors for a variety of cell types *in vitro* and are implicated as mediators of allergic asthma and other inflammatory diseases characterized by vasoconstriction. In addition, 15-H(P)ETE and 15-HETE have been identified as immunosuppressive agents.[10]

In addition, these and possibly other products and intermediates of the lipoxygenase pathway have been implicated in tumor promotion.[11] Inhibitors of arachidonate metabolism, *e.g.*, dexamethasone, can also inhibit tumor growth, and agents which increase arachidonate release, *e.g.*, EGF, can promote tumor growth. In addition, inhibitors of lipoxygenase, *e.g.*, phenidone, inhibit the induction of ornithine decarboxylase.[5]

In recent years, there have been numerous reports of effects of carotenoids on enhancement of immune response and inhibition of tumor production. Enhancement of lymphocyte proliferation, tumoricidal capacity and graft-vs-host reactions by β-carotene have been reported.[7,8] In addition, α-carotene, β-carotene and canthaxanthin have been associated with increased mitogenic response[9,12] and enhanced cytokine production and responsiveness.[13,14] Further, retinoids have immunoenhancement action in some systems.[15] Therefore, we have been interested in the reactions of carotenoids with lipoxygenases and in particular, the fate of carotenoids and carotenoid products in these reactions.

METHODS

β-Carotene solubilized in tetrahydrofuran was added to micelles formed by sonicating linoleic acid solubilized in ethanol in 0.2 M sodium borate (pH 9.0). The reaction was initiated by addition of soybean lipoxygenase. Diene formation was followed spectrophotometrically at 234 nm.

Enzymatic reactions were terminated by addition of organic solvent. Reaction mixtures were divided into parts A and B. To mixture A, hexane was added (1:1 v/v) and the mixture vortexed, and centrifuged at 600 × g for two minutes. The mixture was then extracted three times in hexane. The combined products were evaporated to dryness with N_2 and stored at $-70°C$ until HPLC analysis.

Mixture A was injected without further purification onto a Waters Radial Pak C_{18} cartridge and eluted isocratically with methanol:tetrahydrofuran 90:10 at 2.2 ml/min and monitored by photodiode ray detection using a Hewlett Packard model 1040 A photodiode array detector.

Organic peroxides were extracted as previously described.[16] To one ml of mixture B was added 0.15 ml of 100% ethanol (v/v) and 0.02 ml formic acid (pH 3.5). The mixture was then filtered through a one-ml C_{18} sample extraction column (Alltech) which had previously been treated with 2.0 ml ethanol and 2.0 ml water. The column was then washed with 2.0 ml H_2O followed by 2 ml 15% ethanol and 2.0 ml hexane. Lipid hydroperoxides were eluted with 1 ml methyl formate and dried under N_2, and immediately analyzed on HPLC using a modification of

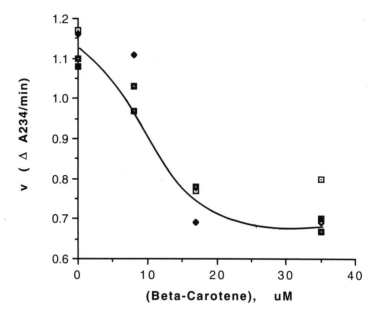

FIGURE 1. Inhibition of the rate of soybean lipoxygenase catalyzed diene formation by micellar preparations of β-carotene. Preparations of β-carotene were added to the enzyme reaction mixture at pH 9 as described in Methods. Conjugated diene formation was followed spectrophotometrically at 234 nm over the linear course of the reaction. *Points* represent single experiments performed on five separate days.

previous methods.[17] Products were eluted from a Waters Radial Pak C_{18} column with acetonitrile:water (75:25 v/v) at a flow rate of 3.0 ml/min and detected at 234 nm using a Milton Ray Model SM 4000 UV detector.

RESULTS

We recently reported that β-carotene inhibits the reaction of soybean lipoxygenase and linoleic acid[18] as measured by conjugated diene formation. As shown in FIGURE 1, the rate of diene formation is inhibited in a dose-dependent fashion by increasing concentrations of β-carotene in the physiological range (~8–35 μM). Rates were measured during the linear portion of the reaction (2–3 minutes), taking care to avoid the early, nonlinear portion of the reaction.

Although diene absorbance at 234 nm is routinely used to assay soybean lipoxygenase activity, it is an indirect measurement. In addition, as carotenoid products formed during the course of the reaction also absorb at 234 nm, at high concentrations of β-carotene these may significantly inflate the 234-nm absorbance, resulting in an underestimation of the inhibition of lipoxygenase activity. Thus we have measured the effect of β-carotene on lipid hydroperoxide products and have previously reported that the putative 13-hydroperoxide as quantitated on HPLC is inhibited with increasing concentrations of β-carotene.[18] In addition, as shown in FIGURE 2, when β-carotene and hydroperoxide products are extracted from the same reaction mixtures and injected onto HPLC, increasing concentrations of linoleic acid result in increased production of lipid hydroperoxide and a corresponding loss in β-carotene as measured spectrophotometrically.

In the presence of soybean lipoxygenase and linoleic acid, we observe a significant decrease in UV absorbance (A_{452}) of β-carotene over the course of the reaction.[18] However, in the presence of enzyme alone, changes in β-carotene absorption spectra were not different from controls, suggesting that β-carotene alone is not a substrate for the enzyme.

In addition to inhibiting the production of lipid peroxyl radical products of the lipoxygenase reaction, β-carotene is metabolized to a number of products in the course of the reaction. We have now isolated three major fractions of β-carotene products of the reaction; a hydrophobic fraction (which includes carotenoids and carotenoid epoxides) and two fractions which are more polar than retinol. The

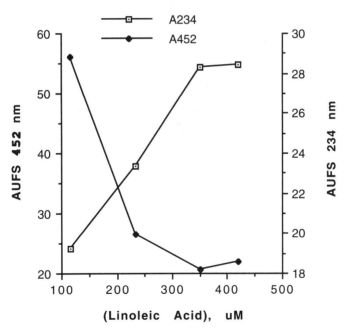

FIGURE 2. β-Carotene and lipid hydroperoxide products of the reaction of soybean lipoxygenase (2500 U), β-carotene (35 μM) and varying concentrations of linoleic acid for five minutes at 30°C. Enzymatic reaction mixtures were prepared as described in Methods, and the products extracted and separated using HPLC. Data are expressed as the area of arbitrary units (AUFS) under the curve representing the peaks of interest and are the average of two experiments performed on separate days. Differences between duplicates were ≤22%.

hydrophobic fraction (FIG. 3) appears to contain the same products or products similar to those previously reported by others using chemical methods.[19,20] We could demonstrate no qualitative differences between the enzymatic and nonenzymatic reactions, although quantitatively the enzymatic reaction produced more products. The polar fractions include a number of products with UV absorbance characteristics of retinoids. We are currently isolating and chemically characterizing these and investigating their biological activity in cellular systems.

DISCUSSION

Cooxidation reactions of carotenoids are potentially significant to carotene action in biological systems. By inhibiting H(P)ETE production, carotenoids may result in diminution of production of eicosanoid products, which function in inflammatory processes and tumor promotion. In addition, by acting as modulators of retinoic acid action, carotenoid cleavage products are potentially important to cell regulatory processes.

Collectively, our results to date support the hypothesis that β-carotene inhibits the production of products of soybean lipoxygenase by reacting with the peroxyl radical intermediate rather than directly with the enzyme. In the absence of lipid substrate, oxidation of β-carotene is not different from autoxidation controls. However, in the presence of fatty acid (linoleic or arachidonic acid) substrate, β-carotene inhibits the production of lipid hydroperoxide products and is itself oxidized to a variety of products of unknown structure. In addition, β-carotene oxidation is stimulated by the addition of linoleic acid substrate. Removal of catalytic concentrations of peroxyl radical by β-carotene as an explanation is inconsistent with the stimulation of oxidation of β-carotene by linoleic acid and by the enzyme. However, our results do not rule out the hypothesis that carotene is delivered differently to the enzyme *in vivo*, *e.g.*, via a binding protein, and this could account for lack of enzyme binding *in vitro*.

The effects of antioxidants other than β-carotene on soybean lipoxygenase have been studied. α-Naphthol, α-tocopherol, BHT, NDGA and Trolox are all effective inhibitors of soybean lipoxygenase, with BHT being the most effective (90% at 0.6 μM). Vitamin E required much higher concentrations (3.0 mM) to show similar inhibition (85%).[21] Although we did not test β-carotene in these concentrations, in the presence of almost 100-fold less concentrations (70 μM) β-carotene, we observed a 40% inhibition in A_{234} by 5 minutes (data not presented). Although the mechanisms by which these various agents act are undoubtedly diverse and therefore direct comparisons cannot be made, these data indicate that inhibition by β-carotene *in vitro* is comparable to that of the more potent biological inhibitors of lipoxygenase action.

The potential biological actions of cooxidation products of carotenoids are of great interest. Our results show that carotenoids are cooxidized in this system to products with spectral and chromatographic characteristics of retinoids. Retinoic acid as well as newly discovered retinoic acid isomers activate nuclear receptors of the steroid superfamily and regulate protein synthesis.[22] Also, retinoids bind to these receptors as heterodimers, thereby modulating the activity of other retinoid and steroid receptors. Such mechanisms are of potential importance to the biological actions of carotenoids in immune function and tumor prevention. In addition, other carotenoids, *e.g.*, crocin and canthaxanthin, undergo cooxidation by soybean lipoxygenases.[3] In preliminary experiments (data not presented), we

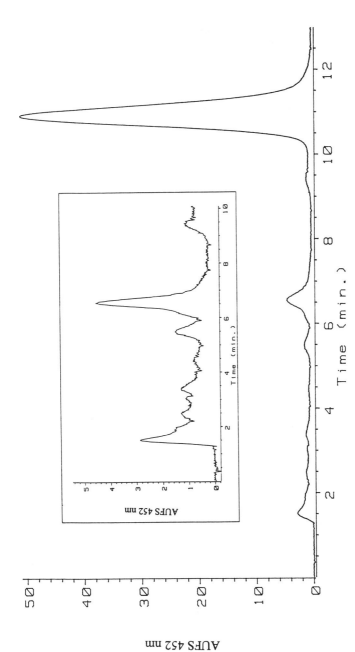

FIGURE 3. HPLC chromatograph of hydrophobic cooxidation products of the reaction of β-carotene with soybean lipoxygenase and linoleic acid. Enzymatic reaction mixtures were prepared as described in Methods, the products extracted, separated using HPLC and detected at 452 nm. *Inset* shows an expanded view of products eluted in the early portion of the chromatogram. Data are expressed as arbitrary units (AUFS).

have demonstrated inhibition of lipoxygenase activity by lutein, a hydroxylated carotenoid, and by bixin, a water soluble, dicarboxylic acid carotenoid. Thus, all dietary carotenoids potentially participate in cooxidation reactions *in vivo*, modulating the production of lipid hydroperoxides and resulting in cooxidation products of possible biological significance.

In summary, the cooxidation of carotenoids by mammalian lipoxygenases has the potential to explain, at least in part, some of the poorly characterized biological actions of carotenoids in immune function and tumor progression. In addition to modulating the production of lipoxygenase products, carotenoid cooxidation products could participate in previously uncharacterized biological reactions.

ACKNOWLEDGMENTS

The authors appreciate technical assistance from John Forage, Nadja Wehmeyer and David Sanders.

REFERENCES

1. GARDNER, H. W. 1977. Lipid enzymes: lipases, lipoxygenases, and "hydroperoxidases". *In* Autoxidation in Food and Biological Systems. M. G. Simic & M. Karel, Eds. 447–504. Plenum Press. New York.
2. SUMNER, J. B. & R. J. SUMNER. 1940. The coupled oxidation reactions of carotene and fat by carotene oxidase. J. Biol. Chem. **134:** 531–533.
3. KLEIN, B. P., D. KING & S. GROSSMAN. 1985. Cooxidation reactions of lipoxygenase in plant systems. Adv. Free Radical Biol. Med. **1:** 309–345.
4. YAMAMOTO, S. 1991. "Enzymatic" lipid peroxidation: reactions of mammalian lipoxygenases. Free Radical Biol. Med. **10:** 149–159.
5. PAPATHEOFANIS, F. J. & W. E. M. LANDS. 1985. Lipoxygenase mechanisms. *In* Biochemistry of Arachidonic Acid Metabolism. W. E. M. Lands, Ed. 9–39. Nijhoff, Ningham, M. A. Kluwer Academic Publishers. Boston.
6. HALEVY, O. & D. SKLAN. 1987. Inhibition of arachidonic acid oxidation by beta-carotene, retinol and alpha-tocopherol. Biochem. Biophys. Acta **918:** 304–307.
7. BENDICH, A. 1989. Carotenoids and the immune response. J. Nutr. **119:** 112–115.
8. BENDICH, A. 1989. Antioxidant nutrients and immune functions. *In* Antioxidant Nutrients and Immune Functions. A. Bendich, M. Phillips & R. P. Tengerdy, Eds. 1–12. Plenum Press. New York.
9. BENDICH, A. & S. SHAPIRO. 1986. Effect of beta-carotene and canthaxanthin on the immune response of the rat. J. Nutr. **116:** 2254–2262.
10. SCHEWE, T. & H. KUHN. 1991. Do 15-lipoxygenases have a common biological role? TIBS **16:** 369–373.
11. FISCHER, S. M., G. D. MILLS & T. J. SLAGA. 1982. Inhibition of mouse skin tumor promotion by several inhibitors of arachidonic acid metabolism. Carcinogenesis **3:** 1243–1245.
12. ALEXANDER, M., H. NEWMARK & R. G. MILLER. 1985. Oral beta-carotene can increase the number of OKTr⁺ cells in human blood. Immunol. Lett. **9:** 221–224.
13. PRABHALA, R. H., H. S. GAREWAL, F. L. MEYSKENS, JR. & R. R. WATSON. 1990. Immunomodulation in humans caused by beta-carotene and vitamin A. Nutr. Res. **10:** 1473–1486.
14. ABRIL, E. R., J. A. RYSKI, P. SCUDERI & R. R. WATSON. 1989. Beta-carotene stimulates human leukocytes to secrete a novel cytokine. J. Leukocyte Biol. **45:** 225–261.
15. ROSS, A. C. 1992. Vitamin A status: relationship to immunity and the antibody response. Proc. Soc. Exp. Biol. Med. **200:** 303–320.
16. BENEDETTO, C. 1987. *In* Prostaglandins and Related Substances: a Practical Approach. 47. Oxford. Washington, DC.

17. ELING, T., A. ALLY & R. WARNOK. 1982. Separation of arachidonic acid metabolites by high-pressure liquid chromatography. Methods Enzymol. **86:** 511–517.

18. CANFIELD, L. M., J. W. FORAGE & J. G. VALENZUELA. 1992. Carotenoids as cellular antioxidants. Proc. Soc. Exp. Biol. Med. **200:** 260–265.

19. KENNEDY, T. A. & D. C. LIEBLER. 1991. Peroxyl radical oxidation of β-carotene: formation of β-carotene epoxides. Chem. Res. Toxicol. **4:** 290–295.

20. HANDELMAN, G. J., F. J. G. M. VAN KUUK, A. CHATTERJEE & N. I. KRINSKY. 1991. Characterization of products formed during the autoxidation of β-carotene. Free Radical Biol. Med. **10:** 427–437.

21. PANGANAMALA, R. V., J. S. MILLER, E. P. GWEBU, H. M. SHARMA & D. G. CORNWELL. 1977. Differential inhibitory effects of vitamin E and other antioxidants on prostaglandin synthetase, platelet aggregation and lipoxidase. Prostaglandins **14:** 261–271.

22. LEID, M., P. KASTNER & P. CHAMBON. 1992. Multiplicity generates diversity in the retinoic acid signalling pathways. TIBS **17:** 427–433.

Studies on the Ability of Dietary Supplementation with β-Carotene to Protect Low-Density Lipoprotein from Oxidative Modification

JOSEPH L. WITZTUM,[a] PETER D. REAVEN,[a] AND
SAMPATH PARTHASARATHY[b]

[a]Division of Endocrinology and Metabolism
Department of Medicine, 0682
University of California, San Diego
La Jolla, California 92093-0682

[b]Department of Gynecology and Obstetrics
School of Medicine
Emory University
Atlanta, Georgia 30322

Much evidence now supports the hypothesis that oxidation of low-density lipoprotein (LDL) enhances the atherogenicity of LDL (reviewed in Refs. 1–3). Oxidized LDL is more atherogenic because it has enhanced uptake in macrophages and can lead to foam cell formation, but in addition it has many other properties that theoretically make it pro-atherogenic. For example, it is chemotactic for monocytes and T-lymphocytes, it inhibits the motility of macrophages, it is cytotoxic, it is immunogenic, and it can adversely affect coagulation and the vasomotor properties of coronary arteries. In addition, oxidized LDL can alter gene expression in arterial cells in ways that may favor the atherogenic process.[4]

In vitro LDL does not become oxidized until its endogenous content of antioxidants has been depleted. As emphasized by Esterbauer *et al.*,[5] initiation of conjugated diene formation and depletion of the unsaturated fatty acids of LDL does not occur until the near complete consumption of most of the endogenous antioxidants in LDL, including vitamin E, β-carotene, and other compounds such as ubiquinol-10. In addition, several studies have suggested that addition of β-carotene *in vitro* inhibits oxidation of LDL.[6-8] It is because of these observations that one would predict that β-carotene plays an antioxidant role in protecting LDL from oxidative stress. Furthermore, since dietary supplementation with β-carotene is known to lead to considerable degrees of enrichment of β-carotene in the LDL, it seemed logical that dietary supplementation would indeed confer increased protection to LDL against oxidative stress. Furthermore, enrichment with both β-carotene and vitamin E would be expected to produce synergistic protection.[9] Thus we hypothesized that supplementation of β-carotene alone and in combination with vitamin E, and vitamin C, would increase the resistance of LDL to oxidation.

In order to test this hypothesis, we initiated a prospective double-blind trial to investigate the ability of supplementation with β-carotene, α-tocopherol and vitamin C to protect LDL from oxidative modification.[10] Vitamin C was used as it is known to help regenerate vitamin E and maintain it in a reduced state. In

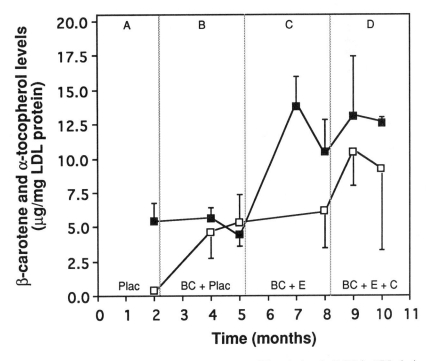

FIGURE 1. Line plot showing content of β-carotene (□) and vitamin E (■) in LDL during various periods of study. During Period A subjects received a double placebo. During Period B subjects took β-carotene (60 mg/day) and during Period C they also took vitamin E (1600 mg/day). During Period D they took β-carotene, vitamin E and vitamin C (2 g/day). (From Reaven *et al.*[10] Reprinted by permission from *Arteriosclerosis and Thrombosis*.)

this protocol, as shown in FIGURE 1, subjects were given a double placebo for β-carotene and for α-tocopherol for a period of 2 months. Then, β-carotene (60 mg/day) was administered for a 3-month period (Period B), followed by a 3-month period of supplementation with both β-carotene and vitamin E (1600 mg/day) (Period C). During a third 3-month period (Period D), vitamin C was added, and finally at the end of this intervention period both β-carotene and vitamin C were discontinued and subjects were maintained on vitamin E alone for 5 months. Twice during each of the study periods, and 5 months after the discontinuation of the β-carotene, LDL was isolated from plasma of subjects and its susceptibility to oxidative modification determined.

The basal level of β-carotene in LDL was 0.26 μg/mg/LDL protein and after 3 months of supplementation with 60 mg/day β-carotene levels increased nearly 20-fold, achieving levels of 5.0 μg/mg protein. When vitamin E (1600 mg/day) was added, the levels of β-carotene in plasma, and in LDL, did not change but during the period of vitamin C supplementation (2 g/day), β-carotene levels rose significantly in plasma, as well as in LDL (9.91 μg/mg LDL protein). Nearly all of the subjects participating in this study experienced some degree of yellowing of their skin during the β-carotene supplementation.

Each isolated LDL was subjected to oxidative stress mediated by exposure to either endothelial cells, or by exposure to a standard concentration of copper, a known catalyst of lipid peroxidation. When LDL undergoes oxidative modification, new epitopes are developed on its surface which are recognized by scavenger receptors on macrophages leading to enhanced uptake. Despite a nearly 20-fold enrichment of β-carotene, LDL isolated from β-carotene-supplemented subjects did not have enhanced protection against oxidative stress (FIG. 2). They showed equal degrees of uptake and degradation by macrophages as did control LDL. Similarly, when the β-carotene-enriched LDL were tested for extent of lipid peroxidation, as judged by thiobarbituric acid reactive substances (TBARS) formation, no protection was observed. In contrast during the subsequent 3-month period, when vitamin E was supplemented (Period C), and vitamin E levels in LDL rose nearly 2-1/2-fold, significant protection to the LDL was demonstrated, both as measured by decreased lipid peroxidation and by decreased macrophages uptake. Furthermore, even though β-carotene levels in the LDL rose still further during the vitamin C supplementation period as noted above, these LDL showed no further protection in the *in vitro* assays than was observed during Period C,

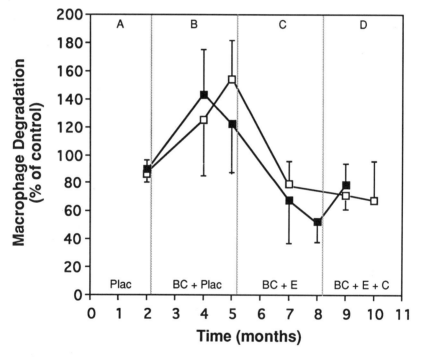

FIGURE 2. Line plot demonstrating effects of vitamin supplementation on the susceptibility of LDL to *in vitro* oxidative modification. During each study period LDL was isolated and subjected to oxidative stress by exposure to endothelial cells (□) or copper sulfate (■) and then the extent of macrophage uptake determined. The results are expressed as a percent of modification of control LDL samples performed simultaneously at each time point. (From Reaven *et al.*[10] Reprinted by permission from *Arteriosclerosis and Thrombosis*.)

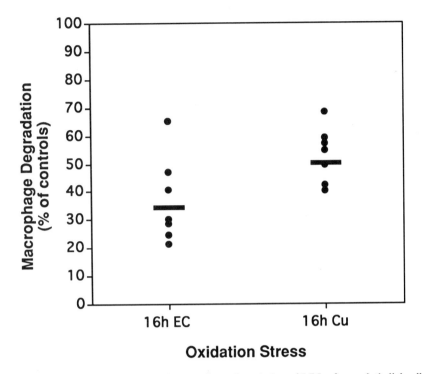

FIGURE 3. Plot showing extent of macrophage degradation of LDL after endothelial cell (EC)- or copper (Cu)-mediated oxidation. Shown are values for LDL isolated from subjects taking only vitamin E (1600 mg/day) and displayed as a percent of the macrophage degradation of control LDL. (From Reaven *et al.*[10] Reprinted by permission from *Arteriosclerosis and Thrombosis.*)

when vitamin E was supplied. These data strongly suggested that β-carotene provided no direct antioxidant protection to the LDL. To confirm that the protection seen during the vitamin E supplementation period (Period C) was due solely to vitamin E, and not to some delayed effect of β-carotene, or some interaction between the two, vitamin E was continued but the β-carotene and vitamin C were discontinued for a period of 5 months, at which time the content of β-carotene in the LDL had returned to basal levels. When LDL were isolated from subjects at this time and then tested for susceptibility to oxidation, all of the protective effect noted during Period C was retained, confirming that it was the vitamin E alone that provided the antioxidant activity (FIG. 3).

These results suggested that even a 20-fold enrichment of LDL with β-carotene did not provide enhanced protection to LDL against susceptibility to oxidative stress. These results are consistent with the report of Princen *et al.*,[11] who also demonstrated that a similar degree of enrichment of β-carotene in LDL did not protect LDL from lipid peroxidation *in vitro*. Thus, a 16- to 35-fold enrichment of β-carotene levels in LDL failed to provide any protective effect. It might be argued that in the high concentrations supplied in these studies, β-carotene (or its metabolites) might actually be acting as a pro-oxidant. In recent studies, we fed β-carotene at more modest levels, so that levels of enrichment in LDL of 2.5-, 8.5- and 14-fold were achieved above LDL isolated from placebo-fed subjects. However, in these LDL no enhanced protection was observed either.[12]

These data appear to differ from several studies which have reported that supplementation of LDL *in vitro* with β-carotene could inhibit the susceptibility of that LDL to oxidative modification.[6-8] The reasons for this discrepancy are not clear. In the *in vitro* studies, the addition of β-carotene to LDL was achieved by solubilization of β-carotene in organic solvents and there was no documentation that the β-carotene was found in the core of the LDL particle, as occurs in LDL enriched by oral supplementation. In those studies in which LDL was reported to be protected by β-carotene, measurements of β-carotene in the LDL were not made. In artificial systems, in which β-carotene was used to enrich liposomes, the degree of enrichment achieved was comparable to that present in LDL after ingestion of large doses of β-carotene, as used in our study. For example, Palozza and Krinsky found approximately 10 nmol β-carotene/mg microsomal protein after adding microsomes to β-carotene-coated tubes.[13] However, even that level of β-carotene enrichment did not inhibit microsomal oxidation.[13] In our studies, even with supplementation of 60 mg/day, only 5–6 β-carotene molecules were incorporated into each LDL particle. This is apparently not sufficient to provide protection. Interestingly, this is equivalent to the number of α-tocopherol molecules present in a given LDL particle isolated from subjects not receiving vitamin E supplementation. Indeed, only when α-tocopherol levels are increased to 10–12 molecules per LDL particle is significantly increased protection against oxidation achieved, and it is possible by analogy that one would have to increase the LDL content of β-carotene nearly 40–60 fold above basal levels to achieve protection, assuming β-carotene was as effective as vitamin E, which it does not appear to be. These data suggest that at a practical level it may not be possible to provide increased antioxidant protection directly to LDL by supplementation with β-carotene. Of course, it should be considered that in the basal state β-carotene still might provide some degree of protection to LDL and that this might only be revealed in LDL which is depleted of β-carotene, as might occur in states of malabsorption.

These results do not necessarily imply that β-carotene may not have an important role in protecting humans against coronary artery disease. Indeed, a number of epidemiologic studies suggest that enhanced intake of β-carotene reduces the risk of coronary artery disease, particularly in smokers.[14-15] Furthermore, in the preliminary report of the Physicians' Health Study it was noted that for physicians who had coronary artery disease at the time of entrance into the study, and who were given β-carotene, 50 mg, every other day, the incidence of new coronary events was reduced by nearly 50%.[16] This study has only been reported in abstract form and we eagerly await the final result of this long-standing trial. However, our data suggest that if β-carotene does indeed have a protective role against coronary artery disease, then it is not achieving this through its ability to directly protect LDL. The possibility remains that it does affect the ability of cells to oxidatively modify LDL. Parthasarathy, for example, has demonstrated that if macrophages are preincubated with a water-soluble analog of probucol, which is a highly potent antioxidant, then these cells have a decreased ability to oxidatively modify LDL.[17] Similarly, Navab *et al.*[18] have demonstrated that β-carotene can modify the ability of a co-culture of smooth muscle cells and endothelial cells to modify LDL. In their assay system, smooth muscle and endothelial cells are co-cultured and if LDL is added, it becomes oxidized and stimulates the generation of chemotactic substances for-monocytes. If LDL is preincubated with β-carotene and then added to their system, no apparent protection is noted, as the number of adherent monocytes to the co-culture is not changed. In contrast, if the smooth muscle and endothelial cell co-culture is preincubated with β-carotene, *prior* to the addition of the LDL, then the number of adherent monocytes is greatly diminished, consistent with a decrease in the oxidative modification of LDL. These data strongly support the notion that β-carotene could be influencing the ability of cells to modify LDL. Clearly further studies to test this hypothesis are warranted. For example, it will be important to determine if monocytes/macrophages isolated from patients consuming large doses of β-carotene have a decreased ablity to oxidatively modify LDL.

In summary, β-carotene is a normal constituent of LDL which, along with other endogenous antioxidants, is consumed before LDL undergoes the propagation phase of lipid peroxidation and subsequent protein modification that leads to macrophage uptake. It is possible that a minimal threshold level is required for basal protection. However, oral supplementation of β-carotene with up to 60 mg/day, such that levels in LDL were increased up to 20–30-fold, failed to increase the protection of LDL to oxidative challenge when tested *in vitro*. Thus, data do not support a role for oral supplementation to directly protect LDL. It is possible, however, that doses of oral β-carotene greater than 60 mg/day might achieve greater degrees of supplementation and that protection might be observed at that level, but this remains to be tested. Similarly, it is possible that β-carotene might exert a protective effect by reducing the ability of arterial wall cells to oxidize LDL. Since epidemiologic data as well as the preliminary results of an intervention trial support a protective role of β-carotene, we continue to feel that the use of β-carotene in clinical trials, both at a primary and secondary intervention level, is appropriate. Only prospective clinical trials can directly test the hypothesis that β-carotene supplementation, by inhibiting the oxidation of LDL, has a role in protection against coronary artery disease.

REFERENCES

1. STEINBERG, D. & J. L. WITZTUM. 1990. Lipoproteins and atherogenesis. Current concepts. J. Am. Med. Assoc. **264**(23): 3047–3052.
2. WITZTUM, J. L. & D. STEINBERG. 1991. Role of oxidized low density lipoprotein in atherogenesis. J. Clin. Invest. **88**(6): 1785–1792.
3. WITZTUM, J. L. 1993. Role of oxidised low density lipoprotein in atherogenesis. Br. Heart J. **69**(Suppl. 1): S12–S18.
4. PARHAMI, F., Z. T. FANG, A. M. FOGELMAN, A. ANDALIBI, M. C. TERRITO & J. A. BERLINER. 1993. Minimally modified low density lipoprotein-induced inflammatory responses in endothelial cells are mediated by cyclic adenosine monophosphate. J. Clin. Invest. **92**(1): 471–478.
5. ESTERBAUER, H., J. GEBICKI, H. PUHL & G. JURGENS. 1992. Free Radical Biol. Med. **13**(4): 341–390.
6. JIALAL, I., E. P. NORKUS, L. CRISTOL & S. M. GRUNDY. 1991. Beta-carotene inhibits the oxidative modification of low density lipoprotein. Biochim. Biophys. Acta **1086**: 134–138.
7. PHILIPPOT, J. R., S. P. VERMA & P.-S. LIN. 1986. Uptake of irridated human low density lipoprotein by cultured Chinese hamster V79 cells. Biochem. Biophys. Res. Commun. **138**(2): 938–944.
8. NARUSZEWICZ, M., E. SELINGER & J. DAVIGNON. 1992. Oxidative modification of lipoprotein (a) and the effect of β-carotene. Metabolism **41**(11): 1215–1224.

9. PALOZZA, P. & N. I. KRINSKY. 1992. Beta-carotene and α-tocopherol are synergistic antioxidants. Arch. Biochem. Biophys. **297**(1): 184–187.
10. REAVEN, P. D., A. KHOUW, W. BELTZ, S. PARTHASARATHY & J. L. WITZTUM. 1993. Effect of dietary antioxidant combinations in human. Protection of LDL by vitamin E but not by β-carotene. Arterio. Thromb. **13**(4): 590–600.
11. PRINCEN, H. M., G. VAN POPPEL, C. VOGELEZANG, R. BUYTENHEK & F. J. KOK. 1992. Supplementation with vitamin E but not β-carotene *in vivo* protects low density lipoprotein from lipid peroxidation *in vitro*. Effect of cigarette smoking. Arterio. Thromb. **12**(5): 554–562.
12. REAVEN, P. D., E. FERGUSON, M. NAVAB & F. POWELL. Susceptibility of low density lipoprotein to oxidative modification in humans: effects of variations in β-carotene concentration and oxygen tension. Submitted.
13. PALOZZA, P. & N. I. KRINSKY. 1991. The inhibition of radical-initiated peroxidation of microsomal lipids by both α-tocopherol and β-carotene. Free Radical Biol. Med. **2**: 407–414.
14. GAZIANO, J. M., J. E. MANSON, L. G. BRANCH *et al.* 1992. A prospective study of β-carotene in fruits and vegetables and decreased cardiovascular mortality in the elderly (abstract). Am. J. Epidemiol. **136**: 985.
15. RIMM, E. B., M. J. STAMPFER, A. ASCHERIO, E. GIOVANNUCCI, G. A. COLDITZ & W. C. WILLET. 1993. Vitamin E consumption and the risk of coronary heart disease in men. N. Engl. J. Med. **328**: 1450–1460.
16. GAZIANO, J. M., J. E. MANSON, P. M. RIDKER, J. E. BURING & C. H. HENNEKENS. 1990. Beta-carotene therapy for chronic stable angina (abstract). Circulation **82**(Suppl. III): III-201.
17. NAVAB, M., S. S. IMES, S. Y. HAMA, G. P. HOUGH, L. A. ROSS, R. W. BORK, A. J. VALENTE, J. A. BERLINER, D. C. DRINKWATER, H. LAKS & A. M. FOGELMAN. 1991. Monocyte transmigration induced by modification of low density lipoprotein in cocultures of human aortic cells is due to induction of monocyte chemotactic protein 1 synthesis and is abolished by high density lipoprotein. J. Clin. Invest. **88**: 2039–2046.
18. PARTHASARATHY, S. 1992. Evidence for an additional intracellular site of action of probucol in the prevention of oxidative modification of low density lipoprotein. Use of a new water-soluble probucol derivative. J. Clin. Invest. **89**(5): 1618–1621.

Serum Reference Values for Lutein and Zeaxanthin Using a Rapid Separation Technique[a]

MARIA STACEWICZ-SAPUNTZAKIS,[b]

PHYLLIS E. BOWEN, AND

JULIE A. MARES-PERLMAN

[b]Department of Nutrition and Medical Dietetics
University of Illinois at Chicago
M/C 517
1919 West Taylor Street, Room 640
Chicago, Illinois 60612
and
University of Wisconsin-Madison
Madison, Wisconsin 53705

Human serum contains about 10 major carotenoids, which are absorbed from diet through intestinal mucosa. The most prominent ones include β-carotene, lycopene and lutein.[1] β-Cryptoxanthin and α-carotene are usually less conspicuous, but may be very significant in some populations consuming a non-Western diet. In most published assays the lutein peak usually includes zeaxanthin, which is structurally very similar (α-dihydroxycarotene vs β-dihydroxycarotene). In light of new findings about the specific accumulation of lutein and zeaxanthin in primate macula[2] it seems important to develop a simple assay separating the two dihydroxy-carotenoids in serum or tissue samples.

Nonfasting serum samples were obtained from 160 participants in the Beaver

TABLE 1. Fat Soluble Vitamins and Carotenoids in Serum of BDES Subjects (n = 160)

	Mean ± SD	Range
Retinol (μg/dl)	64.3 ± 17.5	29.7 –119.5
Retinyl palmitate (μg/dl)	7.3 ± 14.3	0.0 –102.0
γ-Tocopherol (mg/dl)	0.31 ± 0.16	0.03– 1.00
α-Tocopherol (mg/dl)	1.38 ± 0.54	0.63– 3.40
β-Carotene (μg/dl)	19.0 ± 13.6	2.2 – 80.0
α-Carotene (μg/dl)	4.8 ± 3.7	0.3 – 24.0
Lycopene (μg/dl)	29.3 ± 16.3	0.9 – 79.8
β-Cryptoxanthin (μg/dl)	9.5 ± 7.2	0.0 – 46.9
Lutein + zeaxanthin (μg/dl) (common peak method)	15.7 ± 7.7	2.3 – 50.0
Lutein (μg/dl)	11.5 ± 5.8	2.0 – 38.2
Zeaxanthin (μg/dl)	3.0 ± 1.7	0.0 – 11.0
Lutein + zeaxanthin (μg/dl) (sum of separate values)	14.5 ± 7.0	2.0 – 49.2
Ratio: lutein/zeaxanthin	4.1 ± 1.6	1.6 – 10.6

[a] This research was supported by National Institutes of Health National Eye Institute Grants ROIEY08012 and UIOEY06594.

Dam Eye Study (BDES), all Caucasians, with mean age of 70.5 ± 10 years. The serum was extracted and the fat soluble vitamins and carotenoids assayed according to a previously published HPLC method[1] on a monomeric C_{18} column separating retinol, γ-tocopherol, α-tocopherol, β-carotene, α-carotene, lycopene,

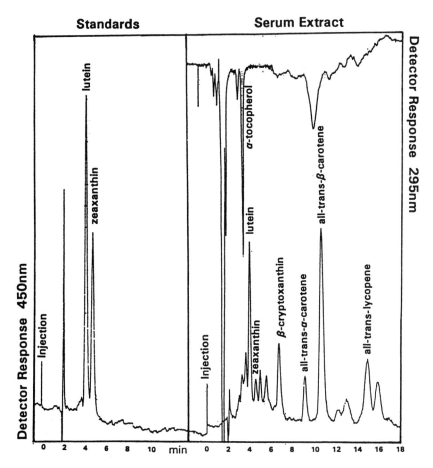

FIGURE 1. Lutein and zeaxanthin separation. *Column:* 5 μm Vydac 201TP5415 150 × 4.6 mm. Column temperature controlled at 20°C. *Mobile phase:* MeOH/ACN (85:15), 0.01% CH_3COONH_4. *Detection:* 450 nm 0.005 AUFS for carotenoids; 295 nm 0.01 AUFS for α-tocopherol (recovery indicator). *Flow Rate:* 1 ml/min. *Injection:* 10 μl. *Run time:* 20 min.

β-cryptoxanthin and lutein together with zeaxanthin (in one peak). The same extract was then chromatographed on a polymeric C_{18} column to separate lutein and zeaxanthin. The chromatographic condition and separation are shown in FIGURE 1. Since the internal standard retinyl acetate, added during extraction, did not separate well from retinol and the solvent front, endogenous α-tocopherol was used as a recovery indicator for lutein and zeaxanthin. The results of both methods are shown in TABLE 1. The mean serum lutein level was 11.5 ± 5.7 μg/dl, and the mean zeaxanthin level was 3.0 ± 1.7 μg/dl. These results correlated well with the mean combined lutein-zeaxanthin level of 15.7 ± 7.7 μg/dl by common peak assay ($r = 0.97$), which indicates reliability of our new method. Lutein levels in serum always exceeded zeaxanthin levels (on average four times), which reflects the prevalence of lutein in the diet. This Midwest population had 15% lower content of both carotenoids than a similar East Coast population in our previous study.[1]

In conclusion, the described method of lutein and zeaxanthin separation appears to be well suited to routine assays of these carotenoids in serum, tissue or diet, because it is simple, sensitive and correlates well with the earlier method. It could be applied in clinical trials, epidemiological surveys and individual assessment of dietary deficiencies, which could be useful in certain ophthalmological diseases.

REFERENCES

1. STACEWICZ-SAPUNTZAKIS, M., P. E. BOWEN, J. W. KIKENDALL & M. BURGESS. 1987. Simultaneous determination of serum retinol and various carotenoids; their distribution in middle-aged men and women. J. Micronutr. Anal. **3:** 27–45.
2. HANDELMAN, G. J., D. M. SNODDERLY, A. J. ADLER, M. D. RUSSET & E. A. DRATZ. 1992. Measurements of carotenoids in human and monkey retinas. *In* Methods in Enzymology. L. Packer, Ed. Vol. **213:** 220–230. Academic Press. San Diego, CA.

Purification of a Carotenoid-Binding Protein from the Midgut of the Silkworm, *Bombyx mori*

ZEINAB E. JOUNI AND MICHAEL WELLS

Department of Biochemistry
University of Arizona
Biological Sciences West Building
Room 440
Tucson, Arizona 85721

INTRODUCTION

Carotenoids cannot be synthesized by animals and, therefore, must be acquired through exogenous sources. In many insects, absorption of dietary carotenoids is selective with a preference for carotenes in Orthoptera and Phasmida, and for xanthophylls in Lepidoptera, as in the case of the silkworm, *Bombyx mori*, the subject of this study.[1] The mechanisms by which carotenoids are transported from the lumen of the midgut into lipophorin (high density lipoprotein) and from lipophorin into the silk gland, where the cocoon is produced, are unknown. There appear to be three genes involved in the transport of carotenoids from the diet through midgut and into silk glands, two of which are proposed to be carotenoid-binding proteins.[2] Cocoons of wild-type *Bombyx mori* are yellow in color due to carotenoid pigments.[3] Interestingly, there are three known mutants which produce white cocoons.[4] Genetic analysis has revealed that two mutations are in midgut-expressed proteins, while the third mutation is in a silk gland-specific protein.[2] Currently we are using these mutants as a model system to examine, at the molecular level, the pathways by which dietary carotenoids are absorbed and transported to their final destination.

METHODS

The $100,000 \times$ g supernatant from a *Bombyx mori* midgut homogenate was subjected to KBr density centrifugation to remove lipophorin. The carotenoid-binding protein was purified from the lipophorin-free fraction by a combination of ammonium sulfate fractionation, gel filtration, chromatofocusing, and anion exchange chromatography, following the manufacturer's instructions (Pharmacia).

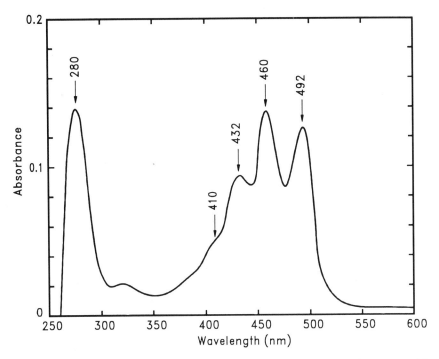

FIGURE 1. Light absorption spectrum of the *Bombyx mori* midgut purified carotenoid-binding protein in phosphate buffer (pH 7.0).

RESULTS AND DISCUSSION

The light absorption spectrum of the purified carotenoid-binding protein is characterized by having three absorbance maxima in the visible spectrum at 432, 460 and 492 nm, which represents a significant red shift (about 20 nm) compared to the spectrum of lutein in hexane (FIG. 1). The prosthetic group of the purified protein has been identified as primarily trans-lutein (FIG. 2). The lutein-protein complex is water soluble and more stable than the carotenoid or protein alone. Preliminary data indicate that lutein binds to the hydrophobic sites of the protein, forming a carotenoprotein which has certain similarity to other complexes that play important roles in physiology, such as retinol-binding protein[5] and fatty acid-binding protein.[6]

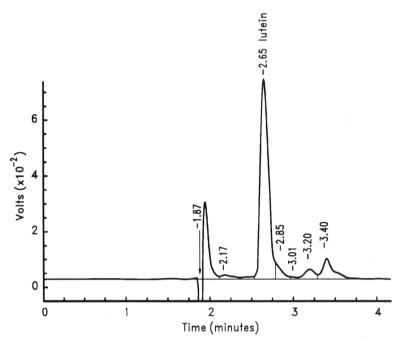

FIGURE 2. HPLC chromatogram of the major carotenoids from the *Bombyx mori* midgut purified carotenoid-binding protein. Carotenoids were isocratically eluted and detected at 452 nm.

REFERENCES

1. KAYSER, H. 1985. *In* Comprehensive Insect Physiol. Biochem. Pharma. G. A. Kerkut & L. I. Gilbert, Eds. Vol. 10, Chap. 11. Pergamon Press, Inc. New York.
2. TAZIMA, Y., Ed. 1978. The Silkworm: an Important Laboratory Tool. National Institute of Genetics. Mishima, Japan.
3. KAWAI, N. 1976. Hormonal effects on carotenoid uptake by the silk gland in the silkworm, *Bombyx mori*. J. Insect Physiol. **22:** 207–216.
4. NAKAJIMA, M. 1963. Bull. Fac. Agr. Tokyo Univ. Agr. Technol. (Japanese) 8: 1.
5. NEWCOMER, M. E., T. A. JONES, J. AQVIST, J. SUNDELIN, U. ERIKSSON, L. RASK & P. A. PETERSON. 1984. The three-dimensional structure of retinol-binding protein. EMBO J. **3:** 1451–1454.
6. SMITH, A. F., K. TSUCHIDA, E. HANNEMAN, T. C. SUZUKI & M. A. WELLS. 1992. Isolation, characterization, and cDNA sequence of two fatty acid binding proteins from the midgut of *Manduca sexta* larvae. J. Biol. Chem. **267:** 380–384.

Provitamin A Activities and Physiological Functions of Carotenoids in Animals

Relevance to Human Health

HARALD WEISER AND ALFRED W. KORMANN

F. Hoffmann-La Roche, Ltd
Building 64/444
4002 Basel, Switzerland

Carotenoids are widely used as food colorants. In contrast to β-carotene and its apo-8' derivatives with established provitamin A activities, the majority of the carotenoids is considered to have no physiological functions. Due to a lack of systematic studies of effects other than pigmentation, we investigated the possibility of such carotenoid functions with two different animal models. This included a comparative evaluation (*all-trans* β-carotene as standard) of the provitamin A activity of zeaxanthin, lutein and lycopene by epithelial protection tests with vitamin A-deficient female rats. In addition, properties of zeaxanthin were also investigated by growth tests with day-old chicks on diets with graded levels of zeaxanthin and a minimal vitamin A supplement or without any vitamin A.

METHODS

Provitamin A activity was assessed by epithelial protection tests. Ovariectomized HotIbm:ROHO(spf) rats (12/group) on a vitamin A-deficient diet and with established vaginal keratinization (squamous cells only) were treated with four oral doses of carotenoid for 2 days. Total doses per rat are indicated in TABLE 1. The duration in days for a complete reversal of vaginal cornification was evaluated by 4-point parallel line assays and expressed as relative activity in comparison to the standard.[1]

Growth tests[2] were performed with day-old chicks (10/group) on a vitamin A- and carotenoid-free diet supplemented with 450 IU vitamin A plus 0, 36 or 72 mg zeaxanthin, or with 36, 72 or 144 mg zeaxanthin per kg for 39 days. Chicks on a diet with 6,000 IUA per kg served as positive controls. Body weight gains were recorded weekly. At termination of the trial, 15,15'-dioxygenase activity in duodenal mucosa extracts was measured by a method adapted from Ref. 3 (1 unit = 1 pmol retinal formed/mg protein · hour, β-carotene as substrate), and retinol[4] and zeaxanthin levels in plasma and liver were determined by HPLC methods. For zeaxanthin analyses, samples were purified by sorbent extraction on BondElut-C8 prior to injection onto a HPLC system with a Lichrosorb Si6O column and acetone/n-hexane 19:81 as mobile phase.[5]

RESULTS AND DISCUSSION

In comparison to *all-trans* β-carotene, approximately 20 times higher doses of the other carotenoids were required to achieve the same effect on vaginal

TABLE 1. Provitamin A Activity of Oral Zeaxanthin, Lutein and Lycopene in Comparison to β-Carotene Determined by Epithelial Protection Tests with Female Vitamin A-Deficient Rats (12/Group)

Carotenoid Applied	Total Dose per Rat (μmol)	Days Required to Reverse Keratinization (Means $\pm$ SEM)	Relative Activity, % (Confid. Limits p 0.05)
β-Carotene	0.093	20.75 $\pm$ 0.35	100
	0.186	34.00 $\pm$ 0.36	
Zeaxanthin	1.86	19.33 $\pm$ 0.31	4.32 (4.14–4.52)
	3.72	30.00 $\pm$ 0.39	
Lutein	1.76	22.00 $\pm$ 0.35	5.13 (4.91–5.36)
	3.52	33.18 $\pm$ 0.42	
Lycopene	1.86	18.08 $\pm$ 0.40	4.17 (3.97–4.38)
	3.72	30.08 $\pm$ 0.45	

keratinization. This led to relative activities of 4.3% for zeaxanthin, 5.1% for lutein, and 4.2% for lycopene (TABLE 1). Therefore, these carotenoids have a small but significant provitamin A activity. This is particularly interesting with regard to lycopene, because it is an acyclic compound with a polyene chain whereas both zeaxanthin and lutein have an identical polyene part and rings with a hydroxy group. It may be added that analogous trials have been carried out to link these values to vitamin A. *all-trans* β-Carotene displayed a relative activity of 75% in comparison to retinyl acetate (not shown).

Growth tests with chicks demonstrated that zeaxanthin supplements increased body weight gain and also retinol and zeaxanthin levels dose-dependently, particularly in the presence of small amounts of dietary vitamin A (TABLE 2). However, a relative vitamin A deficiency was present if a vitamin A-free diet was fed, because even the highest zeaxanthin dosages failed to elevate plasma and liver levels of vitamin A to those of the positive controls. As expected, zeaxanthin induced duodenal 15,15'-dioxygenase activities. It can be concluded that high amounts of dietary zeaxanthin accelerate weight development of chicks but that

TABLE 2. Mean Body Weights, Intestinal 15,15'-Dioxygenase Activities, and Retinol and Zeaxanthin Levels in Plasma and Liver of Day-Old Chicks (10/Group) Fed Diets Containing Zeaxanthin and/or Vitamin A for 39 Days

Supplement per kg Diet		Final Body Weight, kg	Dioxygenase Activity (Units)	Retinol in		Zeaxanthin in	
Vitamin A	Zeaxanthin			Plasma μg/L	Liver μg	Plasma mg/L	Liver mg
450 IU		1.342	148.6	70.8	1.0	0.0	0.0
450 IU	36 mg	1.455	226.8	125.0	4.6	21.7	0.91
450 IU	72 mg	1.477	403.9	142.0	9.2	29.4	1.84
	36 mg	1.036	457.2	31.4	0.0	20.5	0.61
	72 mg	1.292	358.9	60.1	1.0	29.5	1.90
	144 mg	1.375	380.6	137.6	4.2	39.3	3.00
6000 IU		1.464	217.6	938	1415	0.0	0.0

normal values are obtained only if zeaxanthin is combined with a minimal vitamin A supply.

The known similarities of carotenoid metabolism and functions in animals and man suggest that the observed physiological effects are also relevant for human nutrition and health. High dietary zeaxanthin supplements appear to be similar to β-carotene with regard to complementing *in vivo* activities of vitamin A (see the following poster "β-Carotene supplements cannot meet all vitamin A requirements of vitamin A-deficient rats," H. K. Biesalski and H. Weiser).

REFERENCES

1. WEISER, H. & G. SOMORJAI. 1992. Int. J. Vitam. Nutr. Res. **62:** 201–208.
2. WEISER, H. 1989. Z. Ernährungswiss. **28:** 103–129.
3. GOODMAN, D. S., H. HUANG, M. KANAI & T. SHIRATORI. 1967. J. Biol. Chem. **242:** 3543–3554.
4. RETTENMAIER, R. & W. SCHÜEP. 1992. Int. J. Vitam. Nutr. Res. **62:** 312–317.
5. OBERLIN, B. & D. HESS. Personal communication.

β-Carotene Supplements Cannot Meet All Vitamin A Requirements of Vitamin A-Deficient Rats

HANS K. BIESALSKI[a] AND HARALD WEISER[b,c]

[a]University of Mainz
6500 Mainz, Germany
and
[b]F. Hoffmann-La Roche, Ltd
Building 64/444
4002 Basel, Switzerland

Herbivores such as rabbits consume very little or no vitamin A, but they are able to convert β-carotene efficiently to vitamin A.[1] On the other hand, can β-carotene also meet all vitamin A requirements of vitamin A-depleted omnivores? This question was addressed by trials with daily oral administration of three different doses of *all-trans* β-carotene to vitamin A-deficient rats for 8 weeks and subsequent determination of retinol and retinyl esters in several tissues. In addition, another group received 9-*cis* β-carotene to permit a preliminary comparison with the effects of *all-trans* β-carotene.

METHODS

Young male nude rats (Ibm:RORO-n(spf); 10/group) were fed a vitamin A-deficient diet for 4 weeks. Then, they received daily oral doses of 0.15, 0.45 or 1.35 mg emulsified *all-trans* β-carotene or 1.35 mg 9-*cis* β-carotene for 8 weeks. A control group on 1.45 μg retinyl acetate per day was also included. This dose covers the minimal requirement of rats and represents approximately 5% of the normal vitamin A intake. At trial termination, levels of vitamin A compounds in several tissues and plasma were determined by HPLC.[2,3]

RESULTS

TABLE 1 and FIGURE 1 summarize the results of this study. Levels of retinol and retinyl esters in tissues of untreated vitamin A-deficient rats were not determined because the levels of the group on 1.45 μg retinyl acetate were close to or below the detection limit (TABLE 1).

In comparison to rats on the small dose of retinyl acetate, 0.15, 0.45 or 1.35 mg *all-trans* β-carotene increased liver levels of retinol dose-dependently in an approximately linear fashion. Similarly, retinyl ester levels rose very strongly after treatments with *all-trans* β-carotene. A daily dose of 1.35 mg 9-*cis* β-carotene

[c] Corresponding author.

also increased liver retinol and retinyl ester levels but to a lesser extent than all doses of *all-trans* β-carotene.

The trend observed in liver was completely reversed in kidney (TABLE 1). In comparison to the group on 0.15 mg *all-trans* β-carotene, higher doses lowered kidney levels of retinol by 5–19%, and those of retinyl esters by 45%. The treatment with 1.35 mg 9-*cis* β-carotene had the same effect on these levels as 0.15 mg *all-trans* β-carotene.

In lung, levels of retinol and particularly those of retinyl esters rose dose-dependently. Generally, β-carotene administration led to a vitamin A storage in this tissue which followed a similar pattern as in liver although the dose-related differences of lung levels were not as large as those in liver. As in liver, application of 1.35 mg 9-*cis* β-carotene had a similar influence on lung retinol and retinyl esters as 0.15 mg *all-trans* β-carotene (TABLE 1).

TABLE 1. Retinol and Retinyl Ester Levels in Liver, Kidney and Lung of Vitamin A-Deficient Male Rats (10/Group) on Daily Oral Doses of 1.45 μg Retinyl Acetate, 0.15, 0.45 or 1.35 mg *all-trans* β-Carotene, or 1.35 mg 9-*cis* β-Carotene for 8 Weeks

Compound Applied	Daily Dose	Tissue Levels (μg/g Dry Weight; Means ± SEM) Retinol		Retinyl Esters	
Liver					
Retinyl acetate	1.45 μg	0.28	± 0.06	0.15	± 0.02
trans β-Carotene	0.15 mg	13.0	1.52	43.6	6.43
	0.45 mg	51.8	4.37	234	23.6
	1.35 mg	77.4	6.54	852	98.6
9-*cis* β-Carotene	1.35 mg	20.4	3.43	82.6	12.2
Kidney					
Retinyl acetate	1.45 μg	0.89	± 0.12	not detectable	
trans β-Carotene	0.15 mg	1.83	0.33	4.58	± 0.81
	0.45 mg	1.74	0.28	2.58	0.36
	1.35 mg	1.48	0.17	2.53	0.15
9-*cis* β-Carotene	1.35 mg	1.89	0.14	3.93	0.17
Lung					
Retinyl acetate	1.45 μg	not detectable		0.046	± 0.020
trans β-Carotene	0.15 mg	0.811	± 0.130	4.68	0.77
	0.45 mg	0.918	0.139	6.83	0.99
	1.35 mg	1.043	0.141	8.51	1.24
9-*cis* β-Carotene	1.35 mg	0.408	0.064	4.46	0.58

Vitamin A storage in trachea (FIG. 1), another respiratory tissue, contrasted sharply with that of lung. Rats on the small vitamin A dose had levels of 64 ng/g retinol and 425 ng/g retinyl esters in tracheal mucosa. Retinol levels were 7–8-fold higher in the *all-trans* groups and 5 times higher in the 9-*cis* β-carotene group. Levels of retinyl esters, however, were 45% lower in rats on 0.15 mg *all-trans* β-carotene and dropped to undetectable levels in the groups on higher doses. On the other hand, 1.35 mg 9-*cis* β-carotene led to a retinyl ester level of 323 ng/g (FIG. 1).

In plasma, the daily dose of 1.45 μg retinyl acetate increased mean retinol levels from 55 to 274 μg/L. In contrast, treatment with 0.15, 0.45 or 1.35 mg *all-trans* β-carotene resulted in mean plasma levels of 630, 570 and 416 μg/L, *i.e.*, an inverse dose-response was observed. The group on 1.35 mg 9-*cis* β-carotene had a mean retinol level of 611 μg/L.

It should be noted that levels of retinol and retinyl esters in kidney, lung and trachea were at least 10-fold lower than those in liver, the major tissue for vitamin A storage. Levels of retinoic acids were below the detection limit in these tissues and in plasma.

DISCUSSION AND CONCLUSIONS

Our study demonstrated that oral *all-trans* β-carotene supplements lead to dose-dependent increases of vitamin A stores in liver and lung of vitamin A-deficient male rats. Similarly, a treatment with *all-trans* β-carotene also repleted

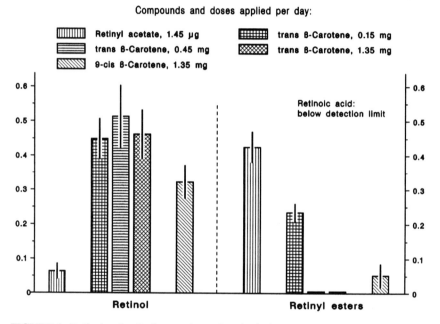

FIGURE 1. Retinol and retinyl esters in trachea (μg/g dry wt.; means ± SEM) of vitamin A-deficient rats after oral application of β-carotene isomers for 8 weeks.

retinol and retinyl ester levels in kidney despite a distinct tendency towards an inverse dose-response relation (TABLE 1).

On the other hand, a completely different pattern was evident in plasma and particularly in tracheal mucosa. The group on 0.15 mg *all-trans* β-carotene had plasma retinol levels in the normal range despite strongly diminished vitamin A liver stores. Higher doses of *all-trans* β-carotene led to lower plasma retinol levels but to an improved transfer of vitamin A to peripheral tissues (TABLE 1), perhaps due to a stronger induction of 15,15'-dioxygenase activities by the lowest β-carotene supplement than by the higher doses. Because all retinol and retinyl ester levels were endpoint determinations, it appears that the high levels of retinyl esters in peripheral tissues resulted in a feedback effect and a corresponding down regulation of plasma retinol levels. A similar phenomenon has been observed after intravenous administration of retinyl esters.[4]

In contrast to the other tissues, an increasing supply of *all-trans* β-carotene led to a marked reduction of retinyl esters in tracheal mucosa. It may be speculated that the tracheal uptake of retinyl esters is primarily based on chylomicrons, whereas other tissues depend mainly on circulating retinol which is subsequently esterified.

Retinyl ester stores in nonhepatic tissues have an important function, because they permit a certain degree of independence of these tissues from circulating retinol, *i.e.*, in case of lowered plasma retinol levels.[5] For a sensitive target tissue such as trachea, this compensation of a fluctuating retinol supply is particularly relevant, because a depletion of retinyl esters in trachea rapidly leads to visible morphological changes, to impaired biological functions, and consequently to an increased incidence of respiratory diseases, especially infections.[6]

In summary, the results presented lead to the conclusion that β-carotene supplements are not able to meet all vitamin A requirements. A minimal intake of vitamin A is essential to restore and maintain normal levels of this vitamin in target tissues such as tracheal mucosa.

REFERENCES

1. KORMANN, A. W., G. RISS & H. WEISER. 1989. J. Appl. Rabbit Res. **12:** 15–21.
2. BIESALSKI, H. K. & H. WEISER. 1989. J. Clin. Chem. Clin. Biochem. **27:** 65–74.
3. BIESALSKI, H. K. & H. WEISER. 1990. J. Micronutr. Anal. **7:** 97–116.
4. GERLACH, T., H. K. BIESALSKI, H. WEISER, B. HAEUSSERMANN & K. BAESSLER. 1989. Am. J. Clin. Nutr. **50:** 1029–1038.
5. BIESALSKI, H. K. 1990. Methods Enzymol. **189:** 83–91.
6. STOFFT, E., H. K. BIESALSKI, U. NIEDERAUER, A. ZSCHÄBITZ & H. WEISER. 1992. Int. J. Vitam. Nutr. Res. **62:** 134–142.

Effect of Vitamin A and β-Carotene Intake on Dioxygenase Activity in Rat Intestine

T. VAN VLIET,[a,b] F. VAN SCHAIK,[a] H. VAN DEN BERG,[a]
AND W. H. P. SCHREURS[a,b]

[a]TNO Toxicology and Nutrition Institute
P.O. Box 360
3700 AJ Zeist, The Netherlands
and
[b]University of Amsterdam
Department of Experimental Zoology
Kruislaan 320
1098 SM Amsterdam, The Netherlands

INTRODUCTION

For a better understanding of the protective effect of carotenoids in certain types of cancer and cardiovascular disease, more knowledge on absorption and metabolism is needed. The purpose of our project is to investigate β-carotene uptake and cleavage and dietary factors affecting metabolism. The vitamin A content of the diet is one of the factors described to affect β-carotene cleavage activity; a low vitamin A intake has been found to induce intestinal cleavage activity.[1,2] In a pilot experiment with hamsters we found a 2.3-fold increase in cleavage activity in hamsters fed a diet low in vitamin A (400 IU/kg) compared to a normal diet.

The aim of the present study is to investigate not only the effect of a low vitamin A intake but also of a high vitamin A intake and β-carotene supplementation on β-carotene metabolism in rats.

MATERIALS AND METHODS

Animal Study

Newly weaned male Wistar rats (n = 105) were given semisynthetic diets with different amounts of vitamin A (added as retinyl palmitate oil) with or without β-carotene (water-soluble beadlets) as shown in FIGURE 1. After 18 weeks 60 rats were sacrificed and small intestine, liver, lungs, spleen, kidneys, adrenals and testes collected for determination of β-carotene cleavage activity (intestine, liver and lungs) and of vitamin A, vitamin E and β-carotene contents. Another 30 rats were used for a lymph cannulation experiment.

Dioxygenase Assay

The proximal 60 cm of the small intestine was removed and flushed with ice-cold 0.9% NaCl. The mucosa was scraped off in 2.5 ml 0.1 M potassium phosphate

220

buffer, pH 7.7, containing 4 mM $MgCl_2$, 30 mM nicotinamide and 1 mM dithiothreitol. After homogenization a 9,000 *g* supernatant (S9) was prepared, frozen in liquid nitrogen and stored at $-80°C$. Incubation was carried out with 3 μg β-carotene and S9 equivalent to 4.4 mg protein in 2 ml 0.1 M potassium phosphate buffer, pH 7.7, containing 15 mM nicotinamide, 2 mM $MgCl_2$, 1.7 mM sodium dodecyl sulfate, 5 mM glutathione, 6.0 mM sodium taurocholate and 0.2 g/l L-α-phosphatidylcholine. After 1 hour incubation at 37°C in the dark samples were extracted and analyzed using HPLC as described.[3]

RESULTS

The tissue samples collected at the end of the study are currently being analyzed. Preliminary data obtained for intestinal β-carotene cleavage activity are

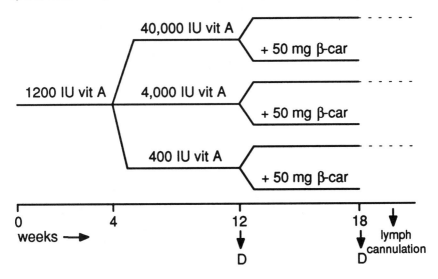

FIGURE 1. Design of animal study with amounts of vitamin A and β-carotene expressed per kg diet. (D: dissection.)

given in FIGURE 2. One-way analysis of variance was used to test mean differences. Only the dioxygenase activity of rats fed a high and those fed a low vitamin A diet without β-carotene differed significantly ($p < 0.01$).

CONCLUSION

β-Carotene cleavage activity measured using the dioxygenase assay seems to increase in rats fed a diet containing only 400 IU/kg vitamin A, and to decrease in rats fed a diet rich in vitamin A (40,000 IU/kg). β-Carotene supplementation resulted in lower cleavage activity in the groups with 400 and 4,000 IU vitamin A, while no effect of supplementation was seen in rats fed a diet with 40,000 IU vitamin A.

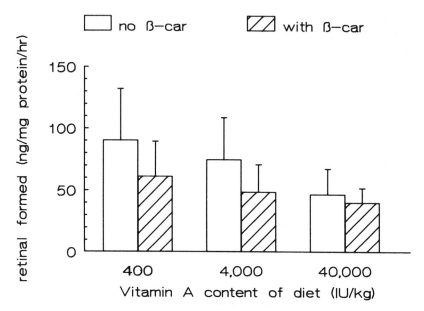

FIGURE 2. Dioxygenase activities in the intestines of rats fed diets with different amounts of vitamin A and β-carotene (mean ± SD, n = 10).

REFERENCES

1. GRONOWSKA-SENGER, A. & G. WOLF. 1970. J. Nutr. **100:** 300–308.
2. VILLARD, L. & C. J. BATES. 1986. Br. J. Nutr. **56:** 115–122.
3. VAN VLIET, T., F. VAN SCHAIK, J. VAN SCHOONHOVEN & J. SCHRIJVER. 1991. J. Chromatogr. **553:** 179–186.

Uptake and Metabolism of β-Carotene Isomers in Rats

HARALD WEISER,[a] GEORGES RISS,[a] AND
HANS K. BIESALSKI[b]

[a]F. Hoffmann-La Roche, Ltd
Building 64/444
4002 Basel, Switzerland
and
[b]University of Mainz
6500 Mainz, Germany

β-Carotene contains several conjugated double bonds. Therefore, it exists as the *all-trans* form or as different *cis* isomers. The specificity of enzymes, receptors, etc. suggests that the metabolism and functions of such isomers are influenced by their structural differences. Accordingly, we determined tissue levels of β-carotenes and vitamin A metabolites after oral application of 9-*cis* or 13-*cis* β-carotene to vitamin A-deficient ovariectomized rats, and these analytical parameters were supplemented by epithelial protection tests with similar rats to evaluate a biological function of both *cis* β-carotenes.

METHODS

During 10 weeks, ovariectomized Hotlbm:ROHO(spf) rats on a vitamin A-deficient diet received 0.15 or 0.45 mg emulsified 9-*cis* or 13-*cis* β-carotene by stomach tube 5 times per week. A control group received a weekly dose of 100 IU vitamin A. Tissue and plasma levels of β-carotenes and vitamin A compounds were measured at trial termination. Total retinyl esters were analyzed by retinol assays prior to and after ester hydrolysis. Retinol, *all-trans*, 9-*cis* and 13-*cis* β-carotene were determined in comparison to external standards by a reverse-phase HPLC system (precolumn Spherisorb ODS2, column Vydac-C18 501TP54, water/MeOH/n-butanol 26:874:100, detection at 325 and 450 nm) adapted from Ref. 1. Analysis of retinoic acids was done by normal-phase HPLC.[2]

Epithelial protection tests were performed with similarly vitamin A-depleted and ovariectomized rats (12/group) of the same breed. Two oral doses of *all-trans* (standard), 9-*cis* or 13-*cis* β-carotene were applied twice daily during two consecutive days to rats with vaginal smears consisting of squamous cells only. Treatment effects, *i.e.*, the duration for a complete reversal of vaginal keratinization, were recorded in days and then statistically evaluated by 4-point parallel line assays.[3]

RESULTS

The results in TABLE 1 show that 9-*cis* and 13-*cis* β-carotene were differently metabolized and stored. Treatment with the 9-*cis* form led to liver levels of 25–26

223

TABLE 1. Liver Levels of β-Carotene Isomers, Retinol and Retinyl Esters, and Plasma Retinol Levels of Female Rats on a Vitamin A-Deficient Diet after a 10-Week Treatment with 9-*cis* or 13-*cis* β-Carotene (means, SEM, 10–12/group)

Liver Levels after Treatments (nmol/g dry wt.)	Control Rats (Treated with 100 IUA/week)[a]	β-Carotene Treatments (5 doses/week)			
		9-*cis*		13-*cis*	
		0.15 mg	0.45 mg	0.15 mg	0.45 mg
all-*trans* β-Carotene	—	8.44	9.06	7.84	11.97
		2.46	1.64	1.96	1.95
9-*cis* β-Carotene[b]	—	26.10	25.63	n.d.	n.d.
		3.65	3.15		
13-*cis* β-Carotene[b]	—	n.d.	n.d.	11.30	14.74
				1.69	2.60
Retinol	5.67	15.91	30.12	23.36	47.15
	0.71	0.94	2.11	1.66	3.63
Retinyl esters (sum)	2.54	300.2	619.2	395.7	1181.4
	0.80	54.7	72.6	54.6	178.9
Plasma retinol (μmol/L)	0.500	1.020	0.905	1.029	0.957
	0.022	0.072	0.069	0.073	0.066

[a] 1 IU vitamin A = 0.3 μg retinol; − = not assayed.
[b] Assumptions: small amounts of these isomers were not optimally separated; n.d. = not detectable.

nmol *cis* β-carotene, and those of the 13-*cis* β-carotene groups were 11–15 nmol. Levels of *trans* β-carotene were similar in all groups. In comparison to the 9-*cis* β-carotene groups, liver retinol and retinyl ester levels of the 13-*cis* β-carotene groups were approximately doubled.

These studies were complemented by epithelial protection tests with similarly vitamin A-depleted and ovariectomized rats of the same breed, *i.e.*, the potency of the *cis* β-carotenes was determined as the ability to reverse vaginal cornification (TABLE 2). Mean relative activities were 0.26 for 9-*cis* β-carotene and 0.42 for 13-*cis* β-carotene in comparison to *all-trans* β-carotene.

TABLE 2. Relative Provitamin A Activity of 9-*cis* and 13-*cis* β-Carotene in Comparison to *all-trans* β-Carotene Determined by Epithelial Protection Tests with Vitamin A-depleted and Ovariectomized Rats (12/Group)

β-Carotene Isomer	Total Dose per Rat (nmol)	Days Required to Reverse Keratinization (Means ± SEM)	Relative Activity (Confid. Limits p 0.05)
all-*trans*	93.12	22.75 ± 0.48	1.00
	186.25	30.00 ± 0.30	
9-*cis*	325.9	19.33 ± 0.39	0.26 (0.24, 0.28)
	651.8	26.17 ± 0.32	
all-*trans*	93.12	20.08 ± 0.29	1.00
	186.25	27.58 ± 0.54	
13-*cis*	186.24	19.17 ± 0.32	0.41 (0.38, 0.43)
	372.48	28.92 ± 0.33	

DISCUSSION

Our studies with ovariectomized rats showed that 9-*cis* and 13-*cis* β-carotene are metabolized to vitamin A compounds, and that they are able to cure epithelial keratinization related to vitamin A deficiency. To gain a deeper insight into these phenomena, it would be advantageous to expand such investigations by administration of other β-carotene *cis* isomers and additional biochemical and functional parameters. Therefore, trials with oral application of 9-*cis* β-carotene to male rats and determination of metabolites have been initiated. An exploratory study revealed different patterns of retinol and retinyl ester levels in liver, kidney, lung, trachea and other tissues (see fourth poster "β-Carotene supplements cannot meet all vitamin A requirements of vitamin A-deficient rats," H. K. Biesalski and H. Weiser).

In addition, the result for 9-*cis* β-carotene as shown in TABLE 2 has been confirmed by a growth assay with vitamin A-deficient male rats. It led to a mean relative activity of 0.23 for 9-*cis* β-carotene. Furthermore, epithelial protection tests have been performed with other β-carotene isomers (unpublished observations). Finally, future investigations should also include analyses of metabolites to explore an asymmetric cleavage of β-carotenes.

In summary, our trials with 9-*cis* and 13-*cis* β-carotene revealed an inverse relationship between the corresponding liver levels of *cis* β-carotene and the potency to cure epithelial cornification. Additional metabolic studies and functional tests with these β-carotene isomers and others such as 15-*cis*, 9,9-*dicis*, 9,15-*dicis* and 13,15-*dicis* will show whether this is a general property of *cis* and *dicis* β-carotenes.

REFERENCES

1. BEN-AMOTZ, A., S. MOKADY & M. AVRON. 1988. Br. J. Nutr. **59:** 443–449.
2. PARAVICINI, U. & A. BUSSLINGER. 1983. J. Chromat. **276:** 359–366.
3. WEISER, H. & G. SOMORJAI. 1992. Int. J. Vitam. Nutr. Res. **62:** 201–208.

Transport of Newly-Absorbed Beta-Carotene by the Preruminant Calf[a]

T. L. BIERER, N. R. MERCHEN, D. R. NELSON,
AND J. W. ERDMAN, JR.

Department of Food Science
University of Illinois
448 Bevier Hall
905 S. Goodwin Avenue
Urbana, Illinois 61801

The objective of the current work is to study the time-course lipoprotein transport of β-carotene and other carotenoids following a single oral dose of 20 mg of the carotenoid in the preruminant calf. Newborn calves were fed a carotenoid-free milk replacer for one week. Externalized portal and thoracic duct catheters were surgically implanted. Calves were fed 20 mg β-carotene as 10% water soluble beadlets (provided by Hoffmann-LaRoche, Inc., Nutley, NJ) dissolved in a small amount of Ensure (Ross Laboratories, Columbus, OH) followed by a normal morning meal. Serial blood samples were taken by jugular puncture. A few of the calves were given ^{14}C-labeled β-carotene (Hoffmann-LaRoche, Inc.) in addition to the 20 mg β-carotene. These calves were killed at 24 hours by an overdose of barbiturates followed by exsanguination. Serum lipoprotein fractions were isolated by sequential ultracentrifugation according to the method of Havel *et al.*[1] Carotenoids were extracted and β-carotene content was determined by HPLC.[2] β-Carotene in chylomicron (CM) and very low density lipoprotein (VLDL) was detected in the first two hours post dosing with a peak in each at about 6 hours (FIG. 1). β-Carotene levels returned to baseline by 24 hours. At 24 hours, low density lipoprotein (LDL) levels were beginning to taper off while high density lipoprotein (HDL) fractions were still sharply rising. A comparison of jugular and portal vein serum showed no significant absorption of β-carotene directly through the portal vein. Lymphatic β-carotene peaked at six hours post dosing with another smaller peak occurring three hours following the second carotenoid-free meal, suggesting a surge of carotenoid through the intestine induced by the second meal (FIG. 2).

^{14}C-labeled vitamin A peaked in the jugular serum at 10 hours. Serum ^{14}C-labeled β-carotene peaked at 24 hours. ^{14}C-labeled β-carotene, retinol and retinyl esters were found in the liver.

In a second study, canthaxanthin (CX), in 10% water-soluble beadlets (Hoffmann-LaRoche, Inc.), was incorporated into the morning meal and fed to three calves. Serial time points show a serum CX peak at nine hours. This is considerably shorter than the 24-hr peak for β-carotene reported earlier by our laboratory.[2] The magnitude of the maximal CX serum concentration was about tenfold lower than that of a similar dose of β-carotene. We have also noted lower CX serum uptake in the ferret.[3]

[a] Supported by CSRS-USDA under Agreement #91-37200-6273.

226

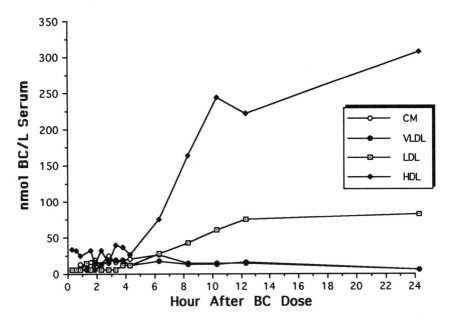

FIGURE 1. Time course β-carotene concentrations in calf serum lipoproteins fractions following an oral dose of 20 mg β-carotene as water soluble beadlets just prior to a morning meal.

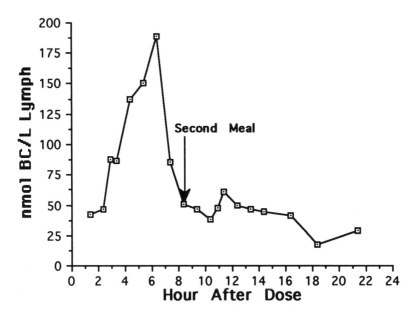

FIGURE 2. Time course β-carotene concentrations in lymph from the thoracic duct of a calf following an oral dose of 20 mg β-carotene as water soluble beadlets just prior to a morning meal.

REFERENCES

1. HAVEL, R. J., H. A. EDER & J. H. BRAGDON. 1955. The distribution and chemical composition of ultracentrifugally separated lipoproteins in human serum. J. Clin. Invest. **34:** 1345–1353.
2. POOR, C. L., T. L. BIERER, N. R. MERCHEN, G. C. FAHEY, JR., M. R. MURPHY & J. W. ERDMAN, JR. 1992. Evaluation of the preruminant calf as a model for the study of human carotenoid metabolism. J. Nutr. **122:** 262–268.
3. WHITE, W. S., K. M. PECK, T. L. BIERER, E. T. GUGGER & J. W. ERDMAN, JR. 1993. Interactive effects of oral β-carotene and canthaxanthin in ferrets. J. Nutr. **123:** 1405–1413.

Evaluation of the Bioavailability of Natural and Synthetic Forms of β-Carotenes in a Ferret Model

WENDY S. WHITE,[a] KATRINA M. PECK,[b]
EDWARD A. ULMAN,[c] AND
JOHN W. ERDMAN, JR.[b]

[a]Department of Food Science and Human Nutrition
Iowa State University
1111 LeBaron Addition
Ames, Iowa 50011

[b]Department of Food Science
University of Illinois
Urbana, Illinois 61801

[c]Research Diets, Inc.
New Brunswick, New Jersey 08901-2721

INTRODUCTION

The objectives were to use the domestic ferret (*Mustela putorius furo*) as a model: 1) to compare the bioavailability of all-*trans*-β-carotene in a natural food source, carrot juice, and in beverages that contained synthetic β-carotenes, and 2) to compare the bioavailability of all-*trans*- and mono-*cis*-β-carotene components of the β-carotene-fortified beverages. In this context, bioavailability is defined as the extent to which dietary β-carotenes are available for intact absorption and accumulation in serum and tissues.

MATERIALS AND METHODS

Male, descented ferrets, aged 8 weeks, were obtained from Marshall Farms (North Rose, NY) and given free access to a low-carotenoid, low-vitamin A purified diet (Diet D93011, Research Diets, Inc., New Brunswick, NJ). The diet was previously formulated in our laboratory and shown to produce excellent food intake and adequate growth.[1] After an initial 16-day feeding period on the purified diet, ferrets were randomly assigned to one of three groups. For a 10-day period, they ingested 1.5 μmol of all-*trans*-β-carotene daily from either: 1) *carrot juice* [filtered to remove pulp and diluted 50% (v/v) with tap water], 2) *test beverage* [CWS (cold water-dispersible) 1% (w/w) β-carotene beadlets (Hoffmann-La Roche, Inc., Nutley, NJ) in a commercial formulation of 20% (v/v) fruit juices (apple, white grape, and pineapple juices)], or 3) *control beverage* (CWS 1% β-carotene beadlets in water). The beverages were prepared at the Miami Valley Laboratories of The Procter & Gamble Company (Cincinnati, OH). The all-*trans*-β-carotene concentration of each (18 μmol/L) was determined by HPLC analysis with a wide-pore, polymeric C_{18} analytical column (Vydac 201TP5415, Hesperia,

229

TABLE 1. Serum and Tissue All-*Trans*-β-Carotene Concentrations of Ferrets after a 10-Day Period of Beverage Ingestion[a,b]

Group	Serum (μmol/L)	Liver (nmol/g)	Adrenal (nmol/g)
Carrot juice (n = 7)	0.305 ± 0.135^c	2.00 ± 1.04^c	0.83 ± 0.98^c
Test beverage (n = 8)	0.972 ± 0.127^d	10.27 ± 0.97^d	6.54 ± 0.92^d
Control beverage (n = 7)	1.081 ± 0.135^d	9.38 ± 1.04^d	4.56 ± 0.98^d

[a] From White et al.[1] Reprinted by permission from the American Institute of Nutrition.
[b] Shown are group means ± SEM calculated from the pooled SD for the model.
[c] Significantly different from ferrets that ingested the test or control beverages ($p < 0.02$).
[d] Significantly different from ferrets that ingested the carrot juice ($p < 0.02$).

CA).[1] At the end of the 10-day treatment period, blood was collected by cardiac puncture under ketamine hydrochloride: xylazine anesthesia. The ferrets were killed and their livers and adrenals removed.

RESULTS AND CONCLUSIONS

Accumulations of all-*trans*-β-carotene in the sera, livers, and adrenals of ferrets that consumed the carrot juice were significantly lower ($p < 0.02$) as compared with those of ferrets that consumed the test or control beverages (TABLE 1). There were no significant differences of liver vitamin A concentrations or liver vitamin A stores among the three treatment groups.

A *cis*-isomer component of the CWS β-carotene beadlet-fortified test and control beverages was tentatively identified as a mono-*cis*-β-carotene by analysis of its UV/visible absorbance spectrum obtained by HPLC with photodiode array detection. The mono-*cis*-β-carotene was not quantitated because identification was tentative and standards were not available. The relative content of the mono-*cis*- and all-*trans*-β-carotenes was expressed according to their HPLC chromatogram peak area count ratio (TABLE 2). The mono-*cis*-/all-*trans*-β-carotene peak

TABLE 2. HPLC Chromatogram Peak Area Count Ratios of Mono-*Cis*- and All-*Trans*-β-Carotenes in Beverages and Tissues of Ferrets[a]

Group	Area Counts of Mono-*Cis*-Peak/Area Counts of All-*Trans*-Peak		
	Beverage[b]	Liver[c]	Adrenal[c,d]
Test beverage	0.65 ± 0.03	0.44 ± 0.02^e	0.13 ± 0.01^f
Control	0.72 ± 0.02	0.39 ± 0.02^e	0.12 ± 0.01^f

[a] From White et al.[1] Reprinted by permission from the American Institute of Nutrition.
[b] Values are means of triplicate extractions ± SEM.
[c] Values are group means ± SEM calculated from the pooled SD for the model.
[d] The mono-*cis*-β-carotene peak could not be quantitated in the adrenal tissue extracts of two animals in each group.
[e] Significantly different from mono-*cis*-/all-*trans*-β-carotene peak area count ratios in adrenal tissues of ferrets, as compared within groups ($p = 0.0001$).
[f] Significantly different from mono-*cis*-/all-*trans*-β-carotene peak area count ratios in liver tissues of ferrets, as compared within groups ($p = 0.0001$).

area count ratios were higher in each CWS β-carotene beadlet-fortified beverage than in the liver and adrenal tissues of ferrets that ingested the beverage; the mono-*cis*-isomer was not measurable in serum. When the mono-*cis*-/all-*trans*-β-carotene peak area count ratios were compared between liver and adrenal tissues of ferrets that ingested the test or control beverages, the ratios were significantly higher in liver tissues within each treatment group ($p = 0.0001$).

It is concluded that: 1) all-*trans*-β-carotene is less bioavailable from a carrot juice filtrate than from β-carotene beadlet-fortified beverages, and 2) geometric isomers of β-carotene differ in their apparent bioavailability for ferrets.

REFERENCE

1. WHITE, W. S., K. M. PECK, E. A. ULMAN & J. W. ERDMAN. 1993. The ferret as a model for evaluation of the bioavailabilities of all-*trans*-beta-carotene and its isomers. J. Nutr. **123:** 1129–1139.

Distribution of β-Carotene and Vitamin A in Lipoprotein Fractions of Ferret Serum

Effect of β-Carotene Supplementation

JUDY D. RIBAYA-MERCADO, JOSE LOPEZ-MIRANDA,
JOSE M. ORDOVAS, MICHAEL C. BLANCO,[a]
JAMES G. FOX,[a] AND ROBERT M. RUSSELL

U.S. Department of Agriculture
Human Nutrition Research Center on Aging
at Tufts University
711 Washington Street
Boston, Massachusetts 02111
and
[a]Division of Comparative Medicine
Massachusetts Institute of Technology
Cambridge, Massachusetts 02139

Like humans, ferrets (*Mustela putorius furo*) absorb significant amounts of intact β-carotene and store this compound in tissues.[1] Unlike humans however, high concentrations of vitamin A esters (primarily retinyl stearate, and also retinyl palmitate) circulate in ferret blood.[1,2] In fasting humans, little or no retinyl esters are found in blood; vitamin A circulates in human blood primarily as retinol bound to retinol binding protein.[3] In this study, we investigated the distribution of β-carotene, vitamin A and cholesterol in lipoprotein- and nonlipoprotein fractions of ferret versus human serum. We also studied whether supplementation of ferret diets with β-carotene induces changes in the distribution of β-carotene and vitamin A in these serum fractions.

METHODS

Six 8-month-old male ferrets (Marshall Farms, North Rose, NY) were fed a basal diet of dry cat food (Purina Cat Chow, Ralston Purina, St. Louis, MO) moistened with water, with or without 80 μg of β-carotene added (as 824 μg of β-carotene beadlets, Hoffmann-La Roche, Nutley, NJ) /g wet diet. For baseline measurements, blood was obtained from jugular veins of overnight-fasted ferrets. After 3 wk, fasted ferrets were killed with carbon dioxide and blood was obtained by cardiac puncture.

Serum lipoproteins and the lipoprotein-deficient serum fraction (LPDS) were prepared from freshly drawn ferret sera by density gradient ultracentrifugation at 10°C.[4] Lipoprotein fractions of densities <1.006 g/ml (VLDL), 1.006 to 1.063 g/ml (LDL), and 1.063 to 1.21 g/ml (HDL) were isolated. For comparison, lipoproteins and LPDS were similarly prepared from freshly drawn serum from an over-

TABLE 1. Distribution of β-Carotene, Retinyl Esters, Retinol, and Cholesterol in Lipoprotein and Lipoprotein-Deficient Fractions of Ferret Serum at Baseline and after 3 Wk of Feeding Diets with or without Added β-Carotene[a]

| | Controls | | β-Carotene-Fed | |
	At Baseline	After 3 Wk	At Baseline	After 3 Wk
β-Carotene (μmol/L)				
VLDL	0 (0%)	0 (0%)	0 (0%)	0.08 ± 0.05 (4.3%)
LDL	0 (0%)*	0 (0%)*	0 (0%)*	0.13 ± 0.06 (6.4%)
HDL	0.004 ± 0.0004 (100%)*	0.004 ± 0.003 (100%)*	0.003 ± 0.002 (100%)*	1.73 ± 0.71 (86.8%)
LPDS	0 (0%)*	0 (0%)*	0 (0%)*	0.05 ± 0.003 (2.5%)
Total retinyl esters (μmol/L)				
VLDL	0.6 ± 0.2 (8.5%)	0.5 ± 0.4 (6.8%)	0.2 ± 0.2 (1.6%)	6.8 ± 4.2 (32.7%)
LDL	2.7 ± 1.2 (37.2%)	0.6 ± 0.3 (7.9%)	2.9 ± 2.8 (23.2%)	7.6 ± 2.2 (36.5%)
HDL	3.9 ± 2.6 (54.0%)	7.0 ± 2.2 (84.5%)*	9.2 ± 3.9 (74.7%)*	6.4 ± 4.0 (30.4%)
LPDS	0.02 ± 0.02 (0.3%)	0.06 ± 0.02 (0.8%)	0.07 ± 0.03 (0.5%)	0.07 ± 0.02 (0.4%)
Retinyl stearate (μmol/L)				
VLDL	0.3 ± 0.1 (8.1%)	0.2 ± 0.2 (6.4%)	0.1 ± 0.1 (1.3%)	3.7 ± 2.3 (37.2%)
LDL	1.3 ± 0.6 (36.6%)	0.3 ± 0.2 (8.0%)	1.5 ± 1.4 (22.6%)	3.1 ± 0.4 (31.6%)
HDL	2.0 ± 1.4 (55.3%)	3.7 ± 1.2 (85.0%)*	5.0 ± 2.1 (75.8%)*	3.0 ± 2.0 (30.8%)
LPDS	0 (0%)	0.03 ± 0.02 (0.6%)	0.02 ± 0.01 (0.3%)	0.04 ± 0.01 (0.4%)
Retinyl palmitate (μmol/L)				
VLDL	0.3 ± 0.1 (9.5%)	0.2 ± 0.2 (7.7%)	0.1 ± 0.1 (1.8%)	2.4 ± 1.4 (31.0%)
LDL	1.1 ± 0.5 (38.7%)	0.3 ± 0.1 (8.5%)	1.1 ± 1.1 (25.1%)	3.1 ± 0.5 (40.4%)
HDL	1.5 ± 1.1 (51.8%)	2.5 ± 0.8 (83.2%)*	3.3 ± 1.4 (72.7%)*	2.1 ± 1.5 (28.3%)
LPDS	0 (0%)	0.02 ± 0.01 (0.6%)	0.02 ± 0.01 (0.4%)	0.02 ± 0.01 (0.3%)

continued

TABLE 1. Continued

	Controls		β-Carotene-Fed	
	At Baseline	After 3 Wk	At Baseline	After 3 Wk
Retinyl oleate (μmol/L)				
VLDL	0.02 ± 0.01 (8.4%)	0.03 ± 0.02 (8.1%)	0.01 ± 0.01 (2.1%)	0.3 ± 0.2 (27.0%)
LDL	0.11 ± 0.05 (41.2%)	0.02 ± 0.01 (7.2%)	0.1 ± 0.1 (23.7%)	0.4 ± 0.1 (35.6%)
HDL	0.1 ± 0.1 (50.4%)	0.3 ± 0.1 (84.7%)	0.4 ± 0.2 (74.2%)	0.4 ± 0.02 (36.4%)
LPDS	0 (0%)	0 (0%)	0 (0%)	0.004 ± 0.002 (0.3%)
Retinol (μmol/L)				
VLDL	0 (0%)	0 (0%)	0 (0%)	0 (0%)
LDL	0 (0%)	0.02 ± 0.01 (1.5%)	0.01 ± 0.01 (1.1%)	0.04 ± 0.04 (3.7%)
HDL	0.07 ± 0.01 (6.7%)	0.09 ± 0.03 (7.8%)	0.11 ± 0.01 (8.1%)	0.2 ± 0.1 (13.8%)
LPDS	1.0 ± 0.1 (93.3%)	1.0 ± 0.2 (90.7%)	1.2 ± 0.3 (90.8%)	1.0 ± 0.2 (82.5%)
Cholesterol (μmol/L)				
VLDL	129 ± 15 (3.8%)	121 ± 9 (3.1%)*	198 ± 9 (4.7%)	164 ± 9 (4.2%)
LDL	414 ± 83 (12.0%)	526 ± 96 (13.8%)	569 ± 91 (13.6%)	457 ± 57 (11.8%)
HDL	2896 ± 30 (84.2%)	3172 ± 168 (83.1%)	3414 ± 230 (81.7%)	3250 ± 236 (84.0%)
LPDS	0 (0%)	0 (0%)	0 (0%)	0 (0%)

[a] Values are means ± SEM for 3 ferrets per group. Numbers in parentheses represent % of total values. VLDL = very low density lipoproteins; LDL = low density lipoproteins; HDL = high density lipoproteins; LPDS = lipoprotein-deficient serum. An * denotes significant difference ($p \leq 0.05$) from β-carotene-fed ferrets after 3 wk, using ANOVA and the Dunnett t test.

TABLE 2. Distribution of Carotenoids (β-Carotene, Lycopene, α-Carotene), Retinoids (Retinol, Retinyl Esters) and Cholesterol in Lipoprotein and Lipoprotein-Deficient Fractions of Human Serum[a]

| | Carotenoids | | | Retinoids | | | |
	β-Carotene (μmol/L)	Lycopene (μmol/L)	α-Carotene (μmol/L)	Retinol (μmol/L)	Retinyl Palmitate (μmol/L)	Retinyl Oleate (μmol/L)	Cholesterol (μmol/L)
VLDL	0.04 (5.1%)	0.03 (4.3%)	0 (0%)	0 (0%)	0.05 (35.7%)	0.02 (14.3%)	414 (8.4%)
LDL	0.54 (69.4%)	0.59 (75.5%)	0.003 (75.0%)	0 (0%)	0.09 (64.3%)	0.07 (50.0%)	3336 (67.9%)
HDL	0.20 (25.5%)	0.16 (20.2%)	0.001 (25.0%)	0.03 (2.9%)	0 (0%)	0.05 (35.7%)	1164 (23.7%)
LPDS	0 (0%)	0 (0%)	0 (0%)	1.1 (97.1%)	0 (0%)	0 (0%)	0 (0%)

[a] Numbers in parentheses represent % of total values. VLDL = very low density lipoproteins; LDL = low density lipoproteins; HDL = high density lipoproteins; LPDS = lipoprotein-deficient serum.

night-fasted human volunteer. Cholesterol was measured with an Abbott Diagnostics Spectrum CCX Bichromatic analyzer (Dallas, TX) using enzymatic reagents.[5] Extraction and HPLC procedures for carotenoid and retinoid analyses and procedures for synthesis of standard retinyl esters have been described.[1] To compare values, analysis of variance (ANOVA) and the Dunnett t test in the software StatView II (Abacus Concepts, Inc., Berkeley, CA, 1987) were used. Differences where $p \leq 0.05$ were considered significant.

RESULTS AND DISCUSSION

The major lipoprotein in human serum is LDL; in ferret serum it is HDL.[6] TABLE 1 shows that ferrets fed the basal diet had low serum β-carotene concentrations (0.003 to 0.004 μmol/L), and 100% of it was associated with HDL. After 3 wk of β-carotene feeding, serum β-carotene concentration was greatly increased to 1.73 μmol/L, 86.8% of which was associated with HDL, 6.4% with LDL, 4.3% with VLDL, and 2.5% with LPDS. Although there was a 663-fold increase in serum β-carotene concentration, it was still lower than total retinyl ester concentration. In ferrets not supplemented with β-carotene, most of the retinyl esters were associated with HDL (54.0 to 84.5%); small amounts were found in LDL (7.9 to 37.2%), and smaller amounts in VLDL (1.6 to 8.5%). After 3 wk of β-carotene feeding, retinyl esters were distributed among the various fractions as follows: HDL, 30.4%; LDL, 36.5%; and VLDL, 32.7%. Thus, the increase in β-carotene concentration in serum altered the distribution of retinyl esters and to a lesser extent, of β-carotene distribution in lipoproteins. A possible explanation might be that the HDL molecule contains a limited capacity for carrying β-carotene and retinyl ester molecules. Once this capacity becomes saturated, retinyl esters or β-carotene are carried in other lipoproteins of lower density. As in humans (Ref. 7 and TABLE 2), serum retinol in ferrets was associated with the lipoprotein-deficient fraction (TABLE 1); its concentrations in ferret and human sera were similar. Total cholesterol in ferret serum was associated mostly with HDL; in human serum, it was associated mostly with LDL. β-Carotene supplementation had no effect on the distribution of retinol or cholesterol in the serum fractions. It has been reported that humans transport serum carotenoids mostly in LDL.[7] Our data in TABLE 2 confirm this. The small amounts of retinyl palmitate and -oleate detected in human serum were also associated mostly with LDL; retinyl stearate was not observed in fasting human serum.

In summary, carotenoids, retinyl esters, and cholesterol in ferret serum were associated mostly with HDL; in human serum these compounds were associated mostly with LDL. The supplementation of ferret diets with β-carotene altered the distribution of retinyl esters in lipoproteins so that these compounds became approximately equally distributed in HDL, LDL and VLDL. β-Carotene distribution was also altered somewhat by dietary β-carotene supplementation in that small amounts became associated with other lipoproteins, although the majority remained in HDL.

REFERENCES

1. RIBAYA-MERCADO, J. D., J. G. FOX, W. D. ROSENBLAD, M. C. BLANCO & R. M. RUSSELL. 1992. β-Carotene, retinol and retinyl ester concentrations in serum and selected tissues of ferrets fed β-carotene. J. Nutr. **122:** 1898–1903.

2. SCHWEIGERT, F. J., O. A. RYDER, W. A. RAMBECK & H. ZUCKER. 1990. The majority of vitamin A is transported as retinyl esters in the blood of most carnivores. Comp. Biochem. Physiol **95A:** 573–578.
3. GOODMAN, D. S. 1980. Vitamin A metabolism. Fed. Proc. **39:** 2716–2722.
4. TERPSTRA, A. H. M. & A. E. PELS. 1988. Isolation of plasma lipoproteins by a combination of differential and density gradient ultracentrifugation. Fresenius Z. Anal. Biochem. **330:** 149–151.
5. MCNAMARA, J. R. & E. J. SCHAEFER. 1987. Automated enzymatic standardized lipid analyses for plasma and lipoprotein fractions. Clin. Chim. Acta **166:** 1–8.
6. CRYER, A. & A. M. SAWYERR. 1978. A comparison of the composition and apolipoprotein content of the lipoproteins isolated from human and ferret (*Mustela putorius furo* L.) serum. Comp. Biochem. Physiol. **61B:** 151–159.
7. KRINSKY, N. I., D. G. CORNWELL & J. L. ONCLEY. 1958. The transport of vitamin A and carotenoids in human plasma. Arch. Biochem. Biophys. **73:** 233–246.

Bioavailability of β-Carotene in a Carotenoid Preparation Derived from *Dunaliella bardawil* in Human Male Adults

HIROSHI TAMAI,[a] TAKUJI MURATA,[a]
TAKAO MORINOBU,[a] MITSUHIRO MANAGO,[a]
HIROYUKI TAKENAKA,[b] KATSUHIKO HAYASHI,[b]
AND MAKOTO MINO[a]

[a]*Department of Pediatrics*
Osaka Medical College
2-7 Daigakumachi, Takatsuki
Osaka 569, Japan
and
[b]*Nikken Sohonsha Corporation*
Gifu 501-62, Japan

The biological functions of β-carotene in the living body are not well known, although there is epidemiologic evidence of nutritional β-carotene in relation to the prevention of carcinogenesis,[1,2] and of the antioxidant activity of carotenoids, especially as scavengers of singlet oxygen. Recently, the β-carotene-rich alga *Dunaliella bardawil* was studied as a food supplement of β-carotene. We investigated the bioavailability of a preparation derived from *Dunaliella bardawil* for cell concentration in human adults.

MATERIALS AND METHODS

Sixty mg of β-carotene preparation derived from *Dunaliella bardawil* or placebo were administered once a day for 3 months to 20 human adult male volunteers, who were all healthy nonsmokers. The all-*trans* form and the 9-*cis* form of β-carotene were equally involved in this preparation. Blood was collected by venipuncture using EDTA-2Na as an anticoagulant after overnight fasting, and blood cells were separated by a density-gradient method. All-*trans* β-carotene levels in plasma (PL), red blood cells (RBC), mononuclear cells (MN), and platelets (PLT) were determined by HPLC with an electrochemical detector.[3] Plasma retinol was determined by HPLC with a fluorescencephotometer.

RESULTS AND DISCUSSION

The concentration of all-*trans* β-carotene in PL increased by 4-fold over the baseline after 2 weeks and reached a plateau, while 9-*cis* β-carotene increased only one tenth of the all-*trans* form, although the same concentrations of the all-*trans* and 9-*cis* forms of β-carotene were contained in this *Dunaliella bardawil* preparation. This finding suggests that the 9-*cis* form was hardly absorbed or was stored in the liver and did not increase in plasma (FIG. 1).

The concentration of all-*trans* β-carotene in MN and PLT increased 2- and 3-fold over the baseline after a month, respectively, while those in RBC did not change by administration of this *Dunaliella bardawil* preparation. 9-*cis* β-Carotene did not increase in circulating blood cells (FIG. 2).

These results suggest that β-carotene derived from *Dunaliella bardawil* was actually absorbed, transferred to tissues, and increased in cells as well as in plasma. This increased concentration of β-carotene in mononuclear cells may act as an immunomodulator for preventing cancers.

Neither side effects nor toxicity were documented in all the volunteers on the basis of the findings of the questionnaire and the clinical screening test.

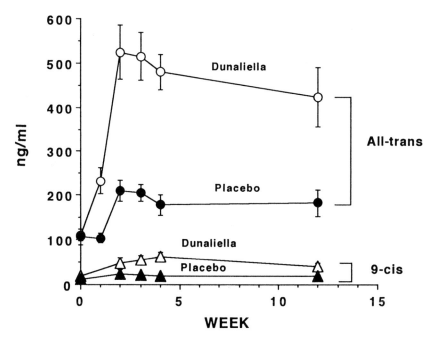

FIGURE 1. Changes in plasma carotene by administration of *Dunaliella bardawil* preparation. Values represent the mean ± SE (n = 10).

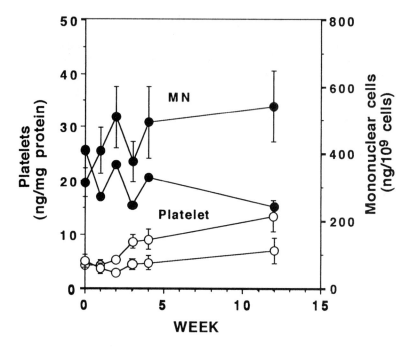

FIGURE 2. Changes in all-*trans* β-carotene of platelets and mononuclear cells. Values represent the mean ± SE (n = 10). The *upper curves* for both cell types were obtained from carotenoid-treated subjects; the *lower curves* were obtained from placebo-treated subjects.

REFERENCES

1. KRINSKY, N. I. 1988. The evidence for the role of carotenes in preventive health. Clin. Nutr. **7:** 107–112.
2. PETO, R., R. DOLL, J. D. BUCKLEY & M. B. SPORN. 1981. Can dietary beta-carotene materially reduce human cancer rates? Nature **290:** 201–208.
3. MURATA, T., H. TAMAI, T. MORINOBU, M. MANAGO, A. TAKENAKA, H. TAKENAKA & M. MINO. 1992. Determination of β-carotene in plasma, blood cells, and buccal mucosa by electrochemical detection. Lipids **27:** 840–843.

Variability of Serum Carotenoids in Response to Controlled Diets Containing Six Servings of Fruits and Vegetables per Day

P. E. BOWEN, V. GARG, M. STACEWICZ-SAPUNTZAKIS,
L. YELTON, AND R. S. SCHREINER

Department of Nutrition and Medical Dietetics (M/C 517)
University of Illinois at Chicago
1919 West Taylor Street
Chicago, Illinois 60612

Serum carotenoid levels (SC) have been proposed as a measure of dietary exposure to fruits and vegetables (FV) in several large diet intervention trials. Yet β-carotene metabolism studies and intervention trials have repeatedly identified low responders (LR), subjects whose serum levels do not appreciably rise with β-carotene dosing. As part of a series of long-term controlled feeding studies which included 5–6 servings of fruits and vegetables per day, a Healthy People 2000 Objective, we were able to (1) assess the proportion of LR, (2) whether low-response was a stable attribute, (3) which carotenoids are sensitive to variability in response and (4) whether SC can serve as a marker of FV exposure in intervention trials and population studies.

We fed 48 healthy, nonsmoking, premenopausal women with plasma cholesterol levels $\geq$50th percentile (Lipid Research Clinics Prevalence Study) as a reference population 5–6 servings of FV per day as part of cholesterol-lowering diets. The study design involved a 40% fat as energy (en%), polyunsaturated : saturated fatty acid ratio (P : S) of 0.5 diet for 1 month followed by 5 months of either a 20en% fat, P : S 2.0, 20en% fat, P : S 0.5 or 30en% fat, P : S 1.0 diet. Each 6-month study was performed in a different year starting in January and ending in June or July. Energy levels were adjusted to maintain body weight throughout each study and diets were consumed in the metabolism laboratory or packed for take-out. Every effort was made to keep the carotenoid content of the diets constant. Although plasma cholesterol decreased by 8% for all diets SC were only marginally affected by the decrease. Furthermore the different diets had no effect on SC. Therefore, we combined the data from the dietary studies for this paper.

The women represented a variety of ethnic groups and 40% had body mass indexes (BMI) >27.5. Their mean age was 32.3 $\pm$ 1.7 yrs. Diets averaged 3 mg/day for lutein/zeaxanthin, 0.5 mg/d cryptoxanthin, 12 mg/d lycopene, 2 mg/d α-carotene and 6 mg/d β-carotene, by chemical analysis of 4-day cycle food aliquots. TABLE 1 presents the SC at baseline, at wks 3 and 4, when women were on the control diet, and at selected weeks when they were consuming the cholesterol-lowering diets. Fourteen (29%) of the 48 women were classified as LR to dietary β-carotene with a clear discontinuity between responders (R) and LR. Low response to dietary carotenoids was a stable characteristic over the entire 6-month controlled feeding period. The differences in serum levels between R and LR (comparing the means of weeks 20 and 24 between R and LR) was most

TABLE 1. Serum Carotenoid Levels in Response to a Diet Containing 5–6 Servings of Fruits and Vegetables per Day (μg/dL)[a]

Carotenoids	Response	Baseline	3 Weeks	4 Weeks	8 Weeks	20 Weeks	24 Weeks	p Values
β-Carotene	responders	20.7 ± 12.4	38.7 ± 15.9	41.4 ± 14.8	43.7 ± 15.0	41.9 ± 18.4	42.6 ± 19.4	<0.0001
	nonresponders	7.1 ± 3.3	14.8 ± 5.2	13.5 ± 3.7	14.6 ± 3.9	14.2 ± 5.1	14.5 ± 5.0	<0.0001
	p values	0.0001	0.0002	0.0002	0.0001	0.0001	0.0001	
α-Carotene	responders	5.2 ± 5.7	10.3 ± 5.4	11.2 ± 10.4	9.9 ± 4.0	9.9 ± 5.6	9.9 ± 5.6	0.0033
	nonresponders	1.6 ± 1.0	5.2 ± 2.1	3.9 ± 1.5	3.9 ± 1.3	3.9 ± 1.8	3.7 ± 1.8	<0.0001
	p values	0.0240	0.0014	0.0160	0.0001	0.0003	0.0002	
Cryptoxanthin	responders	13.6 ± 8.5	32.5 ± 11.5	37.9 ± 11.3	37.4 ± 13.3	33.1 ± 13.6	33.8 ± 16.6	<0.0001
	nonresponders	8.5 ± 4.5	18.1 ± 7.1	18.2 ± 7.3	16.5 ± 6.9	15.3 ± 6.7	17.3 ± 10.3	0.0069
	p values	0.0397	0.0001	0.0397	0.0001	0.0001	0.0001	
Lycopene	responders	25.4 ± 17.6	46.7 ± 17.8	47.1 ± 13.1	42.9 ± 13.7	38.1 ± 13.7	42.4 ± 15.4	<0.0001
	nonresponders	21.9 ± 16.0	35.8 ± 10.7	32.6 ± 13.1	32.0 ± 6.9	30.6 ± 9.5	34.7 ± 6.1	0.0080
	p values	NS	0.0385	0.0015	0.0071	0.0684	0.0778	
Lutein	responders	19.6 ± 6.9	32.3 ± 9.4	31.6 ± 9.4	30.6 ± 9.3	30.0 ± 11.2	29.3 ± 10.2	<0.0001
	nonresponders	14.8 ± 8.8	19.3 ± 5.0	18.4 ± 3.4	18.6 ± 3.4	20.7 ± 5.9	18.1 ± 4.2	0.1242
	p values	0.0493	0.0001	0.0001	0.0001	0.0052	0.0003	
Retinol	responders	43.8 ± 10.7	46.3 ± 10.5	46.1 ± 11.1	48.6 ± 11.3	47.8 ± 11.0	48.4 ± 8.3	NS
	nonresponders	39.4 ± 11.5	44.0 ± 12.3	40.7 ± 11.7	42.8 ± 13.3	45.2 ± 15.1	44.4 ± 12.2	NS
	p values	NS	NS	NS	NS	NS	NS	

[a] Mean ± SD.

pronounced for β-carotene ($\Delta 66\%$), α-carotene ($\Delta 61\%$) and β-cryptoxanthin ($\Delta 51\%$), the provitamin A carotenoids. The differences between R and LR for lutein was intermediate ($\Delta 35\%$) while the differences for lycopene were barely significant ($\Delta 19\%$). There was no difference in retinol levels between the two groups. Diets containing 5–6 servings of FV per day produced serum increases ranging from 90–146% for the provitamin A carotenoids in both R and LR women, because LR women started out with significantly lower carotenoid levels than R women. This increase was evident by wk 3 of each study and was relatively stable thereafter. Increases in serum lutein and lycopene were less dramatic (31–58%) for both R and LR women. Retinol levels did not increase in either group. It may be that these diets did not provide sufficiently higher levels of these carotenoids than these women's usual diets. Nevertheless, it appears that LR women can absorb or maintain circulating levels of lycopene more easily than the provitamin A carotenoids.

Due to the large proportion of LR women in our study group, serum carotenoids cannot be used to assess compliance of an individual to a high FV diet. However, since even the LR women increased their SC levels, groups of individuals would experience rises in SC depending upon the extent of change in their diet. Although LR women had the same percentage increase in SC compared to the R women because of lower baseline SC, they were not able to generate the same circulating levels of carotenoids even after 6 months of FV consumption as the R women on the same diet. Perhaps LR are at greater risk for coronary heart disease, cancer and other diseases because they are unable to generate adequate serum levels of the carotenoids from diet alone. A number of factors such as obesity, lipid-handling and resistance to plasma cholesterol-lowering through lipid-modulated diets can be investigated in this study to further distinguish LR from R women.

Plasma Carotenoid Levels before and after Supplementation with a Carotenoid Complex

ARIANNA CARUGHI AND FRED HOOPER

Neo-Life Company of America
P.O. Box 5012
Fremont, California 94537-5012

Carotenoids may be important cellular antioxidants in animals and man. Interest in the absorption, utilization and metabolism of carotenoids, especially beta-carotene, has been stimulated by several reports from epidemiological studies that suggest these compounds protect against degenerative diseases such as certain cancers, heart disease and macular degeneration.[1] It has been shown that purified beta-carotene raises plasma levels of beta-carotene whereas carotenoid-containing foods increase levels of other carotenoids.[2] Plasma response to supplements containing beta-carotene along with other carotenoids has not been established. In this study we determined changes in beta-carotene, alpha-carotene and lycopene in volunteers given a daily supplement of carotenoids from a carotenoid complex while on a low-carotenoid diet.

Eleven healthy men and women volunteers participated in the study. TABLE 1 shows their characteristics and biochemical indices. Participants ate a diet of natural foods but low in carotenoids for 6 weeks. We estimated that their daily diet would provide less than 0.4 mg of beta-carotene and alpha-carotene and 0 mg of lycopene. After 2 weeks on this low carotenoid diet, they began supplementation with a fruit and vegetable concentrate that provided a total dose of 8.5 mg beta-carotene, 3.5 mg alpha-carotene and 0.5 mg of lycopene per day. Supplementation continued for the next four weeks. Fasting blood samples for carotenoid analysis were collected at the beginning of the study (baseline), after two weeks on the low-carotenoid diet and weekly thereafter. Beta-carotene, alpha-carotene and lycopene levels were quantified using the HPLC method described by Bieri *et al.*[3] Fasting blood samples to determine HDL-cholesterol, LDL-cholesterol and VLDL-cholesterol, total cholesterol and triglyceride values were collected before the beginning, and at the end of supplementation.

During the first two weeks, when volunteers consumed a low-carotenoid diet, the levels of all carotenoids fell significantly (TABLE 2). Alpha- and beta-carotene levels increased significantly after supplementation. Lycopene levels, however, did not increase rapidly during the supplementation period. This is the first study reporting plasma alpha-carotene response to a carotenoid supplement. It shows that carotenoid intake has a rapid and important influence on plasma levels.

Supplements of purified beta-carotene are more effective than fruits and vegetables in raising plasma beta-carotene levels. However, intake of purified beta-carotene does not increase levels of other carotenoids also found in these foods. In this study, supplementation with a carotenoid complex made from fruit and vegetable concentrates significantly increased plasma levels of beta- *and* alpha-carotene. Since carotenoids other than beta-carotene may also offer specific protection against certain degenerative diseases, this type of supplementation may provide an advantageous alternative to supplementing with only beta-carotene.

TABLE 1. Characteristics and Biochemical Indices for the Study Participants before and after Supplementation with a Carotenoid Complex[a]

	Men (n = 4) 45.8 ± 4.7 24.0 ± 1.8		Women (n = 7) 37.9 ± 8.4 21.5 ± 1.0	
Age				
Body Mass Index[b]				
	Before	After	Before	After
	(mg/dL)		(mg/dL)	
Triglycerides	133 ± 54	146 ± 21	65 ± 23	101 ± 18
Cholesterol	233 ± 41	217 ± 44	185 ± 21	185 ± 27
HDL-cholesterol	36 ± 6	31 ± 7	55 ± 16	48 ± 15
VLDL-cholesterol	27 ± 6	29 ± 6	13 ± 4	20 ± 3
LDL-cholesterol	170 ± 41	156 ± 44	117 ± 12	117 ± 13

[a] X ± SD.
[b] Weight (in kg)/stature^2 (in m^2).

TABLE 2. Plasma Carotenoid Concentration in Subjects on a Low-Carotenoid Diet at Baseline and before and after 4 Weeks of Supplementation with a Carotenoid Complex[a]

	Baseline (ng/mL)	Before (ng/mL)	After (ng/mL)
Beta-carotene	462 ± 318	269 ± 177[b]	778 ± 428[b,c]
Alpha-carotene	165 ± 110	99 ± 62[b]	357 ± 168[b,c]
Lycopene	481 ± 193	282 ± 87[b]	305 ± 82

[a] X ± SD (n = 11).
[b] Change significantly different from baseline ($p < 0.05$).
[c] Change significantly different from before supplementation ($p < 0.05$).

REFERENCES

1. MATHEWS-ROTH, M. M. 1990. Recent progress in the medical applications of carotenoids. Pure Appl. Chem. **63:** 147–156.
2. MICOZZI, M. S., E. D. BROWN, B. K. EDWARDS et al. 1992. Plasma carotenoid response to chronic intake of selected foods and beta-carotene supplements. Am. J. Clin. Nutr. **55:** 1120–1125.
3. BIERI, J. G., E. D. BROWN & J. C. SMITH. 1985. Determination of individual carotenoids in human plasma by high performance liquid chromatography. J. Liq. Chromatogr. **34:** 44–48.

Free Radical Scavenging of Lutein in Vitro[a]

M. CHOPRA,[b,e] R. L. WILLSON,[c] AND D. I. THURNHAM[d]

[b]Dunn Nutritional Laboratory
Medical Research Council
Downhams Lane
Milton Road
Cambridge CB4 1XJ, United Kingdom

[c]Department of Biochemistry
Brunel University
Uxbridge, Middlesex UB8 3PH, United Kingdom

[d]Human Nutrition Group
Department of Biology and Biomedical Sciences
University of Ulster at Coleraine
Coleraine BT52 1SA, Northern Ireland

INTRODUCTION

Lutein is one of the most common xanthophyll carotenoids in our diet and is as abundant as β-carotene in most green and yellow vegetables.[1] In the British population, lutein forms 20–40% of the total carotenoid components in the plasma.[2] Its structure is very similar to that of α-carotene except that it has two hydroxyl groups in the terminal ionone rings. The presence of these functional groups should make it slightly more hydrophilic and may influence its antioxidant properties. In the present study we have looked at the oxy, sulfur (RS·) and peroxy (ROO·) radical scavenging activity of lutein in vitro.

METHODS

Oxy and Sulfur Radical Scavenging Activity of Lutein

A gamma radiolysis study was undertaken in which radicals were generated using a cobalt 60 type source at 1 K rad/min. The solvent was 75 : 25 methanol : water. Under our experimental conditions, mainly methanol radicals and a small amount of hydroxyl and superoxide ion will be produced. These would lead to the generation of RS· in the presence of sulfur compounds. Lutein was exposed to gamma radiolysis for one hour in the presence and absence of glutathione (GSH). Aliquots were removed every 15 min and the decrease in absorbance at 445 nm was measured spectrophotometrically.

[a] This study was funded by Nestec Switzerland.

[e] Address correspondence to Dr. M. Chopra, Human Nutrition Group, Department of Biological and Biomedical Sciences, University of Ulster at Coleraine, Coleraine BT52 1SA, Northern Ireland.

Effect of Lutein on Azo-Initiated Peroxidation of Linoleic Acid

Azo-initiated peroxidation of methyl linoleic acid (LA) was followed by measuring oxygen consumption in the presence and absence of antioxidants. Final concentrations in the electrode cell were 133 mmol/l LA, 13.3 mmol/l AMVN and 10 and 25 μmol/l lutein. For comparison the effect of β-carotene and Trolox on azo-initiated oxidation of LA was also investigated.

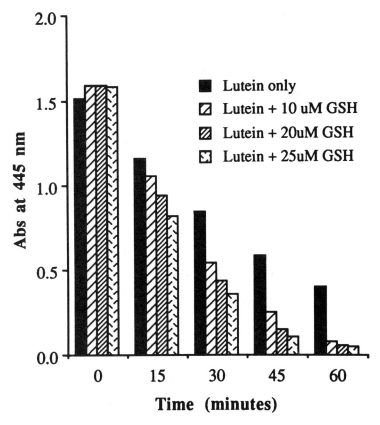

FIGURE 1. Gamma radiolysis of lutein in methanol : water (75 : 25). Final concentration of lutein was 10 μmol/l, and that of GSH was 10, 20 and 25 μmol/l.

RESULTS AND DISCUSSION

Results of this study show that lutein can scavenge toxic oxygen species *in vitro*. Under our experimental conditions it reacts faster with sulfur radicals than oxy radicals (FIG. 1). It inhibited the azo-initiated peroxidation of LA at concentra-

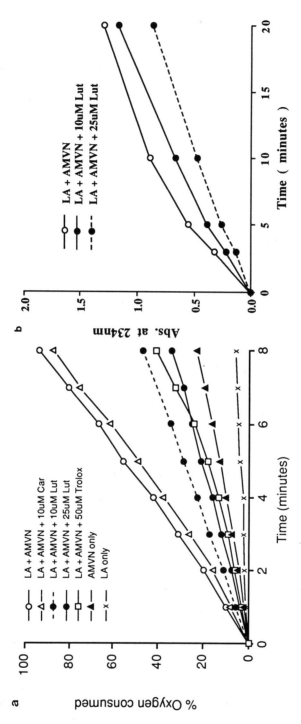

FIGURE 2. The effect of lutein on AMVN-initiated peroxidation of LA followed by measuring (a) oxygen consumption and (b) diene conjugate formation. Final concentration of LA was 133 mmol/l, and that of AMVN was 13.3 mmol/l. Incubation temperature was 50°C.

tions as low as 10 μmol/l, when oxidation was followed by measuring oxygen consumption (FIG. 2a) and diene conjugate formation at 234 nm (FIG. 2b). β-Carotene (10 μmol/l final) showed a small inhibitory effect on oxygen consumption. Trolox (vitamin E analogue) showed no effect at 10 μmol/l and significant inhibition at 50 μmol/l. Stoichiometry of peroxy radical scavenging of α-tocopherol and its hydrophilic homolog Trolox has been reported to be 2 : 1.[3,4] From this the rate of peroxy radical generation by AMVN can be calculated to be approximately 25×10^{-6} mol/minute in our assay system. Since we were measuring oxygen consumption every minute and Trolox reacts very fast with peroxy radicals this can explain why Trolox showed no significant effect on oxygen consumption at the concentration of 10 μmol/l. Lutein inhibited the oxygen consumption at a constant rate in our assay system. This suggests that lutein scavenges radicals more slowly than Trolox but can inhibit peroxidation for a longer time and at lower concentrations.

ACKNOWLEDGMENT

Lutein was a gift from Linexa, Quito, Ecuador.

REFERENCES

1. HEINONEN, M. I., V. OLLILAINEN, E. K. LINKOLA, P. T. VARO & P. E. KOIVISTOINEN. 1989. Carotenoids in Finnish foods: vegetables, fruits, and berries. J. Agric. Food Chem. **37:** 655–659.
2. THURNHAM, D. I. & P. S. FLORA. 1988. Do higher vitamin A requirements in men explain the difference between the sexes in plasma provitamin A carotenoids and retinol? Proc. Nutr. Soc. **47:** 181A.
3. NIKI, E., T. SAITO, A. KAWAKAMI & Y. KAMIYA. 1984. Inhibition of oxidation and methyl linoleate in solution by vitamin E and vitamin C. J. Biol. Chem. **259:** 4177–4182.
4. TSUCHIYA, M., G. SCITA, H.-J. FREISLEBEN, V. E. KAGAN & L. PACKER. 1992. Antioxidant radical-scavenger activity of carotenoids and retinoids compared to α-tocopherol. Methods Enzymol. **213:** 460–472.

all-*trans* Retinoic Acid: a Dose-Seeking Study in Solid Tumors

H. C. PITOT IV, J. RUBIN, J. S. KOVACH, A. J. SCHUTT,
AND P. C. ADAMSON[a]

Medical Oncology Mayo Clinic
Rochester, Minnesota 55905
and
[a]*Pediatric Branch*
National Cancer Institute
Bethesda, Maryland

Retinoids exert a wide range of biological effects, including prevention of head and neck cancers.[1] We conducted a phase I study in advanced solid tumors to determine the maximum tolerable dose (MTD) of daily all-*trans* retinoic acid (TRA). Pharmacokinetic sampling after chronic administration was performed to determine bioavailability on a subgroup of patients because of previous reports of decreasing plasma concentration after prolonged administration.[2,3] Patient eligibility criteria included histologic proof of advanced solid tumors with no more conventional therapy available. All patients had normal hematologic profiles and essentially normal serum chemistries. Thirty-four patients were treated with a median age of 65 years (range 28–78). The ECOG performance score was 0 or 1 in 30 patients. One-half the patients had metastatic colorectal carcinoma. All patients had to have recovered from previous chemotherapy or radiotherapy.

Patients were treated in groups of 3 with escalating dose levels. TRA was divided into 2 doses and administered with an 8-oz. glass of whole milk. The gelatin capsule was supplied by Hoffmann-La Roche through the National Cancer Institute. Patients were evaluated initially at 3 weeks and then every 4 weeks. A subgroup of 6 patients underwent pharmacokinetic sampling after the patients had received 4 weeks of therapy. Sampling was performed on days 28 and 29 at 30-minute intervals and continued for a total of 7 hours. Three patients took the divided dose on day 28 with pharmacology studies performed after the morning dose. A single daily dose was given on day 29 with subsequent sampling. The other 3 patients took the single daily dose on day 28 and the divided dose on day 29. The plasma concentration of TRA was measured by a modified HPLC method.[4]

Toxicity was generally mild (TABLE 1). Virtually all patients experienced some cheilitis and xerosis. There were elevations in serum lipids in nearly all patients, but this was not clinically significant and required no dose modification. Dose-limiting toxicity was reached at 195 mg/m^2. Toxicities experienced at this level included severe dermatitis and headache. Pharmacology sampling showed peak levels following the 78-mg/m^2 dose on either day 28 or day 29 were relatively low when compared to previously reported studies.[2,5] The observed plasma concentrations were quite variable from patient to patient (TABLE 2). The increases in the area under the plasma concentration curves after the double dose were unpredictable and ranged from <1.2 times increased to > a 10-fold increase (mean 4.7-fold increase). No patient obtained a complete or partial response. Twenty-five patients had stable disease with a median time of 56 days on treatment (range 36–199).

In conclusion, the maximum tolerated dose of TRA taken orally on a daily

TABLE 1. Toxicity

Dose (mg/m²)	Patients	Cheilitis/ Xerosis	Skin	Epistaxis	Headache	Hepatic	Triglycerides	Other
45	3	3	0	1	1	2	169 → 328 162 → 478 98 → 157	nausea — 1
56	3	2	0	0	1	2 1 (gr. 2)	79 → 201 153 → 420 165 → 315	
70	3	3	0	1	1 (gr. 2)	2	222 → 508 173 → 399 60 → 255	nausea/vomit — 1 anorexia — 1 alopecia — 1 bone pain — 1 cuticle loss — 1 leukopenia (gr. 1) — 1
87	3	3	0	1	1 (gr. 1) 1 (gr. 2)	3	184 → 234 103 → 281 230 → 493	nausea — 1 fatigue — 1 leukopenia (gr. 1) — 1
100	3	3	1 (gr. 3)	3	0	3	217 → 624 164 → 315 152 → 247	anorexia — 1 stomatitis — 1 alopecia — 1
125	3	3	0	1	2 (gr. 1)	3	103 → 135 314 → 767 73 → 140	alopecia — 2 stomatitis — 1
156	3	3	0	1	2 (gr. 1)	2	228 → 520 175 → 224 104 → 93	nausea — 1 folliculitis — 1 leukopenia (gr. 1) — 1
195	5	3	2 (gr. 3)	1	2 (gr. 3)	3 1 (gr. 2)	171 → 1001 64 → 55 141 → 370 103 → 246 185 → NA	nausea — 1 vomiting — 2 alopecia — 1 anorexia — 1
156	8	7	1 (gr. 2)	2	4 (gr. 1) 2 (gr. 2) 1 (gr. 3)	6	207 → 374 82 → NA 116 → 326 71 → 213 327 → 590 148 → 394 119 → 160 248 → 608	stomatitis — 2 bone pain — 4 nausea — 5 vomiting — 3 anorexia — 3 diarrhea — 2

TABLE 2. Plasma Concentrations of TRA

Patient	Peak Plasma Concentration (μM)		AUC^a (μM $\times$ Min)	
	78 mg/m^2	156 mg/m^2	78 mg/m^2	156 mg/m^2
1	0.4	0.4	58.8	67.0
2	0.13	0.9	11.7	133.4
3	1.2	1.0	139.8	173.4
4	0.17	0.6	16.5	51.9
5	0.42	3.0	54	52.1
6	0.07	0.095	13.7	9.5

^{a} Area under the plasma concentration-time curve.

basis is 156 mg/m^2. The dose-limiting toxicities on this schedule are dermatitis and severe headache. The plasma concentrations are quite variable from patient to patient. There was no antineoplastic activity observed.

REFERENCES

1. HONG, W. K., S. M. LIPPMAN, L. M. ITRI *et al.* 1990. N. Engl. J. Med. **323**(12): 795–801.
2. SMITH, M. A., P. C. ADAMSON, F. M. BALIS *et al.* 1992. J. Clin. Oncol. **10**(11): 1666–1673.
3. MUINDI, J., S. R. FRANKEL, W. H. J. MILLER *et al.* 1992. Blood **79**(2): 299–303.
4. PENG, Y. M., M. J. XU & D. S. ALBERTS. 1987. J. Natl. Cancer Inst. **78**(1): 95–99.
5. MUINDI, J., S. R. FRANKEL, C. HUSELTON *et al.* 1992. Cancer Res. **52**(8): 2138–2142.

Beta-Carotene and Cervical Dysplasia Trials in Australia

D. MACKERRAS,[a] P. BAGHURST,[b] C. FAIRLEY,[c]
L. IRWIG,[a] E. WEISBERG,[d] AND J. SIMPSON[a]

[a]Department of Public Health, A27
University of Sydney
Sydney, New South Wales 2006, Australia

[b]CSIRO
Adelaide, South Australia 5000, Australia

[c]Monash University
Melbourne, Victoria 3181, Australia

[d]Family Planning Association of New South Wales
Ashfield, New South Wales 2131, Australia

There is much interest in the role of dietary antioxidants in protecting against various cancers. However, several large case-control studies have had conflicting findings regarding the effect of beta-carotene and vitamin C on the risk of *in situ* and invasive cervical cancers.[1-3] In Australia, three ongoing randomized controlled trials are investigating the effect of beta-carotene on lower grade cervical abnormalities. The participants in all trials are women who have chosen to have regular colposcopic follow-up rather than immediate ablative therapy.

In Sydney, the independent effects of 30 mg synthetic (all *trans*) beta-carotene and 500 mg vitamin C versus placebo on the 2-year progression and regression rates of grade I cervical intraepithelial neoplasia (CIN I) are being investigated using a double-blind factorial design. Eligibility is based on the assessment of colposcopic, cytological and histological findings. There is a one-month run-in phase to assess compliance before randomization occurs. Participants are contacted monthly by telephone and interviewed in person at their 6-monthly colposcopic assessment. A progression endpoint is reached if the clinician recommends treatment owing to increased severity of the lesion. A regression endpoint is reached when the woman is discharged from the Colposcopy Clinic following two consecutive normal assessments. To date, 114 women have been randomized and among these, seven progression and three regression endpoints have occurred.

In Adelaide, a combined dose of 15 mg beta-carotene (derived from the alga *Dunaliella salina*) and 300 mg vitamin C versus a placebo containing 200 mg lecithin is being tested in women with CIN I. Length of time between colposcopy assessments is left to the clinician's discretion but is no longer than six months. Progression and regression endpoints are based on clinicians' decisions to recommend treatment or discharge respectively. To date, 65 participants have been recruited.

In Melbourne, the effect of 30 mg beta-carotene (derived from *Dunaliella salina*) versus a placebo containing 200 mg lecithin on the changes in human papilloma virus over one year is being studied. Genital samples are collected at 0, 6 and 12 months using tampons and analyzed using quantitative Southern blot and polymerase chain reaction methods. To date, 90 participants have been recruited.

All studies collect a variety of information concerning other risk factors such as smoking, sexual history and dietary intake using a semiquantitative food frequency questionnaire. Blood samples are taken regularly in the Adelaide and Melbourne studies to assess compliance.

REFERENCES

1. BROCK, K. E., G. BERRY, P. A. MOCK & L. A. BRINTON. 1988. Nutrients in diet and plasma and risk of *in situ* cervical cancer. J. Natl. Cancer Inst. **80:** 580–585.
2. HERRERO, R., N. POTISCHMAN, L. A. BRINTON, W. C. REEVES, M. M. BRENES, F. TENORIO, R. C. DE BRITTON & E. GAITAN. 1990. A case-control study of nutrient status and invasive cervical cancer. 1. Dietary indicators. Am. J. Epidemiol. **143:** 1335–1346.
3. ZIEGLER, R. G., L. A. BRINTON, R. F. HAMMAN, H. F. LEHMAN, R. S. LEVINE, K. MALLIN, S. A. NORMAN, J. F. ROSENTHAL, A. C. TRUMBLE & R. N. HOOVER. 1990. Diet and the risk of invasive cervical cancer among white women in the United States. Am. J. Epidemiol. **132:** 432–445.

Carotenoids and Vitamin A in Prevention, Adjuvant Cancer Therapy, Mastalgia Treatment, and AIDS-Related Complex

LEONIDA SANTAMARIA AND
AMALIA BIANCHI-SANTAMARIA

Camillo Golgi Institute of General Pathology
Tumor Center and Institute of Pharmacology II
University of Pavia
27100 Pavia, Italy

PROGRESS REPORT

Current developments in research on the chemopreventive/therapeutic action by carotenoids (CARs), as carried out in our Institute–Tumor Center have so far (1989–1993) produced the following original data.

Protection against Chemical Genotoxic Agents

The supplementation of CARs in humans protects against chemical genotoxic agents as demonstrated by the reduction of micronuclei induced by bleomycin in cultured lymphocytes.[1] The method consisted of supplementation of normal human volunteers (age 25–35, both sexes) to reach about 5 μg/dL blood carotenoid concentration. Then, lymphocytes from CARs-supplemented and control subjects were cultured *in vitro* in the presence of bleomycin to produce chromosome breakage.

Immunostimulation by β-Carotene

The immunostimulation by β-carotene in mice and rats increases survival after transplantation of ascites tumors along with a dramatic increase in the number of liver mastocytes and other immunocompetent cells (FIG. 1). This increase in mastocyte number was quantified in a 23 : 1 β-carotene-supplemented vs control increased ratio.[2] The immunostimulation was obtained by feeding BALB/c mice with a β-carotene-enriched diet[3] one month before tumor transplantation.

Adjuvant Cancer Therapy

The supplementation of β-carotene 80 mg/day as adjuvant to radiotherapy in nonsurgically treatable human lung cancer cases, but with good performance status, leads to an increase (1.5–3 times more) in overall survival with respect to expected median survival.[4] This was observed in a pilot study on patients who complied well with the above treatment.

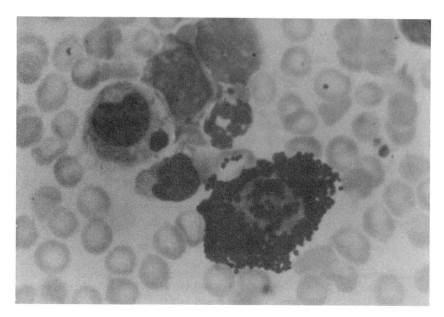

FIGURE 1. Liver imprinting from female Wistar rat having undergone Yoshida tumor transplantation, and serial tumor sampling until day 23 after transplantation. May Grunwald Giemsa staining, 1000×. Evidence of 3 cancer cells with presence of immunocompetent cells including a mastocyte.

Mastalgia Treatment

The treatment of premenstrual cyclical mastalgia, associated with benign breast disease (BBD) or otherwise, using β-carotene continuous daily administration at low dosage (20 mg/day) and intermittent retinyl acetate at high dosage (150,000–300,000 I.U./day) for seven days just before periods (FIG. 2) produces

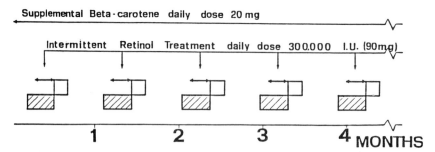

FIGURE 2. Scheme of combined β-carotene continuous and retinol intermittent (premenstrual–seven days) supplementation in cyclical mastalgia. ↔ 7-day premenstrual retinol treatment; □ 5-day menstrual period (28-day cycle); ▨ premenstrual cyclical mastalgia (~10 days).

marked pain relief and sometime recovery with no vitamin A side effects at all.[5] This clinical experimental approach was attempted in an effort to modulate the beneficial effect on mastalgia by vitamin A at high dosage, a therapy that, unfortunately, had to be dropped because of retinol toxicity.[6]

Possible Activity of β-Carotene in Patients with the AIDS-Related Complex (ARC)

In a pilot single blind study, β-carotene supplementation produced, in ARC patients under current treatment, apparent recovery from asthenia, fever, nocturnal sweating, diarrhea, and loss in weight, and led as a result to an improvement in general health and working efficiency, but not to an improvement in multiple district lymphoadenopathies. Nevertheless, β-carotene appeared to prevent progress to AIDS and, in addition, to lower the effective dosage of AZT used in one case of ARC developed into AIDS, producing a recovery from opportunistic infections and an inhibition of Kaposi sarcoma diffusion, in line with a twofold rise in CD4 counts.[8]

CONCLUSIONS

On the whole, the above data concerning protection against chemical genotoxic agents, immunostimulation by β-carotene, and adjuvant cancer therapy demonstrated that CARs are powerful oxygen free radical quenchers,[3,7] able to exert not only chemopreventive, but also therapeutic effects, through anticlastogenic and immunostimulatory mechanisms. The data concerning mastalgia treatment refer to ongoing studies, started as early as 1989, to relieve and/or recover from pain in cyclical mastalgia by β-carotene plus intermittent retinol acetate. This original treatment scheme demonstrated that the therapeutic effect should well be due to the following mechanisms: a) a synergism between β-carotene and retinyl acetate, thus totally avoiding retinol toxic side effects; b) an antiinflammatory effect of β-carotene likely by antioxidant action; and c) a possible antioestrogenic and antiprolactinic action by vitamin A. Finally, β-carotene supplementation relieves symptoms in ARC patients preventing progress to AIDS.

REFERENCES

1. BIANCHI, L., A. BIANCHI, F. TATEO, R. PIZZALA, L. STIVALA & L. SANTAMARIA. 1990. Reduction of chromosomal damage by bleomycin in lymphocytes from subjects supplemented with carotenoids. Relevance in bleomycin tumour chemotherapy. Preliminary results. Boll. Chim. Farm. 129(12): 83s–87s.
2. ROVETA, G., A. BIANCHI & L. SANTAMARIA. 1992. Beta-carotene supplementation is effective in modulating host defense as detected in a tumor and host organ imprint assay. Med. Biol. Environ. 20: 193–200.
3. SANTAMARIA, L., A. BIANCHI, A. ARNABOLDI, C. RAVETTO, L. BIANCHI, R. PIZZALA, L. ANDREONI, G. SANTAGATI & P. BERMOND. 1988. Chemoprevention of indirect and direct chemical carcinogenesis by carotenoids as oxygen radical quenchers. Ann. N.Y. Acad. Sci. 534: 584–596.
4. DELL'ORTI, M., A. BIANCHI-SANTAMARIA & L. SANTAMARIA. 1992. Survival increase by beta-carotene supplementation in non-surgically treatable lung cancer. A preliminary study. Med. Biol. Environ. 30(2): 351–355.

5. SANTAMARIA, L. & A. BIANCHI-SANTAMARIA. 1990. Cancer chemoprevention by supplemental carotenoids and synergism with retinol in mastodynia treatment. Med. Oncol. Tumor Pharmacother. **7**(3-3): 153–167.

6. BAND, P. R., M. DESCHAMPS, M. FALARDEAU, J. LADOUCEUR & J. COTE. 1984. Treatment of benign breast disease with vitamin A. Prev. Med. **13**: 549–554.

7. SANTAMARIA, L. & A. BIANCHI-SANTAMARIA. 1991. Free radicals as carcinogens and their quenchers as anticarcinogens. Med. Oncol. Tumor Pharmacother. **8**(3): 121–140.

8. Bianchi-Santamaria, A., S. Fedeli & L. Santamaria. 1992. Short communication: possible activity of beta-carotene in patients with the AIDS related complex. A pilot study. Med. Oncol. Tumor Pharmacother. **9**(3): 151–153.

The Absence of a Synergistic Protective Effect of β-Carotene and Vitamin E on Skin Tumorigenesis in Mice

L. A. LAMBERT, W. G. WAMER, R. R. WEI, S. LAVU,
AND A. KORNHAUSER

US Food and Drug Administration
Center for Food Safety and Applied Nutrition
HFS-128
200 C Street SW
Washington, DC 20204

Epidemiological[1,2] and experimental[3,4] studies have indicated that β-carotene and vitamin E show protective effects against a variety of cancers. We were interested in determining if a dietary combination of β-carotene and vitamin E would result in a synergistic protective effect against chemically-induced skin tumors in mice.

Possible mechanisms for the induction of cancer and other diseases include the effects of free radicals and activated oxygen species which cause cell and tissue damage. These active molecules can be produced as a result of cellular metabolism or from environmental factors such as pollution and certain dietary components. Biological defenses against these active molecules include the enzymes superoxide dismutase, catalase, and peroxidase. In addition there are micronutrients and vitamins such as β-carotene, selenium, zinc, and the vitamins A, C, and E. Vitamin E is important for scavenging free radicals. It intercalates in the lipid bilayers of cell membranes and terminates free radical chain reactions and confines membrane damage. The micronutrient β-carotene is best known for its ability to quench singlet oxygen and scavenge free radicals.

In our study 45 Skh-1 mice were assigned to each of four diet groups: 1. standard, Ralston Purina Rodent Chow, 2. β-carotene (0.5%, all *trans*, crystalline), 3. vitamin E (0.12%, d-α-tocopheryl acid succinate), and 4. β-carotene (0.5%) + vitamin E (0.12%). Diet supplements were blended with ground standard diet, moistened, cut into squares, and dried (50°C).

Skin tumors were generated by topically treating mice with a single application of the initiator, 7,12-dimethylbenz[a]-anthracene (DMBA). This was followed by weekly applications of the promoter, phorbol 12-myristate 13-acetate (PMA). A decrease in the number of skin tumors in supplemented-diet groups as compared to the standard diet group was the measure by which the protective effect of each diet was determined. Mice were observed for tumors each week for 27 weeks after chemical initiation (FIG. 1). Statistically significant decreases in the number of cumulative tumors at week 27 for each diet group were 32% for β-carotene, 25% for vitamin E, and 21% for β-carotene + vitamin E. There were no statistically significant differences in the number of tumors among any of the three supplemented groups. The β-carotene + vitamin E diet group showed a statistically significant delay in the onset of tumors 1–8 which was not observed in any other diet group. In addition, for tumors which eventually regressed, the tumors in this group regressed sooner than those in any other diet group. Analyses of skin showed increased levels for β-carotene and α-tocopherol in animals that received

TABLE 1. α-Tocopherol and β-Carotene in Serum and Skin*

| | Serum and Skin Levels | | | | | |
| | α-Tocopherol | | | β-Carotene | | |
Diet Group	†8 Weeks	24 Weeks	43 Weeks	8 Weeks	24 Weeks	43 Weeks
Standard						
Serum (µg/ml)	§1.37 ± 0.62[a]	0.48 ± 0.07[de]	1.81 ± 0.28[ijk]	NA	NS	NS
Skin (µg/g)	4.27 ± 1.45[bc]	9.11 ± 1.97[fgh]	5.51 ± 1.44[lmn]	ND	0.16 ± 0.09[op]	NS
β-Carotene						
Serum (µg/ml)	NS	NS	0.78 ± 0.36[i]	NA	0.017 ± 0.019	0.061 ± 0.011
Skin (µg/g)	ND	4.62 ± 1.39[f]	2.15 ± 0.71[l]	3.43 ± 1.16	2.41 ± 1.24[o]	0.52 ± 0.08
α-Tocopheryl succinate						
Serum (µg/ml)	2.42 ± 1.58	1.79 ± 0.29[d]	2.64 ± 0.74[j]	NA	ND	ND
Skin (µg/g)	23.0 ± 3.5[b]	47.6 ± 2.4[g]	52.5 ± 24.4[m]	NA	0.29 ± 0.21	ND
β-Carotene + α-toc. succinate						
Serum (µg/ml)	2.65 ± 1.35[a]	2.14 ± 0.60[e]	5.17 ± 1.67[k]	NA	NS	0.041 ± 0.013
Skin (µg/g)	20.8 ± 6.6[c]	50.5 ± 12.8[h]	49.9 ± 4.5[n]	1.54 ± 0.41	1.55 ± 0.41[p]	0.91 ± 0.27

* Female Skh-1 mice received one of 4 diets: 1. standard, Ralston Purina Rodent Chow; 2. β-carotene, 0.5% (all *trans*, crystalline); 3. α-tocopheryl acid succinate, 0.12%; and 4. β-carotene, 0.5% + α-tocopheryl acid succinate, 0.12%. KEY: *a–p*, numbers in the same column (only columns are statistically analyzed) with matching superscript letter show differences that are statistically significant ($p < 0.05$, Student *t* test); †, weeks on specified diet; §, average ± SD, for 5 mice; ND, not detectable; NA, not analyzed; NS, micronutrient level below the limits of detection in some animals. The resulting average is not statistically different from zero.

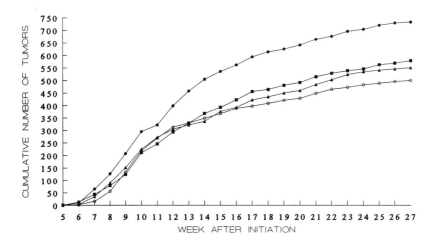

FIGURE 1. Cumulative number of tumors in Skh-1 mice. Tumors resulted from a DMBA-initiated (150 μg/mouse), PMA-promoted (5 μg/mouse, multiple applications) 2-stage tumorigenesis treatment regimen. Mice were fed 10 wk before chemical initiation and for the remainder of the study on one of 4 diets: 1. ● standard, Ralston Purina Rodent Chow; 2. ○ β-carotene 0.5% (all *trans,* crystalline); 3. ▲ vitamin E succinate 0.12%; and 4. ■ β-carotene 0.5% + vitamin E succinate 0.12%. Supplements were mixed with standard chow.

these supplements as compared to the standard diet group (TABLE 1). However, only the vitamin E diet group showed consistent increases in serum levels.

In conclusion, dietary supplementation with β-carotene or vitamin E substantially reduced the number of chemically-induced skin tumors in Skh mice. Mice which received a combination diet of β-carotene and vitamin E, although showing a similar degree of protection against tumors as the animals fed the individual supplements, showed no synergistic effect for a greater protection against this type of tumor.

REFERENCES

1. ZEIGLER, R. G., A. F. SUBAR, N. E. CRAFT, G. URSIN, B. H. PATTERSON & B. I. GRAUBARD. 1992. Does β-carotene explain why reduced cancer risk is associated with vegetable and fruit intake? Cancer Res. **52**(Suppl.): 2060S–2066S.
2. WALD, N. J., S. G. THOMPSON, J. W. DENSEM, J. BOREHAM & A. BAILEY. 1987. Serum vitamin E and subsequent risk of cancer. Br. J. Cancer **56:** 69–72.
3. LAMBERT, L. A., W. H. KOCH, W. G. WAMER & A. KORNHAUSER. 1990. Antitumor activity in skin of Skh and sencar mice by two dietary β-carotene formulations. Nutr. Cancer **13:** 213–221.
4. SHKLAR, G., J. L. SCHWARTZ, D. TRICKLER & S. REID. 1990. Prevention of experimental cancer and immunostimulation by vitamin E (immunosurveillance). J. Oral Pathol. Med. **19:** 60–64.

Influence of Beta-Carotene on Immune Functions

RAO H. PRABHALA, LAIMA M. BRAUNE,
HARINDER S. GAREWAL, AND
RONALD R. WATSON

Department of Microbiology
Chicago College of Osteopathic Medicine
555 31st Street
Downers Grove, Illinois 60515
and
University of Arizona Medical Center
Tucson, Arizona 85724

INTRODUCTION

A role for retinoids and carotenoids in the prevention and treatment of cancer has been suggested on the basis of a great deal of evidence from epidemiological, laboratory and clinical studies.[1] There has been recent interest in exploring the possible contribution of their immunomodulation, in addition to their effects on cellular growth and differentiation, to explain mechanisms for their anticancer effects. The major objective of this investigation is to assess the nature of the changes in the immune functions occurring over time *in vivo* in humans enrolled in a clinical trial using beta-carotene for treatment of oral leukoplakia.

RESULTS AND DISCUSSION

We observed that 13 of the 16 patients (81%) showed a significant increase in natural killer cells after beta-carotene treatment for 2 months. Modest increase in other T-lymphocyte subpopulations was also observed during the same time interval.[2] Following two months of beta-carotene treatment, there was an increase in the cytotoxicity of natural killer cells against K562 target cells. When we sought to identify the mechanisms involved in beta-carotene-induced immunostimulation, we were surprised that beta-carotene-responsive patients (71%)[3] showed higher plasma levels of tumor necrosis factor-alpha (TNF-alpha) in comparison with their nonresponsive counterparts (TABLE 1). We then examined whether beta-carotene alters any surface marker expression by oral epithelial cells, so that they can communicate better with natural killer cells. Recent preliminary data indicates that the expression of intercellular adhesion molecule-1 by oral epithelial cells was significantly increased when they were exposed to TNF-alpha (TABLE 2). These studies indicate that there is a potential clinical application using beta-carotene in the treatment of premalignant lesions like oral leukoplakia and head and neck cancer.

262

TABLE 1. Presence of TNF-Alpha in Plasma Samples from Oral Leukoplakia Patients during Treatment with Beta-Carotene[a]

| Groups (N) | TNF-Alpha Levels (Units/ml) Mean ± SD | |
	Pretreatment (0 Months)	Treatment (2 Months)
Responders (12)	12.6 ± 5.4	124.8 ± 16.5*
Nonresponders (4)	9.8 ± 6.2	14.2 ± 5.5

[a] Plasma levels of TNF-alpha were measured using ELISA kits. *Asterisk* indicates values significantly different from pretreatment responders and from nonresponders (p 0.05).

TABLE 2. Influence of TNF-Alpha on the Expression of HLA-DR and ICAM-1 Antigens on Human Oral Epithelial Cell Line[a]

Markers	TNF-Alpha	% Positive Cells (Mean ± SD)
HLA-DR	−	5.4 ± 2.5
	+	7.8 ± 3.0
ICAM-1	−	10 ± 3.7
	+	38.5 ± 8.8*

[a] Oral epithelial cells were cultured with or without TNF-alpha (100 Units/ml) for five days. After washing, cells were stained with appropriate monoclonal antibodies and analyzed with flow cytometry. Results are presented as mean ± SD of three or more representative experiments. *Asterisk* indicates values significantly changed from untreated controls (p 0.05).

SUMMARY

Recent reports have demonstrated that beta-carotene, a nontoxic carotenoid, is able to stimulate immune functions in humans. The purpose of this study is to understand the mechanisms of immunoenhancement by carotenoids in order to explain their anticancer effects. We have evaluated the clinical efficacy of beta-carotene, given 30 mg/day orally, for treatment of oral leukoplakia patients. Patients who responded to beta-carotene treatment showed increased plasma levels of TNF-alpha. Epithelial cells from these patients were characterized *in vitro*. These results may lead to a better understanding of the therapeutic use of beta-carotene in humans.

REFERENCES

1. MEYSKENS, F. L., JR. 1990. Coming of age—the chemoprevention of cancer. N. Engl. J. Med. **323:** 825–827.
2. PRABHALA, R. H., H. S. GAREWAL, M. J. HICKS, R. E. SAMPLINER & R. R. WATSON. 1991. The effects of 13-*cis*-getenoic acid and beta-carotene on cellular immunity in humans. Cancer **67:** 1556–1560.
3. GAREWAL, H. S., F. L. MEYSKENS, JR., D. KILLEN, D. REEVES, T. A. KIERSCH, H. ELLETSON, A. STROSBERG, D. KING & K. STEINBRONN. 1990. Response of oral leukoplakia to beta-carotene. J. Clin. Oncol. **8:** 1715–1720.

Effect of Beta-Carotene on Cytotoxic Activity and Receptor Expression of Tumor-Specific Lymphocytes

EMMANUEL T. AKPORIAYE,[a] ANN PETERSEN,[a]
PAUL PIERCE,[a] JESUS VALENZUELA,[b]
LOUISE CANFIELD,[b] AND JAMES BENDER[c]

[a]Department of Microbiology and Immunology
[b]Department of Biochemistry
University of Arizona
Tucson, Arizona 85724
and
[c]Baxter HealthCare Co.
Round Lake, Illinois 60073

INTRODUCTION

Numerous studies using animal models of cancer have documented chemo-preventive and immunoenhancing roles for beta-carotene.[1] Although the exact mechanisms of these effects *in vivo* are unknown, the antitumor action of beta-carotene has been attributed to its oxygen radical scavenging properties and/or direct stimulation of immune cells which include T cells, NK cells and macrophages. Attempts to elucidate the mechanisms of carotenoid-mediated potentiation of immune function have led to the use of *in vitro* assays by numerous investigators to study the interactions between beta-carotene and cells of the immune system. The results from these studies have been conflicting. In our studies we examined the ability of beta-carotene to potentiate T cell-mediated antitumor immunity *in vitro*. Our results indicate that beta-carotene treatment of tumor-sensitized splenic T lymphocytes stimulates neither tumoricidal activity, nor the expression of selected activation markers.

MATERIALS AND METHODS

Beta-carotene was dissolved sequentially in tetrahydrofuran (THF) and ethanol. THF was used from a freshly redistilled stock stored under argon gas, or chromatographed on an activated alumina column immediately prior to use. Beta-carotene (Fluka) was dissolved in THF at a concentration of 10 mg/ml, sonicated 20 minutes to facilitate dispersion and diluted 1 : 10 in absolute ethanol. The amount of dispersed beta-carotene was calculated using $E_{1\%}$ of 2620 at 455 nm. Beta-carotene was diluted to 1.0×10^{-7} M in complete RPMI 1640 medium plus antibiotics. All manipulations were performed in the dark. Splenic lymphocytes from mice immunized I.P. with T168 tumor cells were incubated with beta-carotene and/or IL-2 for 72 hours at 37°C in 7% CO_2.

RESULTS AND DISCUSSION

In this study, we examined the ability of beta-carotene to augment the *in vitro* tumoricidal activity of tumor-sensitized T lymphocytes and to stimulate their expression of activation markers. The results indicate that by itself, beta-carotene was unable to activate tumor-specific T lymphocytes. In contrast, IL-2 treatment stimulated tumoricidal activity towards 168 cells and YAC-1 cells (FIG. 1). The addition of beta-carotene to IL-2 cultures did not improve the lytic activity of IL-2-stimulated cells. In order to determine if high dose IL-2 (1000 Units/ml) was masking any potentiation of IL-2 stimulated cytolytic activity by beta-carotene, beta-carotene-treated cultures were stimulated with smaller levels (100 or 10 Units/ml) of IL-2.

At reduced levels of IL-2 stimulation, beta-carotene was still unable to cause any induction of cytotoxic activity above that observed with IL-2 only (data not shown). Similar effects were observed with IL-2 cultures treated with retinoic acid (data not shown). Flow cytometric analysis revealed that beta-carotene treatment of sensitized splenic lymphocytes alters neither the distribution of T cell subsets, nor the expression of activation markers. In contrast, IL-2 treatment resulted in increased expression of IL-2R and not I-A^d. The findings reported here are in agreement with the work of Jyonouchi *et al.*,[2] who recently demonstrated that beta-carotene was unable to stimulate the proliferation, cell surface marker expression, and antibody production of murine lymphocytes. Our findings however differ from those of Prabhala *et al.*[3] using human peripheral blood mononuclear

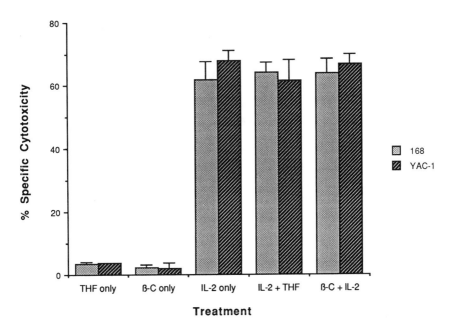

FIGURE 1. Effect of beta-carotene on the tumoricidal activity of T lymphocytes. Splenic lymphocytes were incubated in the presence of beta-carotene and/or IL-2 and were tested for their ability to induce the lysis of 168 tumor cells or NK susceptible YAC-1 tumor cells. Cytotoxic activity was measured using a 4 or 8 hour chromium-51 release assay.

TABLE 1. Effect of Beta-Carotene Treatment on Distribution of T Cell Subsets and Expression of Activation Markers[a]

Treatment	CD4+	CD8+	AGM 1	IL-2R	I-A^d
THF	38%	11%	20%	6%	7%
Beta-carotene	28%	14%	24%	6%	8%
IL-2 + THF	32%	23%	35%	23%	10%
IL-2 + beta-carotene	26%	25%	35%	—	7%

[a] Splenic lymphocytes were assessed for the presence of T cell subsets (and NK cells) by labelling cell suspensions with monoclonal antibodies to CD8, CD4 and Asialo GM1 that recognize T cytotoxic/suppressor, T helper and NK cells, respectively. The expression of IL-2R (p55) and I-A^d (Class II MHC) was determined by staining with anti-IL-2R and anti I-A^d monoclonal antibodies. Cells were analyzed by multi-color flow cytometry.

cells in which they demonstrated increase in NK cells and expression of activation markers (IL-2R, HLA-DR and Transferrin receptors) as a result of *in vitro* beta-carotene treatment. The discrepancy in these studies could be due in part to differences in species, cell types and methodological procedures employed in the assays.

Although we are unable to demonstrate any beta-carotene-mediated anti-tumor effects *in vitro,* numerous studies have documented these effects *in vivo.* While the discrepancies between the *in vitro* and *in vivo* data are not explained by the present data, these studies raise a number of important possibilities about the action of beta-carotene *in vivo*: Firstly, the action of beta-carotene *in vivo* that is independent of provitamin A activity may involve the generation of cleavage products with direct or indirect (via soluble cytokine mediators) immune enhancing properties on T cells. These cleavage products may not be efficiently generated *in vitro.* Secondly, the availability of beta-carotene to immune cells *in vivo* may depend on the presence of a carrier which is not available in *in vitro* systems. The absence of such a carrier *in vitro* would make it impossible to achieve intracellular concentrations of beta-carotene necessary for activation of immune cells. Experiments to test these hypotheses are in progress.

REFERENCES

1. BENDICH, A. & J. A. OLSON. 1989. FASEB J. **3:** 1927–1932.
2. JYONOUCHI, H. *et al.* 1991. Nutr. Cancer **16:** 93–105.
3. PRABHALA, R. H. *et al.* 1989. J. Leukocyte Biol. **45:** 249–254.

Carotenoids Slow the Growth of Small Cell Lung Cancer Cells[a]

L. J. GALLIGAN, C. L. JACKSON, AND L. E. GERBER

Food Science and Nutrition Research Center
University of Rhode Island
530 Liberty Lane
West Kingston, Rhode Island 02892-1802
and
Rhode Island Hospital/Brown University
Providence, Rhode Island 02903

Epidemiological studies have suggested a relationship between carotenoid consumption and decreased incidence of lung cancer. The current research has elucidated some cellular and molecular effects of carotenoids on lung cancer cells.

NCI-H69 small cell lung cancer cells were obtained from American Type Cell Culture (Bethesda, MD) and grown according to their instructions. Cells were cultured at 5×10^4 cells/ml in 10 ml medium. An appropriate concentration of beta-carotene or canthaxanthin beadlet was added as an emulsion in water that had been sequentially filtered through a 0.8-micron and then a 0.2-micron filter for sterilization. Final concentrations of 2 to 20 micromolar were obtained. Appropriate concentrations of retinoic acid were dissolved in acetone and added. Control cultures received an equivalent amount of noncarotenoid-containing beadlets, or an equivalent amount of acetone, or no treatment. The medium was changed and treatments were delivered three times weekly. Change in cell number was monitered by counting in a Coulter Counter. Beta-carotene prevented the growth of the cells in a dose-dependent manner with the 10 and 20 micromolar doses resulting in significantly slowed growth at twelve days (FIG. 1). No other group differed from controls. After twelve days the treatments were withdrawn and the growth of cells previously exposed to beta-carotene did not differ from the growth of control cells.

Further studies compared the effects of alpha-carotene, beta-carotene and retinol. Alpha-carotene and beta-carotene were delivered in THF and the medium was changed twice weekly. Alpha-carotene was as effective as beta-carotene in growth prevention. Flow cytometry of nuclei to determine DNA content showed that carotenoid-treated cells had twice as many cells in a resting stage (G1/G0) as control or retinol-treated cells. Preparation of nuclei and their analysis followed a standard procedure.

Additional studies used unfiltered beta-carotene beadlets, in which higher doses of beta-carotene were required to achieve the same growth reduction as when using filtered beadlets. Twenty micromolar unfiltered beta-carotene beadlets had no effect on the growth of the cells as indicated by cell number or cell cycle stage compared to controls. After 26 days, however, this dose resulted in a decrease in N-myc mRNA of 90% relative to actin expression when compared to controls

[a] This work was supported in part by the Rhode Island Agricultural Experimental Station and the University of Rhode Island Foundation. This paper is Rhode Island Agricultural Experiment Station Publication No. 2901.

(FIG. 2) as determined by Northern Blot analysis[1] followed by densitometry according to manufacturer's instructions (LKB Bromma Ultroscan XL Laser Densitometer). A decrease in c-jun mRNA of 82% relative to GAP was also observed by densitometry using a RT-PCR technique[2] where products were separated on a Pharmacia PhastSystem Phast-gel according to manufacturer's instructions.

The results of these studies taken together show that the administration of alpha- or beta-carotene to the NCl-H69 lung cancer cell line results in a decrease in growth in a dose-dependent manner. This decrease in growth was independent of the manner in which the carotenoid was delivered. Analysis of the cells at several time points after the administration of alpha- and beta-carotene showed that carotenoid-treated cells had a higher percentage of cells in the G1/G0 stage

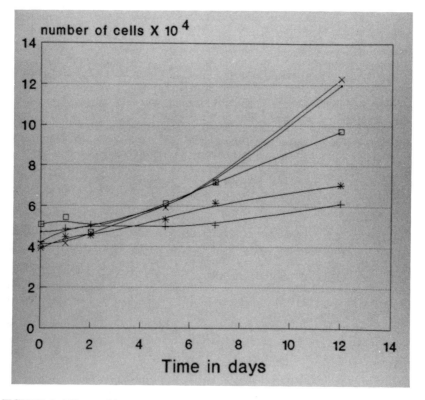

FIGURE 1. Effects of beta-carotene on the proliferation of NCl-H69 cells. Cells were cultured at 5×10^4 cells/ml in 10 ml medium (control, ●), and the following concentrations of beta-carotene beadlets were added to the medium: 2 μM, ×; 5 μM, □; 10 μM, *; and 20 μM, +. The 10- and 20-μM doses of beta-carotene resulted in significantly slowed growth compared to control ($p = 0.05$).

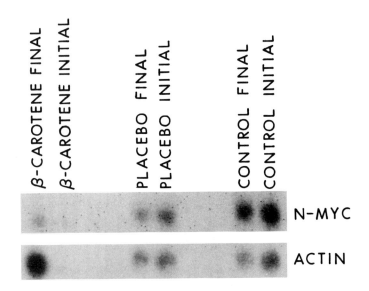

FIGURE 2. Northern blots of mRNA from control, placebo (treated with noncarotenoid-containing beadlets) and 20 micromolar unfiltered beta-carotene beadlets. The *upper panel* shows the blot hybridized with N-myc. The *lower panel* shows the same blot hybridized with actin. Densitometric analysis shows beta-carotene final to have a 90% decrease in N-myc expression compared to controls.

of the cell cycle as compared to control or retinol-treated cells. The decrease in growth was preceded by a decrease in N-myc and c-jun mRNA.

REFERENCES

1. AUSEBEL, F. M., R. BRENT, R. E. KINGSTON, D. D. MOORE, J. G. SEIDMAN, J. A. SMITH & K. STRUHL, Eds. 1990. Current Protocols. 4.1–4.9. Green Publishing Associates, Wiley Interscience. New York.
2. MURPHY, L. D., C. E. HERZOG, J. B. RUDICK, A. T. FOJO & S. E. BATES. 1990. Biochemistry **29:** 10351–10356.

β-Carotene Reduces Paw Swelling in the Rat Adjuvant Arthritis Model, while Increasing IL-1 Production in Peritoneal Macrophages

H. BACHMANN,[a] R. NEMZEK,[b] AND J. W. COFFEY[b]

[a]Vitamin Research
F. Hoffmann-La Roche, Ltd
CH-4002 Basel, Switzerland
and
Preclinical Research
Hoffmann-La Roche, Inc.
Nutley, New Jersey 07110

INTRODUCTION

Adjuvant-induced arthritis (AJA) is a model of immune-mediated arthritis in rats and is widely used in the search for active compounds for the treatment of human rheumatoid arthritis (RA).[1] Histological changes in rat AJA and in human RA follow a similar pattern with massive infiltration of inflammatory cells into the affected tissue.[2] Macrophages, a cell type known to produce large amounts of inflammatory mediators such as eicosanoids, radicals (*e.g.*, superoxide anion and hydrogen peroxide), degradative enzymes (*e.g.*, proteases), interleukins and interferons are prominent in the cellular infiltrates.[3–5] β-Carotene and other carotenoids have been shown to have tissue-protecting properties as scavengers of free radicals.[6] In addition, β-carotene augments the response of rat T lymphocytes to the mitogens, concanavalin A and phytohemagglutinin, and rat B lymphocytes to lipopolysaccharide.[7] A study was initiated to determine antiinflammatory activity of β-carotene in the adjuvant arthritis model. In addition to paw swelling, the production of IL-1 by peritoneal macrophages was also investigated.

MATERIALS AND METHODS

HEPES, FCS (heat inactivated at 56°C), Gentamycin and the cell culture media HBSS and RPMI, were obtained from Gibco or Sigma. Solutions of PMA (1 mM in DMSO), LPS (from *E. coli*, 50 μg/mL) and recombinant rat IFNγ (Amgen, 10^5 U/mL) were prepared, aliquoted as stock solutions, and kept at -20°C until use. Arachidonic acid (AA, 10 mM) in 70% ethanol was prepared before use. Male Lewis rats from Charles River Labs with body weights of 125–150 g were used after a one-week adaptation period. The animals were divided at random into groups, housed individually and fed the experimental diets for a period of 3 weeks (trials I, II) or 2 weeks (trial III) prior to induction of AJA and continued until the end of the experiment. The control group designed as con was fed the semipurified diet described by Shapiro *et al.*[8] The basic diet, supplemented with 200 ppm

TABLE 1. Effect of β-Carotene (bCa) and Placebo (con) on Paw Edema in Rat Adjuvant Arthritis (AJA)[a]

Trial	Treatment		Mean Paw Volume (mL, SEM; N) on				
			Day 12	Day 14	Day 21	Day 27	Day 31
I.	AJA	con	0.73 (0.07;10)	1.18 (0.14;10)	2.74 (0.29;7)	3.37 (0.30;7)	3.73 (0.39;7)
	AJA	bCa	0.46 (0.10;10) −**37%***	0.72 (0.11;10) −**39%****	1.45 (0.13;7) −**47%*****	1.78 (0.20;7) −**47%*****	1.88 (0.19;7) −**50%******
II.	AJA	con		0.62 (0.08;16)	1.19 (0.13;8)		
	AJA	bCa		0.35 (0.09;15) −**44%*****	0.80 (0.26;7) −**33%***		
	—	con		0.11 (0.10;16)	0.34 (0.04;8)		
	—	bCa		0.04 (0.03;16)	0.15 (0.06;8)		
III.	AJA	con		1.46 (0.15;20)	2.24 (0.13;15)	3.13 (0.18;10)	3.63 (0.27;10)
	AJA	bCa		1.39 (0.12;20) −**5%**	2.02 (0.13;15) −**10%***	2.75 (0.27;10) −**12%**	3.03 (0.24;10) −**17%**
	—	con		0.21 (0.01;9)	0.32 (0.04;10)		0.28 (0.04;5)
	—	bCa		0.15 (0.05;5)	0.37 (0.04;5)		

[a] β-Carotene treatment was started in trial I and II three weeks before inducing AJA and was continued until the end of the trial. In trial III, the pretreatment was two weeks. The adjuvant arthritis was induced on day 0 in groups designated as AJA. The animals were injected subcutaneously into the base of the tail with 0.1 mL adjuvant (heat-killed *Mycobacterium butyricum*, 0.52% w/v, in heavy mineral oil containing 0.2% digitonin). Paw volume, measured by water plethysmography, was recorded at the time indicated. Paw volume in mL, calculated as: $(v_1 + v_r)_{dayx} - (v_1 + v_r)_{day0}$, where v_1 is the volume of the left and v_r of the right hind paw.
*$p < 0.05$; **$p < 0.01$; ***$p < 0.001$.

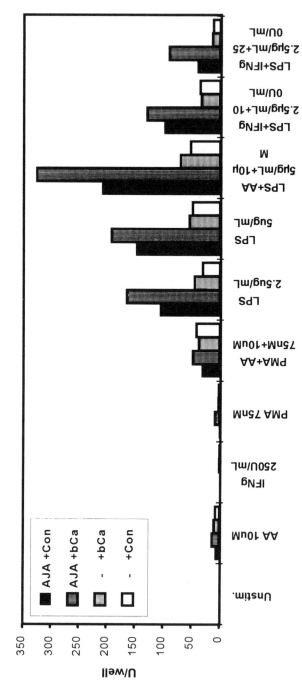

FIGURE 1. Release of IL-1 in normal and arthritic peritoneal macrophages isolated from rats on diets with or without β-carotene (bCa). Experiment from trial II, day 21. Peritoneal exudate cells were recovered using standard sterile techniques. Cells from individual animals were resuspended in RPMI-medium, supplemented with 5% FCS, 50 μg/ml Gentamycin and 25 mM HEPES. Individual samples or pools from different animals were diluted to 2.0 · 10⁶ cells/mL, and 100 μL aliquots were plated into 96-well flat bottom plates. Cells were allowed to adhere for 90 minutes and the nonadherent cells were removed by washing twice with 100 μL sterile warm media. Adherent cells were stimulated for 24 hours with the appropriate stimuli. Supernatants were collected, filtered through 0.2-μm filters and stored at −70°C until analysis. IL-1 activity was determined using the D10.G4 cell proliferation assay.[9] Each bar represents the mean of 2 pools, and each pool contains an equal amount of supernatant from 5 incubations with cells from 5 animals.

β-carotene (as beadlets containing 10% β-carotene, F. Hoffmann-La Roche) was fed to β-carotene groups. The animals had free access to feed and tap water.

RESULTS AND DISCUSSION

Three independent trials were conducted to test the effect of β-carotene on the development of AJA. In trials I and II (3 weeks pretreatment), paw swelling was reduced significantly between days 12 and 30 while, in trial III (2 weeks pretreatment), the reduction in paw swelling did not reach significance (TABLE 1). The effect of β-carotene at a calculated dosage of 15 mg/kg/day (assuming 18 g diet consumed per day) on paw swelling on day 14 was similar to the reduction seen with effective dosages (p.o.) of several established antiinflammatory agents, *e.g.*, phenylbutazone (33 mg/kg, −55%), indomethacin (0.5 mg/kg, −54%), benzoxaprofen (1.8 mg/kg, −50%), and hydrocortisone acetate (33 mg/kg, −50%) (data from ref. [9]). In these studies, β-carotene maintained its potency as an antiinflammatory agent from day 14 through 30, while the established antiinflammatory drugs were sometimes less potent at later times. In this regard, β-carotene resembled the immunoreactive drugs, cyclosporin A, cyclophosphamide, and methotrexate.

The number and the size of peritoneal macrophages was increased in rats with AJA as compared to normal. Both of these parameters were decreased slightly following treatment with β-carotene (data not shown). To assess the functional properties of peritoneal macrophages from arthritic animals, IL-1 production was measured in macrophages from arthritic and normal animals (FIG. 1). Of the stimuli studied, LPS was the most potent, inducing a higher level of IL-1 production in macrophages from arthritic as compared with normal animals. LPS-stimulated IL-1 production tended to be increased in macrophages from β-carotene-treated arthritic animals as compared with arthritic animals receiving the control diet (trial II, day 21).

REFERENCES

1. PEARSON, C. M. 1956. Proc. Soc. Exp. Biol. Med. **91:** 95–101.
2. HOLOSHITZ, J., W. VAN EDEN, A. FRENKEL & I. R. COHEN. 1987. *In* Perspectives on Autoimmunity. 155–165. I. M. Cohen, Ed. CRC Press, Boca Raton, FL.
3. KARNOVSKY, M. L. & J. A. BADWEY. 1986. Methods Enzymol. **132:** 353–394.
4. DRAYER, J. M., S. M. KRAUSE & D. R. ROBINSON. 1976. Proc. Natl. Acad. Sci. USA **73:** 945–949.
5. BROWNING, J. 1987. Immunol. Today **8:** 372–374.
6. BENDICH, A. 1989. Clin. Nutr. **7:** 113–117.
7. BENDICH, A. & J. A. OLSON. 1989. FASEB J. **3:** 1927–1932.
8. SHAPIRO, S. S., D. J. MOTT & L. J. MACHLIN. 1984. J. Nutr. **114:** 1924–1933.
9. LOMBARDINO, J. G. 1985. *In* Chem. and Pharmacol. of Drugs. D. Leduicer, Ed. Vol. **5:** 173–184. Wiley & Sons. New York.
10. KAYE, J., S. PORCELLI, J. TITE, B. JONES & C. A. JANEWAY. 1983. J. Exp. Med. **158:** 836–839.

Carotenoids and Antioxidant Nutrients following Burn Injury[a]

CHERYL L. ROCK,[b] JORGE L. RODRIGUEZ,[b]
RUBINA KHILNANI,[b] DEBORAH A. LOWN,[b]
AND ROBERT S. PARKER[c]

[b]Program in Human Nutrition and Department of Surgery
The University of Michigan
M5539 SPHII
Ann Arbor, Michigan 48109-2029
and
[c]Division of Nutritional Science
Cornell University
Ithaca, New York 14853-0001

Carotenoids are among the circulating antioxidant micronutrients, and plasma levels of these compounds generally reflect dietary intake, when possible confounding factors such as body mass are considered.[1,2] Patients who have suffered burn injury are abruptly withdrawn from food and are fed via enteral formula diet. Until recently, such diets provided essential nutrients (including vitamin C and vitamin E) but have not provided carotenoids. Oxidant damage following burn injury can result in lipid peroxidation and may promote acute lung injury, and antioxidant micronutrients may play a protective role.

The purpose of this study is (1) to identify the dynamic pattern of plasma antioxidant nutrients following burn injury, using high performance liquid chromatography (HPLC) methods, and (2) to evaluate the effect of administering beta-carotene enterally for 21 days following burn injury. Serial carotenoid levels in adipose tissue samples are also being quantified. Outcome variables include measures of lung function and biological indicators of immune function, including interleukin-8 levels in bronchial secretions.

METHODS

Subjects are patients with burn injury who are admitted to The University of Michigan Hospitals: 18–65 years of age, major burn injury (>20% total body surface area [BSA], full thickness [FT]), within two postburn days at recruitment, in a stable clinical state. Patients are fed a low carotenoid enteral formula diet (without additional micronutrient supplementation) within 24–48 hours of admission and treated with a standard protocol of fluid resuscitation, early excision of burned areas, and skin grafting. Blood samples are obtained at baseline and at least twice weekly during the 21-day (three-week) study period. Patients are randomly

[a] Work described in this poster paper was supported in part by a grant from Ross Laboratories.

274

assigned to receive 30 mg/day beta-carotene or placebo capsules (Hoffmann-La Roche, Nutley, NJ).

Plasma levels of vitamin E (alpha- and gamma-tocopherol), retinol, and the predominant carotenoids (beta-carotene, alpha-carotene, lycopene, beta-cryptoxanthin, and lutein) are quantified with HPLC methods.[3,4] Plasma cholesterol and triglycerides are also measured in each blood sample for interpretation of fat-soluble nutrient levels. Plasma vitamin C levels are measured with a derivative spectrophotometric method.[5] Tissue analysis is achieved using the extraction method of Parker.[6] Measures of immune status are obtained by collaborators in the Department of Surgery.

TABLE 1. Selected Plasma Micronutrient Levels (Mean ± SD, n = 12)[a]

Baseline	Week 1	Week 2	Week 3
Beta-Carotene (umol/L)			
P:0.0547 ± 0.0459	0.0832 ± 0.0585	0.0452 ± 0.0356	0.0283 ± 0.0292
B:0.0451 ± 0.0058	0.0892 ± 0.1039	0.0996 ± 0.0368	0.6196
Lycopene (umol/L)			
P:0.2090 ± 0.0931	0.2659 ± 0.1324	0.1295 ± 0.0679	0.0651 ± 0.0546
B:0.1513 ± 0.0663	0.1548 ± 0.0969	0.0935 ± 0.0091	0.2476
Retinol (ug/dL)			
P:8.7595 ± 4.3841	13.191 ± 6.3953	21.750 ± 12.573	20.588 ± 7.9522
B:8.8546 ± 5.5431	9.1792 ± 0.2447	17.554 ± 15.056	30.949
Alpha-Tocopherol (mg/dL)			
P:0.4649 ± 0.1871	0.7238 ± 0.4608	0.8670 ± 0.4337	0.7783 ± 0.4571
B:0.4248 ± 0.0042	0.5831 ± 0.0024	0.6928 ± 0.2330	0.9082
Vitamin C (mg/dL)			
P:0.4430 ± 0.1690	0.8426 ± 0.5560	1.2254 ± 0.6832	0.9876 ± 0.3300
B:0.4098 ± 0.3040	0.8294 ± 0.0984	0.7292 ± 0.1292	1.1268

[a] P indicates placebo group, and B indicates beta-carotene supplemented group.

RESULTS AND CONCLUSIONS

A total of 12 patients (4 females, 8 males) who met study criteria have been recruited, and 8 of these survived the 21-day study period. Descriptive data on these subjects are: 43 ± 15 years, 33.4 ± 8.3 weight[kg]/height[m²] body mass index, 47 ± 18% BSA, 41 ± 21% FT. Descriptive data on selected plasma micronutrients are listed in TABLE 1.

Overall, plasma carotenoid levels were initially low and tended to remain low unless supplemented. Beta-carotene supplementation was not associated with increased plasma retinol levels; instead, increased retinol levels occurred in association with recovery. A time-dependent increase in certain chromatographic peaks was observed, among the more polar carotenoids on the chromatogram, following burn injury. These compounds may be oxidized carotenoid metabolites.

Plasma levels of tocopherols and vitamin C were initially low, compared with normal values, but these levels increase during treatment in association with enteral diets. Correlations between plasma tocopherols and lipid levels were not observed in these patients. Plasma levels of alpha-tocopherol were inversely correlated with interleukin-8 levels ($r = -0.698$) in bronchial secretions.

In conclusion, levels of circulating carotenoids remain low during low carotenoid enteral formula feeding unless supplemented. The dynamic pattern of plasma antioxidant nutrients following burn injury indicates reduced circulating levels and increased risk of medical problems secondary to oxidant stress. Supplementation may be necessary to promote maintenance of antioxidant defense mechanisms in these patients.

ACKNOWLEDGMENTS

The authors wish to express their gratitude to Dr. Hemmige Bhagavan of Hoffmann-La Roche, Inc. (Nutley, NJ) for kindly providing beta-carotene, placebo capsules and carotenoid standards.

REFERENCES

1. MICOZZI, M. S., E. BROWN, B. K. EDWARDS, J. G. BIERI, P. R. TAYLOR, F. KHACHIK, G. R. BEECHER & J. C. SMITH. 1992. Am. J. Clin. Nutr. **55:** 1120–1125.
2. ROCK, C. L., M. E. SWENDSEID, R. A. JACOB & R. W. MCKEE. 1992. J. Nutr. **122:** 128–135.
3. BIERI, J. G., E. D. BROWN & J. C. SMITH. 1985. J. Liquid Chromatogr. **8:** 473–484.
4. BIERI, J. G., T. J. TOLLIVER & G. L. CATIGNANI. 1979. Am. J. Clin. Nutr. **32:** 2143–4149.
5. OMAYE, S. T., J. D. TURNBULL & H. E. SAUBERLICH. 1979. Methods Enzymol. **62:** 3–11.
6. PARKER, R. S. 1988. Am. J. Clin. Nutr. **47:** 33–36.

Beta-Carotene in HIV Infection[a]

GREGG O. COODLEY, HEIDI D. NELSON,
MARK O. LOVELESS, AND CATHI FOLK

*Division of Internal Medicine
and
Division of Infectious Diseases
Oregon Health Sciences University
L475
3181 SW Sam Jackson Park Road
Portland, Oregon 97201-3098*

BACKGROUND

A number of studies have suggested that beta-carotene, a carotenoid with provitamin A (retinol) activity, enhances immune function.[1-3] In 1985, Alexander conducted a trial of beta-carotene supplementation in a group of 10 healthy volunteers over a period of three weeks. He reported that 180 mg a day of beta-carotene (Solatene, Hoffmann-La Roche, Nutley, NJ) resulted in an increase in T helper (CD4) lymphocytes, as well as an increase in the T helper/T suppressor (CD4/CD8) ratio.[4]

Since destruction of the T helper cell population is the major mechanism by which the HIV virus affects the immune system in infected patients, we decided to test whether beta-carotene could increase levels of CD4 cells in HIV-infected patients. We gave 180 mg beta-carotene (Solatene) a day to three HIV-infected patients over a two-week period and observed a mean 89% increase in the numbers of CD4 cells in these patients.[5] Based on this preliminary data, we decided to conduct a double blind placebo controlled trial of beta-carotene in HIV-infected patients.

METHODS

Twenty-one HIV-seropositive patients were recruited from the outpatient clinics at Oregon Health Sciences University. Patients were excluded if they were on other forms of vitamin A supplementation, had preexisting hepatic or renal dysfunction (creatinine >1.5, asparate aminotransferase >2X upper limit of normal) or had an acute opportunistic infection or fever at time of entry. Inclusion criteria included being HIV seropositive and having not changed or started new antiretroviral therapy less than two months prior to entry.

Participating patients were randomized to receive either beta-carotene 180 mg a day (Solatene; Hoffmann-La Roche, Nutley, NJ) or placebo, both divided into three tablets a day for four weeks. At four weeks, patients then crossed over to receive the alternative therapy for the second four weeks. Patients remained on their usual antiretroviral and other therapy during the study. Outcome variables

[a] This study was supported by a grant from Hoffmann-La Roche, Inc., Nutley, NJ.

277

included mean changes and mean percent changes in total white blood cells, total lymphocytes, B lymphocytes, CD4 cells/mm^3, CD4/CD8 ratios and carotene levels, drawn at baseline and at the end of weeks 2, 4, 6, and 8.

RESULTS

Seventeen of the 21 patients beginning the study completed one or both arms (13 completed both, 3 completed beta-carotene only, one completed placebo only). The four patients who dropped out did not appear to differ significantly from those completing the study. Both beta-carotene and placebo were well tolerated, with no patient stopping the study secondary to a medication effect and a slight orange color on beta-carotene being the only reported side effect.

Beta-carotene use was associated with a statistically significant increase in total WBC count ($p = 0.01$), percent change in CD4 count ($p = 0.02$) and percent change in CD4/CD8 ratio ($p = 0.01$) compared to placebo. The absolute CD4 count, CD4/CD8 ratio, total and B lymphocytes all increased on carotene and fell during placebo, although the differences did not reach statistical significance. No significant sequence ($p < 0.05$) effect was detected.

CONCLUSION

Beta carotene appears to have an immunostimulatory effect in HIV-infected patients. Further studies are needed to demonstrate if the benefits of beta carotene will be justified over an extended time period.

The full study was published in the *Journal of the Acquired Immunodeficiency Syndrome* in March, 1993.[6]

REFERENCES

1. BENDICH, A. & S. SHAPIRO. 1986. Effect of beta carotene and canthaxanthin on immune responses of the rat. J. Nutr. **116:** 2254–2262.
2. PRINCE, M. R. 1991. Beta carotene to prevent skin cancer. N. Engl. J. Med. **324:** 924–925.
3. SKLAR, D., T. YOSEFOV & A. FRIEDMAN. 1989. The effects of vitamin A, B-carotene and canthaxanthin on vitamin A metabolism and immune responses in the chick. Int. J. Vitam. Nutr. Res. **59:** 245–250.
4. ALEXANDER, M., M. NEWMARK & R. G. MILLER. 1985. Oral beta carotene can increase the number of OKT4$^+$ cells in human blood. Immunol. Lett. **9:** 221–224.
5. COODLEY, G. 1991. Beta carotene therapy in human immunodeficiency virus infection. Clin. Res. **39**(2): 634a (abstract).
6. COODLEY, G. O., H. D. NELSON, M. O. LOVELESS & C. FOLK. 1993. Beta-carotene in HIV infection. J. Acquir. Immune Defic. Syndr. **6:** 272–276.

Possible Association of Skin Lesions with a Low-Carotene Diet in Premenopausal Women

B. J. BURRI,[a] Z. R. DIXON,[a] A. K. H. FONG,[a]
M. J. KRETSCH,[a] A. J. CLIFFORD,[b]
AND J. W. ERDMAN, JR.[c]

[a]Western Human Nutrition Research Center
United States Department of Agriculture
Agricultural Research Service
Pacific West Area
P.O. Box 29997
Presidio of San Francisco, California 94129

[b]University of California
Davis, California 95817

[c]University of Illinois
Urbana, Illinois 61801

Nine healthy adult women ate a low-carotene diet (10 retinol equivalents (RE)/day) for 68 days, supplemented with a placebo (Placebo Beadlets, Hoffmann-La Roche, Nutley, NJ). Then they were repleted with the same diet supplemented with beta-carotene (Dry Carotene Beadlets, Hoffmann-La Roche; 2500 RE/day) for 28 days. An additional mixed carotene supplement (Carotenoid Complex, Neolife Corp., Fremont, CA) was fed the last week of repletion. The diet was adequate in other nutrients. The women lived on a metabolic unit (MRU) from May to August 1992, with control of diet, exercise and activities.

Seven women developed skin lesions while eating the low-carotene diet. Five had rash and acne (one also had blisters), one had eczema, and one had conjunctivitis and sty. Participants also complained of dry skin, itch, and blurred vision. Changes in the rapid test for dark adaptation between depletion and repletion approached significance (t test, $p = 0.053$). Two cases of acne improved and the conjunctivitis, eczema, and blisters resolved during carotene repletion.

Increased photosensitivity may have caused the lesions.[1] Beta-carotene treatments ameliorate photosensitivity, and both carotene and vitamin A analogs are helpful for people with a variety of skin disorders. Women who developed lesions may have had chronically lower vitamin A or carotene dietary intakes, because they had lower stores of vitamin A than those without (2.2–59.5 vs 60.9–195 μg retinol/g liver, respectively, FIG. 1). Alternatively, the skin lesions may have been secondary to menstrual cycle disruptions. Six women had prolonged menstrual cycles (33 to 70 days), four also had delayed ovulation (22 to 31 days after end of menses).

Living on an MRU can be stressful: at times one to two women in MRU studies develop skin lesions or abnormal menstrual cycles. However, the abnormalities on this study were more numerous and more severe than we have seen in other MRU studies. We believe that our low-carotene diet caused or exacerbated skin lesions in these women. Most people with skin lesions have normal vitamin A

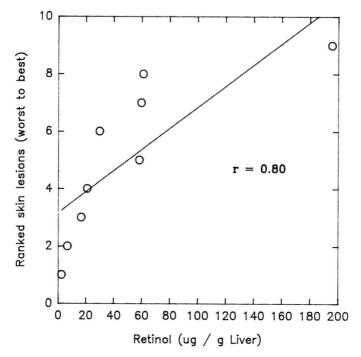

FIGURE 1. Influence of vitamin A status on observed severity of skin lesions (worst to best). Retinol (μg) estimated by stable isotope dilution. Liver (g) estimated from body weight.

and carotene concentrations,[2] but chronically low carotene or vitamin A intakes may contribute to some cases. This requires further study.

REFERENCES

1. MATHEWS-ROTH, M. M. 1986. Biochimie **68:** 875–884.
2. MATSUOKA, L. Y., J. WORTSMAN, G. TANG, R. M. RUSSELL, L. PARKER, R. GELFAND & R. G. MEHTA. 1991. Arch. Dermatol. **127:** 1072–1073.

Anti-Stress Effect of β-Carotene

TOHRU HASEGAWA

Department of Community Health Science
Saga Medical School
Nabeshima, Saga 849, Japan

The primary cause of death in the United States and Europe is ischemic heart disease, which is deeply related to stress.[1-3]

Hirayama reported recently that a person who eats green or yellow vegetables every day shows a lower incidence of stress syndrome (irritation, sleeplessness) than one who does not eat them every day.[4] He suggests that β-carotene, a high level of which is contained in green and yellow vegetables, has the same effect on stress reaction. However, the precise mechanism is not yet known.

We show here that β-carotene suppresses the increase of stress-related hormones such as corticotropin-releasing hormone (CRH), adrenocorticotropic hormone (ACTH), noradrenaline (NA), and adrenaline (AD).

The effect of β-carotene on exhaustive exercise stress was investigated. Twelve healthy male volunteers (18–20 years old) were divided into two groups. One group was control and the other took β-carotene (30 mg/person) two hours before exercise. They exercized with ergometric bicycling with loading of 100 watts to the extent of all-out exhaustion.

Exhaustive exercise induced nonspecific stress reaction (FIG. 1); increases in the plasma levels of ACTH, NA and AD were observed. But β-carotene completely suppressed this increasing secretion of ACTH, NA and AD. In other words, β-carotene completely inhibited the stress reaction induced by the exercise stressor.

Why did β-carotene inhibit the stress reaction? Selye has pointed out[5] that the stressor stimulates the hypothalamic function, which controls the sympathetic nerve system,[6] and also controls the secretion of ACTH in the pituitary through the secretion of CRH.[7] Then we investigated whether the effective site of β-carotene is the hypothalamus by determining the effect of β-carotene on the secretion of CRH.

As is clearly shown in TABLE 1, β-carotene suppressed the secretion of CRH dose-dependently. It is also suggested that the effective site of β-carotene is the hypothalamus, where β-carotene suppressed the secretion of CRH induced by exercise stress, and consequently the secretion of ACTH in the pituitary. As CRH stimulates the sympathetic neuron,[6] β-carotene also inhibited the stimulation of NA and AD secretion through the suppression of CRH secretion.

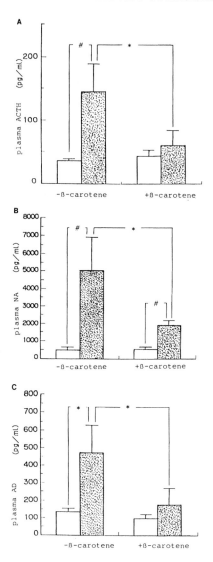

FIGURE 1. The effect of β-carotene on the increasing secretion of **(A)** plasma ACTH, **(B)** plasma NA, and **(C)** plasma AD induced by exhaustive exercise (*clear columns*: before exercise, *shaded columns*: after exercise; #: $p < 0.001$, *: $p < 0.05$). Twelve healthy male volunteers (18–20 years old) were divided into two equal groups. One group was control and the other one took β-carotene (30 mg/person) orally two hours before exercise. They exercized with ergometric bicycling with loading of 100 watts to the extent of all-out exhaustion every 4 minutes. 190–220 Watts was the exhaustive loading. The β-carotene group showed a longer time of performance and a heavier exhaustive loading than control. Their blood was collected before and after exercise. Plasma CRH, ACTH (radioimmunoassay), NA, and AD (HPLC method) were analyzed. The experiment was conducted at 4:30 P.M.

TABLE 1. Dose-Dependent Effect of β-Carotene on the Increase in Plasma CRH Levels Induced by Exhaustive Exercise[a]

	Percent Increase	
Control	315 ± 85	(100%)
+ β-carotene		
6 mg	252 ± 71	(20% inhibition)
30 mg	45 ± 30	(85% inhibition)
60 mg	0	(100% inhibition)

[a] Experimental conditions were as described in FIGURE 1. Before exercise every person showed different CRH levels (9–25 pg/ml plasma). After exhaustion, CRH levels increased. These increasing levels were expressed as the percent increase of the level before exercise. Two hours before exercise, they took the β-carotene. Their body weights were from 65 to 78 kg. Exercise started at 4:30 P.M. Control: n = 12, + β-carotene: n = 4 at each dose.

REFERENCES

1. ORTH-GOMER, K. 1979. J. Psychosom. Res. **23:** 165–173.
2. ROBERTSON, T. L. *et al.* 1977. Am. J. Cardiol. **39:** 239–243.
3. NEWLIN, D. B. *et al.* 1982. J. Psychosom. Res. **26:** 393–402.
4. HIRAYAMA, T. 1992. Personal communication.
5. SELYE, H. 1976. Can. Med. Assoc. J. **115:** 53–56.
6. KUROSAWA, M., A. SATO, R. S. SWENSON & Y. TAKAHASHI. 1986. Brain Res. **367:** 250–257.

β-Carotene Uptake, Metabolism, and Distribution *in Vitro*

W. G. WAMER, R. R. WEI, J. E. MATUSIK,
A. KORNHAUSER, AND V. C. DUNKEL

Food and Drug Administration
Center for Food Safety and Applied Nutrition
HFS-128
200 C Street SW
Washington, DC 20204

INTRODUCTION

In vitro studies of β-carotene are proving increasingly valuable for investigating the mechanism(s) of β-carotene protective effects at the cellular level. In the present study, we characterize the absorption, intracellular distribution and metabolism of β-carotene in BALB/c 3T3 embryonic fibroblasts. The information derived from these measurements is useful in determining the role of retinoids in β-carotene protective effects, and in identifying the intracellular targets of β-carotene protection.

METHODS

BALB/c 3T3 clone A31-1-1 cells were cultured in Eagle's minimum essential medium supplemented with 7.5% fetal bovine serum, antibiotics (100 U/ml penicillin and 100 μg/ml streptomycin), and 2 mM L-glutamine. As required, the medium was supplemented with 3μM β-carotene added as a water dispersible beadlet formulation (Hoffmann-La Roche, Nutley, NJ). Control beadlets containing all components except β-carotene were used in control treatments of cells. At selected times following initial treatment, cell monolayers were collected, extracted, and analyzed for β-carotene by reversed phase HPLC as previously described.[1] Routine analysis of retinol in cell pellets was performed by reversed phase HPLC.[1] Analysis of cell extracts by a distinct, normal phase HPLC method[2] yielded similar results (data not shown). To determine the intracellular location of β-carotene following exposure of cells for five days to β-carotene-supplemented medium, cells were fractionated to obtain membranes and nuclei.[1] Cellular fractions were analyzed for β-carotene by reversed phase HPLC.

RESULTS

The effect of media supplementation with β-carotene (3 μM) or control beadlets on cellular β-carotene and retinol levels is shown in TABLE 1. Cellular accumulation of β-carotene increases rapidly during the first 48 hr of treatment and then appears to plateau thereafter. Cells treated with control beadlets had no detectable levels of β-carotene. After an apparent lag phase, retinol levels were found to significantly

284

TABLE 1. Cellular Levels of β-Carotene and Retinol

Length of Treatment	β-Carotene ng/10⁶ Cells	Retinol ng/10⁶ Cells
4 hours		
β-Carotene	66.4 ± 10.1[a]	1.00 ± 0.09
Control	N.D.[b]	N.A.[c]
1 day		
β-Carotene	241 ± 11	1.26 ± 0.09
Control	N.D.	1.23 ± 0.14
2 days		
β-Carotene	287 ± 2	1.02 ± 0.06
Control	N.D.	N.A.
3 days		
β-Carotene	311 ± 48	2.23 ± 0.22
Control	N.D.	1.27 ± 0.26
5 days		
β-Carotene	306 ± 31	4.68 ± 0.60
Control	N.D.	1.60 ± 0.01

[a] Data are the average ± SD of 3 determinations.
[b] N.D. = not detectable.
[c] N.A. = not analyzed.

increase in β-carotene-exposed cells above those measured in control cells. Retinol levels in cells exposed to β-carotene five days had increased approximately three-fold relative to cells treated with control beadlets. The content of β-carotene in subcellular fractions is presented in TABLE 2. A major portion of intracellular β-carotene is found in the crude membranes. Although the crude nuclear fraction contained significant levels of β-carotene, no detectable levels of β-carotene were found in purified nuclei.

DISCUSSION

In all *in vitro* studies of the mechanism of β-carotene protection, the role of β-carotene's provitamin A activity must be evaluated. The results presented here indicate that the ability to metabolize β-carotene to retinoids is observable *in vitro*.

TABLE 2. β-Carotene Content of Cell Fractions

Cell Fraction	β-Carotene, % Recovered
Crude membranes	70.1 ± 18.5%[a]
Purified membranes (light fraction)	28.7 ± 9.1%
Purified membranes (heavy fraction)	2.1 ± 0.5%
Crude nuclei	23.9 ± 8.6%
Purified nuclei	N.D.[b]
Cytoplasm	0.8 ± 0.2%

[a] Average ± SD of 4 determinations.
[b] N.D. = not detectable.

The methods described here allow measurement of small increases of intracellular retinol without use of radiolabelled β-carotene. The association of β-carotene with cellular membranes indicates that, in this *in vitro* model, membranes may be an important target of β-carotene protection.

REFERENCES

1. WAMER, W. G., R. R. WEI, J. E. MATUSIK, A. KORNHAUSER & V. C. DUNKEL. 1993. Nutr. Cancer **19**: 31–41.
2. LANDERS, G. M. & J. A. OLSON. 1988. J. Chromatogr. **438**: 383–392.

Metabolic Activities of Rat Liver Preparations on Retinol, β-Carotene, and Lycopene[a]

A. NAGAO AND J. A. OLSON

Department of Biochemistry and Biophysics
Iowa State University
3256 Molecular Biology Building
Ames, Iowa 50011

Microsomes, which contain some electron transport and cytochrome P450 systems, play an important role in the oxidative transformation of a large number of substances, such as steroids, fatty acids and xenobiotics.[1] Retinoic acid and retinol were found to be metabolized to polar metabolites, including the 4-hydroxy derivatives, by human, rabbit and rat liver microsomal cytochrome P450 preparations. It is not known whether carotenoids can be oxidized by microsomal enzymes of mammals. In the present study, we examined whether β-carotene and lycopene were oxidatively metabolized by microsomal enzymes of rat liver in a way similar to retinoids.

The ability of rat liver microsomes, which were prepared from normal rats and from phenobarbital (PB)-treated rats, to oxidize retinol to its 4-hydroxy derivative was first measured. In our hands, the specific activities of liver microsomes from untreated and PB-treated rats were 0.13 and 0.15–0.20 nmol/min/mg protein, respectively, as shown in TABLE 1. PB markedly increased the size of the liver and moderately enhanced the 4-hydroxylation of retinol, but to a lesser degree in our studies than in those reported by Leo and Lieber.[2]

When purified β-carotene or lycopene was solubilized in 2% bovine serum albumin (BSA) or was dissolved in peroxide free-tetrahydrofuran (THF), the two carotenoids at 10 μM were found to be stable during aerobic incubation with microsomes. However, both carotenoids were rapidly converted to a large number of oxidation products during solvent extraction, unless antioxidants such as α-tocopherol, n-propyl gallate, or pyrogallol were present in the extracting solvent. Carotenoids were also found to be more efficiently extracted by chloroform/methanol (1 : 2, v/v) than by ethyl acetate following ethanol treatment.

To investigate metabolic transformations, β-carotene and lycopene, which were solubilized in BSA or THF, were separately incubated aerobically at 37°C for 30 min with liver microsomes of PB-treated rats in an incubation mixture containing NADPH, as described in the legend to FIGURE 1. Then, carotenoids were extracted with chloroform/methanol (1 : 2, v/v) containing 1 mM pyrogallol and subjected to HPLC analyses. No C-40 metabolites were found, whether or not NADPH was present (FIG. 1). In this HPLC system, polar carotenoids such as 4,4'-dihydroxy-β-carotene could be separated from the solvent front, and the

[a] Supported by the Japanese International Cooperation Agency; by National Institutes of Health Grant CA-46406; and by United States Department of Agriculture Center for Designing Foods to Improve Nutrition Grant 91-34115-5903.

TABLE 1. Activities of Retinol 4-Hydroxylation in Rat Liver Microsomes

Treatment	Specific Activity (nmol/min/mg Protein)	% Liver Weight/Body Weight
Untreated (9.6 weeks old)	0.133	2.7
0.1% PB[a] in drinking water for 6 days (9 weeks old)	0.155	4.4
0.1% PB in drinking water for 26 days (8 weeks old)	0.149	5.9
PB-ip (5 weeks old)	0.195	5.4

[a] PB, phenobarbital.

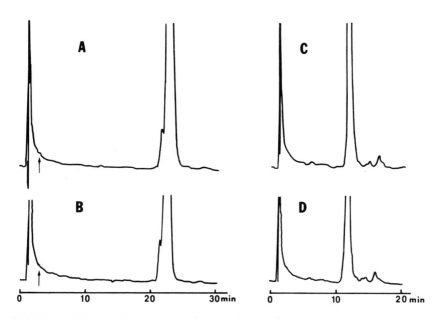

FIGURE 1. HPLC profiles of extracts from incubation mixture of β-carotene and lycopene with rat liver microsomes. β-Carotene or lycopene/BSA (10 μM) was incubated at 37°C for 30 min with liver microsomes (1.8 mg protein/ml), which were prepared from rats treated with an ip injection of phenobarbital, suspended in the following mixture: 1 mM NADPH; 0.1 M Tris-HCl buffer, pH 7.4; 0.15 M KCl; 5 mM MgCl$_2$; 1 mM EDTA. Carotenoids were extracted with chloroform/methanol (1 : 2, v/v) that contained 1 mM pyrogallol and were analyzed with a Nova-Pack C18 column (3.9 × 150 mm) developed with acetonitrile/dichloromethane/methanol (85/5/10, v/v/v) that contained 0.05% ammonium acetate. Carotenoid absorption was monitored at 450 nm. β-Carotene and lycopene eluted at 22.2 min and 11.2 min, respectively. The *arrows* indicate the elution position of 4,4'-dihydroxy-β-carotene. **(A)** β-Carotene in the presence of NADPH; **(B)** β-carotene in the absence of NADPH; **(C)** lycopene in the presence of NADPH; **(D)** lycopene in the absence of NADPH.

presence of at least 20 nM β-carotene in an incubation mixture could be detected. Similarly, carotenoids were not detectably converted to C-40 oxidation products by crude homogenates of rat liver, whether or not dithiothreitol, NAD, or NADPH were present. Because endogenous retinol and retinyl esters were abundantly present, however, carotenoid cleavage activity could not be assessed. Thus, liver microsomes seem to be involved in the catabolism of retinoids but not of β-carotene and lycopene, although β-carotene has a β-ionone ring like retinol. The extraction procedure must be rigorously controlled to avoid artifactual oxidation.

REFERENCES

1. COON, M. J., X. DING, S. J. PERNECKY & A. D. N. VAZ. 1992. FASEB J. **6:** 669–673.
2. LEO, M. A. & C. S. LIEBER. 1985. *J. Biol. Chem.* **260:** 5228–5231.

Plasma β-Carotene Response to Intake of β-Carotene Drink in Normal Men

K. MASAKI, T. DOI, K. YUGE, Y. YOSHIOKA,
AND Y. NAGATA[a]

Saga Research Institute
Otsuka Pharmaceutical Co., Ltd.
Higashisefurimura Kanzakigun
Saga 842-01, Japan

Recent research has revealed that β-carotene exerts direct effects on human health through its antioxidative property.[1,2] However, the Japanese average daily intake of β-carotene is as low as 2.5 mg, far below the recommended intake of 6 mg. Otsuka Pharmaceutical Co., Ltd. has developed a β-carotene-containing drink. This product consists of 3 mg of β-carotene and 5 g of dietary fiber (polydextrose) in its 100-ml bottle. Two studies were designed to evaluate plasma β-carotene response to intake of the product in healthy subjects.

SUBJECTS AND METHODS

Study 1: Male subjects fed low carotenoid diet (0.17–0.46 mg/day) were given 6 mg of β-carotene either from the product or cooked carrots for 7 days, and the change in plasma β-carotene was followed for 3 weeks thereafter. Fasting blood samples were obtained on day −4 before the start of this study (the beginning of the low carotenoid diet), day 0 (the start of administration) and days 1, 2, 3, 6 (the end of administration), and days 7, 8, 9, 10, 13, 17, and 21. Plasma β-carotene was quantified with HPLC.[3]

Study 2: Whether the low plasma β-carotene level in smokers is elevated to that in nonsmokers after intake of the β-carotene drink was assessed under the same condition as in Study 1. The disappearance rate of the administered β-carotene was evaluated based on the decay of plasma β-carotene levels after the end of intake.

RESULTS AND DISCUSSION

In Study 1, subjects fed the β-carotene product showed a higher level of plasma β-carotene as compared with those fed cooked carrots, as shown in FIGURE

---

[a] Corresponding author.

1 (22.4 ± 6.6 µg/dl vs 2.1 ± 1.3 µg/dl, $p < 0.001$, as the maximum change from baseline). We confirmed the findings of previous studies by showing that purified β-carotene is more efficiently absorbed than is a similar amount present in vegetables.[4,5]

In Study 2, daily intake of the product for 7 days in smokers with a low initial level of β-carotene (15.8 ± 5.3 µg/dl) increased its level in plasma (38.3 ± 14.0 µg/dl) to that found in nonsmokers, as shown in FIGURE 2. For the period after administration we calculated a half-life of 7–21 days for β-carotene in smokers and nonsmokers. After the cessation of β-carotene administration, the level of plasma β-carotene declined more rapidly in smokers than in nonsmokers, as shown in FIGURE 2 (t1/2 11.8 ± 1.8 vs 14.9 ± 3.1 days, $p < 0.05$), indicating the possibility that cigarette smoking increases consumption of β-carotene as an anti-oxidant.

CONCLUSION

From the results in Study 1, β-carotene drink is more effective in raising the plasma β-carotene level as compared with cooked carrots.

The cessation of the administration of β-carotene decreased the plasma β-carotene level in Study 2, which suggests the necessity for continuous intake of the drink in order to maintain the proper plasma β-carotene level.

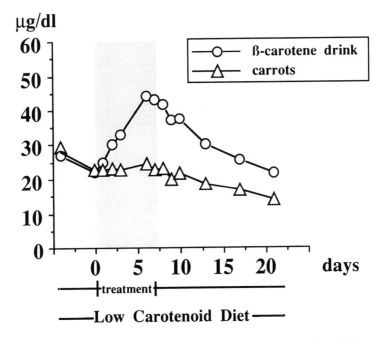

FIGURE 1. Mean plasma β-carotene response to β-carotene drink and cooked carrots. O, β-carotene drink; △, carrots.

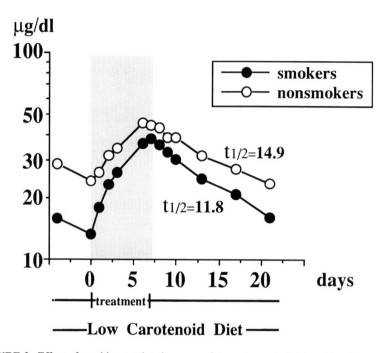

FIGURE 2. Effect of smoking on the clearance of β-carotene administered by β-carotene drink. ●, smokers; ○, nonsmokers.

REFERENCES

1. HIRAYAMA, T. 1979. Diet and cancer. Nutr. Cancer **1:** 67–81.
2. STAHELIN, H. B., K. F. GEY, M. EICHHOLZER & E. LUDIN. 1991. Beta-carotene and cancer prevention: the Basel Study. Am. J. Clin. Nutr. **53**(Suppl. 1): 265S–269S.
3. KAPLAN, L. A., J. A. MILLER, E. A. STEIN & M. J. STAMPFER. 1990. Simultaneous, high-performance liquid chromatographic analysis of retinol, tocopherols, lycopene, and alpha- and beta-carotene in serum and plasma. Methods Enzymol. **189:** 155–167.
4. RAO, C. N. & B. S. N. RAO. 1970. Absorption of dietary carotenes in human subjects. Am. J. Clin. Nutr. **23**(1): 105–109.
5. BROWN, E. D., M. S. MICOZZI, N. E. CRAFT, J. G. BIERI, G. BEECHER, B. K. EDWARDS, A. ROSE, P. R. TAYLOR & J. C. SMITH, JR. 1989. Plasma carotenoids in normal men after a single ingestion of vegetables or purified beta-carotene. Am. J. Clin. Nutr. **49**(6): 1258–1265.

Subject Index

Index of Contributors